Handbook of
Patient Care in
Vascular Surgery

Handbook of Patient Care in Vascular Surgery

Third Edition

John W. Hallett, Jr., M.D.

Professor of Surgery, Mayo Medical School; Director of Vascular
Surgery Fellowship, Mayo Clinic and Mayo Foundation;
Attending Surgeon, St. Mary's Hospital and
Rochester Methodist Hospital, Rochester, Minnesota

David C. Brewster, M.D.

Associate Professor of Surgery, Massachusetts General Hospital
and Harvard Medical School, Boston

R. Clement Darling, Jr., M.D.

Associate Clinical Professor of Surgery, Harvard Medical School;
Senior Surgeon and Former Chief of the Vascular Clinic,
Massachusetts General Hospital, Boston

Little, Brown and Company

Boston   New York   Toronto   London

Third Edition

Library of Congress Cataloging-in-Publication Data
Hallett, John W.
    Handbook of patient care in vascular surgery / John W. Hallett,
Jr., David C. Brewster, R. Clement Darling, Jr. —3rd ed.
        p. cm.
    Rev. ed. of: Patient care in vascular surgery. 2nd ed. c1987.
    Includes bibliographical references and index.
    ISBN 0-316-34053-7
    1. Blood-vessels—Surgery—Handbooks, manuals, etc. 2. Blood
-vessels--Diseases--Handbooks, manuals, etc. I. Brewster, David C.
II. Darling, R. Clement, 1927–   III. Hallett, John W. Patient
care in vascular surgery. IV. Title.
    [DNLM: 1. Vascular Surgery--outlines. 2. Vascular Surgery-
-handbooks. WG 18.2 H186h 1995]
RD598.5.H35 1995
617.4'13--dc20
DNLM/DLC
for Library of Congress   94-47952
                                                                  CIP

Printed in the United States of America
RRD-VA

Editorial: Nancy E. Chorpenning
Production Editor: Marie A. Salter
Copyeditor: Elizabeth Willingham
Indexer: Ann Blum
Production Supervisor: Michael A. Granger
Composition and Production: Silverchair Science+Communications
Cover Designer: Michael A. Granger

Second   Printing

Contents

Preface

In 1982, we introduced the practical *Manual of Patient Care in Vascular Surgery*. This new *Handbook of Patient Care in Vascular Surgery*, the third edition of this book, maintains the enduring principles from the first edition and includes the latest developments in pathophysiology, diagnosis, and treatment. We continue to focus on fundamentals that guide students, residents, technicians, and nurses who work on the front lines of patient care.

Readers who have used previous editions will recognize numerous changes. Each chapter has been updated, and two new chapters have been added on vascular trauma and hemodialysis access. Significant alterations and subtle refinements in diagnosis and therapy have remodelled our current practice. The pressures of health care reform and cost containment have resulted in changes in outpatient and inpatient management and length of hospitalization. We have tried to address both the benefits and risks of these forces on patient care.

In addition, we have deleted voluminous reference lists in favor of limited lists of recommended references and readings, which appear at the end of each chapter. The availability of computerized literature-search systems provides instantaneous access to the latest information on any subject. Thus, our current references emphasize an increasing number of randomized clinical trials in vascular surgical, radiologic, and medical therapy. We have also cited excellent reviews by experts in each area discussed and have included a few well-recognized reference books. Many more articles and books are obviously available and must be consulted for second opinions and additional details on all topics.

Readers of previous editions have offered many suggestions that have been used to enhance this edition of *Handbook of Patient Care in Vascular Surgery*. We thank them for their valuable input. We hope that those who use the new edition will take time to let us know how future editions might be improved.

J.W.H.
D.C.B.
R.C.D.

Acknowledgments

We gratefully acknowledge the contributions of the following individuals, whose efforts were essential to the development and completion of this handbook: Nancy Chorpenning of Little, Brown, for her encouragement to do this project for a third time and for her patience in adjusting deadlines; Marie Salter of Little, Brown and Elizabeth Willingham of Silverchair for expert editorial review of the manuscript; Michael A. Granger of Little, Brown and Thane Kerner of Silverchair for production of the book; the Department of Medical Illustrations at the Mayo Clinic for their new contributions; and Renee Brandt and Diane Richardson for their help in manuscript preparation.

We also extend special thanks to the following colleagues for their thoughtful review and suggestions: Thom W. Rooke, M.D. (Noninvasive Vascular Testing), Anthony W. Stanson, M.D. (Vascular Radiology), William C. Oliver, Jr., M.D. (Anesthesia), and Yvonne Baerga-Varela, M.D. (Early Postoperative Care). Their experience and insights have enhanced these special sections of the handbook.

Finally, J. W. Hallett wishes to acknowledge Margaret Brinkman Hallett, who, more than anyone else, understands what it takes to bring such a project to completion.

Handbook of
Patient Care in
Vascular Surgery

Notice

The views expressed in this book are our own and do not necessarily represent the opinions of the entire staff at the Mayo Clinic or Massachusetts General Hospital.

The indications and dosages of all drugs in this book have been recommended in the medical literature and conform to the practices of the general medical community. The medications described do not necessarily have specific approval by the Food and Drug Administration for use in the diseases and dosages for which they are recommended. The package insert for each drug should be consulted for use and dosage as approved by the FDA. Because standards for usage change, it is advisable to keep abreast of revised recommendations, particularly those concerning new drugs.

Basic Concepts

Management of the simplest or the most complicated vascular problem is based on a limited number of basic principles of arterial and venous diseases. Following these principles, one can consistently provide logical and appropriate patient care. In the first two chapters, we outline and emphasize these basic concepts. Since the scope of this handbook covers primarily atherosclerotic arterial disease and acquired venous disease, we have organized these introductory concepts around the two broad disease groups. These general comments are further subdivided under the headings of the magnitude of the problem, basic anatomy, etiology, pathophysiology, and natural history.

Arterial Disease

I. **Magnitude of the problem.** Arterial diseases are a leading cause of death in the United States and many other countries. Perhaps more important than mortality is the disability that cardiovascular disease causes in so many people. For example, approximately 500,000 Americans have strokes each year. Many of these people are left with a permanent neurologic deficit. The social and economic impact of a stroke can be devastating to both the patient and his or her family. Others are incapacitated by angina pectoris, leg claudication, and ischemic foot lesions.

   Advances in the accurate diagnosis and successful treatment of these arterial problems have been rapid. However, significant progress in prevention has been much slower. This progress may come with better control of risk factors. Currently, too many patients are reluctant to modify their diets, to stop smoking, and to take medications regularly. Thus, arterial disease will remain a leading health problem during the entire career of most physicians alive today.

II. **Arterial anatomy.** Few physicians think of the arterial system as a complex and highly structured organ. Like the heart, arteries must withstand the stress of pulsatile blood flow for many years. Three distinct layers of large- and medium-sized arteries must remain intact for normal function. These layers are the intima, media, and adventitia (Fig. 1-1).

   A. **The intima,** the innermost layer, is a monolayer of flattened endothelial cells with a thin underlying matrix of collagen and elastic fibers. An **internal elastic membrane** separates the intima from the media.

   B. **The media** is a relatively thick middle layer of varying amounts of smooth muscle, collagen, and elastic fibers. The amount of elastic tissue decreases progressively from the thoracic aorta (elastic artery) to the distal medium-sized arteries, such as the femoral or carotid (muscular arteries). In contrast to the intima, the media has a dual source of nourishment. The innermost portion receives its nutrients by diffusion from the circulating blood. The outer regions are nourished by small vessels that penetrate the outer arterial wall. These **vasa vasorum** may be affected by the arteriosclerotic process, leading to degeneration of wall strength. An **external elastic membrane** encloses the outer border of the media and separates it from the adventitia.

   C. **The adventitia,** the outermost layer of an artery, may appear thin and weak. However, its collagenous and elastic structure makes it a key element in the total strength of the arterial wall. In muscular arteries it may be as thick as the media. Primary surgical closure of the arterial wall or anastomosis of a synthetic graft to the vessel must incorporate the adventitia. Failure to include the adventitia may result in a weakened spot and eventual pseudoaneurysm formation.

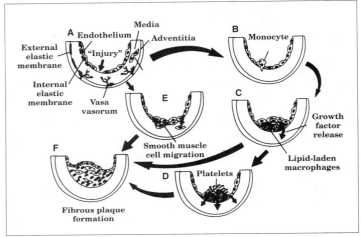

Fig. 1-1. Pathogenesis of atherosclerosis. Advanced atheromatous plaques may arise by at least two pathways. Hypercholesterolemia may induce endothelial "injury" (A). Monocytes attach to injured endothelium (B), secrete growth factors (C), and finally migrate into the subendothelial layer. Lipid-laden macrophages become part of the fatty streak. Endothelial disruption attracts platelets (D) that secrete platelet-derived growth factor (PDGF). Smooth muscle cells in the proliferative atheromatous lesion may also secrete growth factors such as PDGF. Fibrous plaques (F) evolve from fatty streaks. Another pathway for atherosclerosis may involve "injury" (e.g., mechanical, low-density lipoproteins, homocysteine, immunologic, toxins, viruses) to the endothelium, *which initially remains intact* (A to E to F). Increased endothelial turnover results in enhanced growth factor production. Smooth muscle cells are stimulated to migrate into the intimal layer (E). Smooth muscle and "injured" endothelial cells turn up their growth factor production. Atheroma develop from fatty streaks to fibrous plaques that can degenerate eventually into complicated plaques with surface ulceration, hemorrhage, and embolization. (Adapted from R Ross. The pathogenesis of atherosclerosis. *N Engl J Med* 314:488, 1986.)

III. Etiology. The etiology of most arterial diseases today is atherosclerosis. There is some confusion about the terms **atherosclerosis** and **arteriosclerosis.** Arteriosclerosis was introduced originally to describe any arterial disease that caused wall thickening. Atheroma was applied to plaques that contained soft fatty contents. Finally, atherosclerosis was defined by the World Health Organization as a combination of changes in the intima and media. These changes include focal accumulation of lipids, hemorrhage, fibrous tissue, and calcium deposits. The development of atherosclerotic lesions is a complex biochemical and cellular process. The cellular mechanisms are beyond the scope of this handbook. However, the gross appearance and developmental sequence may be divided into three major stages.

   A. Early lesions usually appear as fatty streaks in childhood or young adult life. Their content is primarily lipid;

they also contain macrophage infiltration and some smooth muscle. Cholesterol or its esters are the main lipid components. Some evidence indicates that these early lesions can regress.

B. Fibrous plaques appear in later life. They represent a more permanent lesion and closely follow the development of symptomatic atherosclerosis. Located mainly at arterial bifurcations, fibrous plaques have a lipid core surrounded by a capsule of elastic and collagenous tissue.

C. Complicated lesions usually develop from the fibrous plaque. Necrosis of the plaque may lead to surface ulceration. Thrombi tend to occur at these ulcerated sites. Intramural hemorrhage also may occur, with or without ulceration. The elasticity of the arterial wall is lost as local calcifications accumulate. The atherosclerotic process may narrow the vessel lumen, or the wall may degenerate and dilate, forming an aneurysm.

D. The development of atherosclerosis follows a variable course. In the same patient, one may find a spectrum of early and complicated lesions. Intimal thickening and calcification of arteries apparently are a normal aging process. However, complicated atherosclerosis is a disease process whose natural course is influenced by a number of risk factors. The primary ones appear to be smoking, hypertension, hyperlipidemia, and diabetes mellitus. Failure to control these factors usually leads to accelerated atherogenesis.

IV. Pathophysiology. Basic principles of fluid dynamics (Table 1-1) help explain the physiologic consequences of arterial occlusive and aneurysmal disease. In some patients, both processes coexist.

A. Occlusive disease. Atherosclerosis generally becomes symptomatic by gradual occlusion of blood flow to the involved extremity or organ. Symptoms finally occur when a **critical arterial stenosis** is reached. Blood flow and pressure are not significantly diminished until at least 75% of the cross-sectional area of the vessel is obliterated (Fig. 1-2). This figure for cross-sectional area can be equated with a 50% reduction in lumen diameter. The formula for the area of a circle (area = $3.14 \times \text{radius}^2$) explains the relationship between vessel diameter and cross-sectional area.

Factors other than radius influence critical stenosis but to a lesser extent. These include the length of the stenosis, blood viscosity, and peripheral resistance. Longer stenotic segments reach a critical stenosis earlier. Likewise, flow and pressure across a stenosis diminish sharply when the blood becomes more viscous. In low-resistance situations, flow is increased, but turbulence at a stenosis is also worsened and pressure across the lesion may drop.

Experimental evidence also shows that a series of subcritical stenoses can have an additive effect that is similar to a single critical stenosis. This cumulative effect, however, is not linear. Thus, three subcritical stenoses (30%, 40%, and 10%) may not have the same effect as a single 80% narrowing of a vessel.

Table 1-1. Basic principles of fluid dynamics

Principle	Definition	Equation	Terms of equation
Bernoulli's principle	Expresses the relationship between pressure, gravitational energy, and kinetic energy in an idealized fluid system. In moving blood through arteries, the portion of total fluid energy lost is dissipated mainly in the form of *heat*.	$P_1 + \rho g h_1 + \frac{1}{2}\rho\upsilon_1{}^2 =$ $P_2 + \rho g h_2 + \frac{1}{2}\rho\upsilon_2{}^2 + \text{heat}$	P = pressure $\rho g h$ = gravitational potential energy $\frac{1}{2}\rho\upsilon^2$ = kinetic energy
Poiseuille's law	Describes the relationship between flow and the pressure difference across the length of a tube, its radius, and the fluid viscosity. The most important determinant of flow is obviously *radius*.	$Q = \dfrac{r^4(P_1 - P_2)}{8L\eta}$	Q = flow r = radius of vessel $P_1 - P_2$ = potential energy between 2 points L = distance between 2 points η = viscosity
Reynolds number	A dimensionless quantity that defines the points at which flow changes from laminar (stream-lined) to turbulent (disorganized) flow. If Re > 2000, local disturbances in laminar flow will result in fully developed turbulence. In normal arterial circulation, Re is usually < 2000.	$Re = \dfrac{d\bar{\upsilon}\rho}{\eta}$	Re = Reynolds number d = tube diameter $\bar{\upsilon}$ = velocity ρ = specific gravity η = viscosity
Resistance (rearranged Poiseuille's law)	Analogous to Ohm's equation of electrical circuits (pressure = flow × resistance)	$R = \dfrac{P_1 - P_2}{Q} = \dfrac{8\eta L}{\pi r^4}$	R = resistance $P_1 - P_2$ = pressure drop Q = flow η = viscosity L = length of tube r = radius of tube

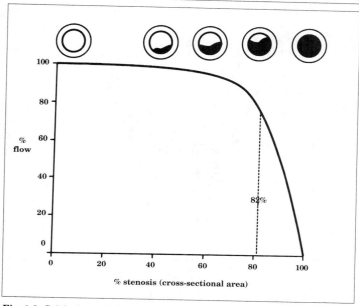

Fig. 1-2. Critical arterial stenosis. Blood flow remains relatively normal across an arterial stenosis until at least 75% of the cross-sectional area is obliterated (50% diameter reduction). (Adapted from AG May et al. Critical arterial stenosis. *Surgery* 54:250, 1963.)

Turbulence has been identified as the most important cause of blood flow and pressure drop across a stenosis. The turbulence occurs in the poststenotic section of the vessel, where kinetic energy is dissipated by these turbulent eddies. The influence of blood flow on the degree of narrowing of a vessel necessary to cause a critical stenosis explains why ankle pressures may be normal at rest but fall sharply with exercise. Exercise increases extremity blood flow. Because increased blood flow across a stenosis causes more turbulence, flow and pressure eventually will decrease. The patient who may have no complaints at rest will experience claudication with exercise. Hence, a stenosis may be noncritical at rest but critical with exercise.

Experimental and clinical observations also indicate that atherosclerotic lesions form near areas of blood flow separation and low shear stress (Fig. 1-3). The layer of blood adjacent to an arterial wall, as blood flows through an artery, is referred to as the **boundary layer**. Although flow in the center of the arterial lumen is rapid and laminar, the area of boundary layer separation has slower, more disturbed currents. These areas of boundary layer separation and low shear force generally occur at the outer wall of arterial bifurcations where atheroma formation is more pronounced.

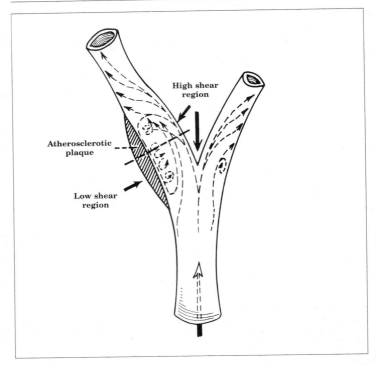

Fig. 1-3. Patterns of low and high shear stress. Atherosclerotic plaques, which usually localize to the outer wall at arterial bifurcations, tend to develop at areas of boundary layer separation and low shear stress. (Modified from CK Zarins et al. Atherosclerotic Plaque Distribution and Flow Profiles in the Carotid Bifurcation. In JJ Bergan, JST Yao (eds), *Cerebrovascular Insufficiency*. New York: Grune & Stratton, 1983.)

B. **Aneurysmal disease.** Aneurysms are the result of degeneration and weakening of the network of protein fibers in the arterial wall. The pathophysiologic mechanisms that result in aneurysm formation are multifactorial (Fig. 1-4) (see Chap. 16). Rupture occurs if the intraluminal pressure exceeds the tensile strength of the wall. The etiology of this wall degeneration and the mechanisms of its dilation and rupture are not fully understood. However, certain observations and hemodynamic principles provide a reasonable explanation.

When a pulse wave arrives at a vessel bifurcation, a portion of the pressure is reflected against the arterial wall proximal to the bifurcation. Minimal reflections occur when the sum of the cross-sectional areas of the daughter arteries (e.g., iliacs) to the parent artery (aorta) is 1.15. With advancing age this ratio decreases, even in aortas without atheromatous change, and so more oscillating pressure is reflected. The result is a partial stand-

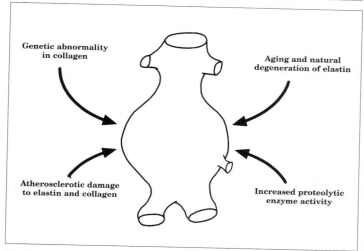

Fig. 1-4. Contributory factors to the multifactorial pathogenesis of arterial aneurysms.

ing wave in the abdominal aorta. These reflective pressure waves at major bifurcations may determine the increased incidence of aneurysms at these locations.

In addition to reflected pressure waves, the paucity of vasa vasorum in the abdominal aorta also may contribute to its susceptibility to aneurysm formation. When arteriosclerosis obliterates vasa vasorum, necrosis of the media results in weakening and vessel dilation. Vasa vasorum are more plentiful in the thoracic aorta, where aneurysms are less common.

Defects in the structural integrity of the vessel collagen and elastic content are found in certain congenital conditions, such as Marfan's syndrome. Whether normal adults who develop aneurysms have an inherited predisposition to arterial dilatation has not been proved but has been clinically observed in some families. The collagen content of an atherosclerotic aneurysm is reduced. Collagen fibers constitute about 25% of an atherosclerotic arterial wall but only 6–18% of an aneurysmal wall.

The risk of aneurysm rupture increases with increased aneurysm size. The stress in the vessel wall increases as the vessel diameter (d) enlarges and its wall thickness (t) decreases. Wall stress is also proportional to intraluminal pressure (P):

Stress = $P \times d/t$

The importance of blood pressure control becomes obvious when this Laplace relationship is examined. In addition, a layer of clot often lines a large aneurysm, but this clot does not necessarily protect against rupture.

V. Natural history. For most patients, atherosclerosis is diffuse and slowly progressive. During early adult life, it usually remains asymptomatic. However, when it becomes symptomatic in one part of the body, a careful history and physical examination will often reveal evidence of significant disease at other sites. Sometimes the asymptomatic disease is more life-threatening. For example, a patient may present with calf claudication but have an unknown abdominal aortic aneurysm palpable on routine physical examination. The diffuse nature of atherosclerosis requires that the initial patient evaluation include a baseline examination of the entire vascular system.

The natural history of atherosclerosis is extremely variable. Some patients are minimally bothered by its presence, while others are totally incapacitated. Although atherosclerosis, like cancer, may follow a malignant course despite therapeutic intervention, the natural history can be altered satisfactorily in most cases by appropriate treatment. Although not curative, properly selected arterial reconstructions can offer excellent palliation of the atherosclerotic process. Subsequent chapters will emphasize specific aspects of the natural history of atherosclerosis so that clinicians can select patients who are most likely to benefit from medical, radiologic, and surgical intervention.

Selected Reading

Clowes AW. Vascular biology—the new frontier. *Cardiovascular Surg* 2:301, 1994.

Gibbons GH, Dzau VJ. The emerging concept of vascular remodeling. *N Engl J Med* 330:1431, 1994.

Ross R. Pathophysiology of Atherosclerosis. In FJ Veith, RW Hobson, R.A Williams, SE Wilson (eds), *Vascular Surgery* (2nd ed). New York: McGraw-Hill, 1994. Pp. 9–20.

Strandness DE Jr, Sumner DS. *Hemodynamics for Surgeons.* New York: Grune & Stratton, 1975.

Yao JST, Pearce WH. *Aneurysms: New Findings and Treatments.* Norwalk, CT: Appleton & Lange, 1994.

Zarins CK, Glagov S. Pathophysiology of Human Atherosclerosis. In FJ Veith, RW Hobson, RA Williams, SE Wilson (eds), *Vascular Surgery* (2nd ed). New York: McGraw-Hill, 1994. Pp. 21–39.

Zierler RE, Strandness DE Jr. Hemodynamics for the Vascular Surgeon. In WS Moore (ed), *Vascular Surgery: A Comprehensive Review* (4th ed). Philadelphia: Saunders, 1993. Pp. 96–107.

Venous Disease

The most common venous disorders are varicose veins, superficial and deep venous thrombosis, pulmonary embolism, and postphlebitic syndrome. Like arterial disease, a limited number of basic principles can explain the physiologic consequences of these different conditions. Proper treatment is based on these concepts.

I. **Magnitude of the problem.** Simple varicose veins affect about 15% of the adult population. They generally are associated with low morbidity and mortality rates. In contrast, acquired deep venous thrombosis and its complications debilitate or kill thousands of patients each year. Pulmonary embolism is the most common lethal pulmonary disease in the United States. Of those patients who survive deep venous thrombosis and pulmonary embolism, the majority eventually will develop postphlebitic syndrome. Current statistics indicate that the incidence of serious venous problems in the United States is increasing.

II. **Anatomy**

A. **Valves.** Of all the anatomic features of veins, the valves play the central role in most venous disorders. Normal venous valves are bicuspid, opening so that blood flows toward the heart and closing to prevent reflux. The greatest number of valves are located in the lower leg. The number decreases as the veins approach the inguinal ligament. A single valve usually is found in the external iliac or common femoral vein, and it is the only valve preventing reflux into the superficial saphenous vein. In approximately one-third of the population, no external or common femoral iliac valves exist. The inferior vena cava is valveless.

B. **Layers.** Like arteries, veins have three wall layers. The composition and function of these layers differ distinctly from the adjacent companion arteries. These differences include (1) a relatively thin wall that is one-tenth to one-third as thick as the artery; (2) less elastic tissue; (3) a media that is predominantly smooth muscle; (4) venules that lack a media and smooth muscle; and (5) an adventitia composed of collagen and elastin that forms the major portion of large veins. Although veins have vasa vasorum, they do not completely penetrate the vein wall, which receives most of its nourishment by diffusion from the bloodstream.

C. Unlike arteries, the veins can be conveniently divided into a **superficial** and a **deep system**. The superficial or surface system has relatively thick-walled and muscular veins. The superficial vein that is most commonly diseased is the greater saphenous vein. Deep veins are thinner and accompany arteries. Some are large and form sinusoids within skeletal muscle. The soleus sinusoids, for example, empty into the posterior tibial vein and are a common site for early deep venous clots. Communicating veins perforate the muscle fascia to connect the deep and superficial systems, and normally, blood flows from the superficial to the deep system. One-way valves in the communicating veins resist reflux of blood from the deep to the superficial system. This normal flow direction is interrupted by valve damage from thrombophlebitis.

D. Musculovenous pump mechanism. When leg muscles contract around intramuscular and surrounding veins, blood is propelled toward the heart. The major reservoirs of this pump are the soleus and gastrocnemius sinusoids. Pressures in excess of 200 mm Hg occur when these calf muscles contract. This mechanism may provide as much as 30% of the energy to circulate blood during strenuous exercise.

III. Etiology

A. Varicose veins. Varicose veins occur when the valve cusps of the saphenous system fail to close properly and the structural integrity of the vein weakens. The result is downward reflux of blood and chronic vein dilation. Many patients with varicose veins appear to have a familial predisposition. It usually is a progressive, functional failure of the valves rather than the absence of enough valves. In other cases, the valvular incompetence is acquired after venous thrombosis has damaged the valves. Fibrous contracture of the valve cusps leads to valvular incompetency.

The presence of multiple small arteriovenous anastomoses in patients with varicose veins has also been demonstrated by angiography, microsurgical dissection, Doppler ultrasound flow detection, and measurement of venous partial oxygen pressure, hemoglobin saturation, and venous oxygen content. It is debatable whether these arteriovenous shunts are the cause or result of varicose veins.

B. Venous thrombosis. Several factors contribute to the etiology of **superficial** and **deep venous thrombosis**. Most physicians recall Virchow's etiologic triad of venous stasis, vein injury, and blood hypercoagulability.

1. Although **venous stasis** in an immobile extremity has been associated with deep venous thrombosis, the mechanism of clot formation has been unclear. Recent evidence indicates that flow patterns through venous valves create a slow, disturbed movement in the deepest part of valve cusps. Flow stagnation in venous valve cusps has been associated with local hypoxia that may lead to endothelial injury and thrombosis.

2. Other studies also document that extensive surgical trauma is associated with excessive dilation of venous smooth muscle in the extremities and focal **endothelial injury**. The results are characteristic endothelial tears that are most frequent at the confluence of side branches with main veins. Leukocytes, not platelets, are the predominant cellular element to initially attach to these endothelial tears. These leukocytes are followed by the attachment of fibrin and platelets. In most patients, the normal fibrinolytic system appears to prevent extensive thrombosis. However, fibrinolytic

activity may be reduced in patients with recurrent idiopathic deep venous thrombosis.

3. **Hypercoagulability** also has been difficult to define but may be important, particularly in the postoperative patient. Shortened platelet survival or increased platelet adhesiveness has been demonstrated in patients with recurrent venous thrombosis. In addition, the increased incidence of thromboembolism in women using oral contraceptives has been associated with low levels of antithrombin III. Recurrent venous thromboembolism has also been correlated with congenital deficiency of protein C, a vitamin K–dependent protein produced in the liver and capable of inactivating clotting factors V and VIII. Protein S, an antithrombotic plasma cofactor of activated protein C, may likewise be decreased in some patients with recurrent venous thromboembolism. Nonetheless, coagulation studies often will be normal. Thus, the etiology of venous thrombosis is probably multifactorial in many patients.

The term **thrombophlebitis** implies an inflammatory or infectious origin. It can occur when the vein has been injured by an intravenous catheter or solution or when a superficial vein clot becomes seeded with bacteria or fungi. However, in many cases no phlebitis exists, so a better term would be **venous thrombosis**.

C. **Pulmonary embolism**. The etiology of **pulmonary thrombi** most commonly is embolism from lower-extremity clots. In rare cases, the pulmonary thrombi may form in situ. Occasionally, they will embolize from other sites, such as the arms or pelvic venous plexus.

D. **Postphlebitic syndrome** eventually follows most severe cases of deep venous thrombosis of the legs (Table 2-1). The leg edema, stasis dermatitis, and ulceration appear to be related to chronic venous hypertension in the superficial veins. It is the direct result of incompetent deep venous valves in the popliteal segment and incompetent communicating veins that perforate the fascia of the calf.

IV. **Pathophysiology**. The physiologic consequences of venous disease relate to two factors: valve insufficiency and vein obstruction (Fig. 2-1).

A. **Normal situation**. Standing still, the normal individual will have a venous pressure at the ankle equal to a column of blood rising to the right heart. This pressure approximates arterial pressure. With calf exercise, the musculovenous pump moves blood from the superficial system through the communicating veins and propels it via the deep system toward the heart. Baseline pressure in the foot veins drops approximately 70%.

B. **Varicose veins**. When patients with varicose veins exercise their legs, foot vein pressures drop only 30–40%. Although blood may move normally from the superficial to the deep system, as much as one-fifth to one-fourth of the total femoral outflow is refluxed into the varicose saphenous system and back down the leg in "circus"

Table 2-1. Postphlebitic syndrome

Years after deep venous thrombosis	% Patients with lower leg swelling	% Patients with leg ulcers
5	45	20
10	72	52
>10	91	79

Source: Modified from H Dodd, FB Crockett. The Post-Thrombotic Syndrome and Venous Ulceration. In H Dodd, FB Crockett (eds), *The Pathology and Surgery of the Veins and Lower Limb*. Edinburgh: Churchill Livingstone, 1976.

> motion. Patients with acquired varicosities after deep venous thrombosis also have incompetent communicating veins. With exercise, their foot vein pressures drop less than 20% of baseline values.
> **C. Venous thrombosis.** The basic problem in venous thrombosis is obstruction of venous outflow. In the supine position, venous pressure in acute thrombosis is about twice normal at the foot level. The extent of the clot and the adequacy of collateral channels determine the amount of limb swelling. If the patient is standing, the venous

Fig. 2-1. Ambulatory venous pressures. Normally leg exercises cause lower-extremity venous pressure to drop approximately 70% because the musculovenous pump propels blood toward the heart and competent venous valves prevent reflux. Varicose veins are associated with a 30–40% venous pressure reduction with exercise, because a portion of deep venous return is refluxed down the incompetent saphenous vein. Deep venous valve incompetence results in a minimal fall in venous pressure when chronic venous insufficiency (postphlebitic syndrome) is present. (Adapted from JL Juergens, JA Spittell Jr, JF Fairbairn II (eds). *Peripheral Vascular Disease*. Philadelphia: Saunders, 1980. P. 788.)

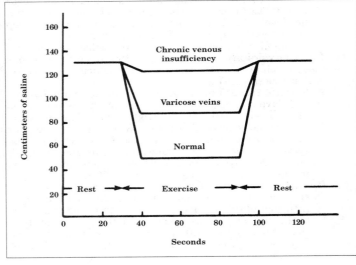

pressure is only mildly elevated, but it changes minimally with exercise.

D. Pulmonary embolism. The main physiologic consequence of acute pulmonary embolism is hypoxemia, which appears to be primarily the result of mechanical blockage of the pulmonary arteries. Some evidence indicates that humoral factors also may contribute to the hypoxic state. The chronic physiologic result can be pulmonary hypertension, chronic hypoxemia, and right heart failure.

E. Postphlebitic syndrome. Two main physiologic abnormalities may occur in patients experiencing postphlebitic syndrome: venous outflow obstruction and valve incompetence. The venous obstruction tends to be less important and to decrease with time, as the deep veins often recanalize over a 3- to 6-month period. Valve incompetence resulting from damage to the valve cusps by the thrombotic process generally is the most important physiologic abnormality. It results in a minimal drop in venous pressure with exercise in the postphlebitic limb, because the musculovenous pump functions poorly when the deep vein valves are incompetent. Chronic edema is the primary manifestation of the high venous pressures. Heavy (40 mm Hg) below-the-knee support hose can assist the limb with venous emptying and help minimize the chronic elevation of venous pressure.

V. Natural history. Although venous diseases can acutely threaten life, they frequently are chronic problems. It is important that both the patient and physician understand this chronicity. In most cases, the natural history can be satisfactorily altered so that the patient remains productive and comfortable.

A. Varicose veins. Varicose veins generally follow a chronic and benign course. For many patients, the main annoyance is their unsightly appearance. They tend to become worse during pregnancy and with obesity, as intraabdominal pressure is increased. Occasionally, superficial thrombophlebitis occurs but is seldom complicated by deep venous extension or embolism. Hemorrhage is rare but can lead to substantial bleeding and occasional shock, especially in elderly debilitated people. For most patients, simple varicose veins cause no more than a tired, heavy feeling of the legs after prolonged standing.

B. Venous thrombosis. The most feared natural consequence of deep venous thrombosis is thromboembolism to the lung. Pulmonary embolism seldom occurs when the clots are located below the knees, but it is not uncommon in cases of iliofemoral thrombosis. Another severe complication is **phlegmasia cerulea dolens**, the result of extensive deep venous thrombosis. It can cause cutaneous gangrene and usually causes a grave prognosis. The natural course for many patients with simple deep venous thrombosis, even without anticoagulation, is gradual resolution of the acute tenderness and swelling. Over a period of several months, the deep veins usually recanalize. However, without appropriate anticoagulation, about 30% of untreated patients have recurrent thrombosis or pulmonary embolism with a high mortality.

C. Pulmonary embolism. Because many episodes of deep venous thrombosis probably go undetected, the incidence of thromboembolism to the lungs is difficult to ascertain. Best estimates indicate a pulmonary embolism rate of about 25% in untreated deep venous thrombosis of the lower limb and 5% in adequately treated patients. Approximately 1 patient in 10 with a symptomatic pulmonary embolus dies within 1 hour. The remaining patients who are adequately treated with anticoagulants usually follow a course of complete resolution and return to good cardiopulmonary function within several weeks. The most important factor leading to a poor prognosis is the presence of preexisting heart disease. A small group of patients develop recurrent emboli and eventually pulmonary hypertension with cor pulmonale.

D. Postphlebitic syndrome. To delineate the natural history of postphlebitic syndrome, patients with previous deep venous thrombosis must be followed for a long period, preferably at least 5–10 years. Within 5 years, approximately 50% have developed chronic induration and stasis dermatitis at the ankle. Nearly 20% have had a venous ulcer. These percentages continue to increase with time. This natural history can be altered by proper elastic leg support hose and surgery in properly selected patients.

Selected Reading

Belcaro G, Christopoulos D, Nicolaides AN. Lower extremity venous hemodynamics. *Ann Vasc Surg* 5:305, 1991.

Bergan JJ, Yao JST (eds). *Venous Disorders*. Philadelphia: Saunders, 1991.

Moneta GL, Dorfman GS. Acute and Chronic Venous Disorders. In DE Standness Jr, A van Breda (eds), *Vascular Diseases: Surgical and Interventional Therapy*. New York: Churchill Livingstone, 1994.

Nicolaides AN, et al. The relation of venous ulceration with ambulatory venous pressure measurements. *J Vasc Surg* 17:414, 1993.

Initial Patient Evaluation

The initial patient interview and physical examination provide information that directs all subsequent diagnostic tests and treatment. Advances in sophisticated techniques of noninvasive vascular testing and imaging have tended to divert attention from the importance of simply talking to and examining the patient. These newer diagnostic tests certainly add valuable hemodynamic and anatomic information to the initial patient evaluation. However, they do not replace the need for a careful history and physical examination as the first step in optimum patient care.

The initial history and physical examination serve several important purposes. First, they enable the clinician to establish a **clinical impression** or preliminary diagnosis. Peripheral vascular diseases generally result in physical changes that are apparent by inspection, palpation, and auscultation. Simple interviewing and examination of the patient often provide enough information to arrive at an accurate clinical impression. More sophisticated diagnostic tests can then be selected to confirm the clinical impression, to establish accurate size or pressure measurements, and to define the vascular anatomy.

Second, the history and physical examination allow the clinician to determine the **urgency for treatment**. Arterial and venous problems usually are easily divided into two groups. Some need emergency care to save life or limb. However, most vascular problems will require elective evaluation and treatment. This determination generally must be made on the basis of patient history and physical examination.

Finally, the initial interview establishes a certain rapport or **relationship** between the patient and physician. All subsequent interactions are influenced by the rapport developed at the initial evaluation. The patient generally wants to know what, if anything, is wrong with his or her health and what treatment is recommended. The physician hopes to gain the patient's trust, reassure the patient, and obtain some understanding of the patient's socioeconomic situation and how his or her illness is affecting it.

This section outlines the basic techniques of the initial vascular examination. The equipment needed for the examination is simple: a stethoscope, blood pressure cuff, tape measure, and funduscope. A portable Doppler unit also is helpful and allows measurement of arterial pressures and evaluation of arterial and venous sounds. With this modest amount of equipment, the clinician can make an accurate diagnosis at the bedside of most patients. The examinations of the arterial and venous systems are discussed individually, although some patients will have combined arterial and venous problems. The discussion is further subdivided into body regions, since the patient's symptoms usually are localized to one area of the body.

Examination of the Arterial System

I. **General examination.** We emphasized earlier that atherosclerotic arterial disease often is diffuse. Therefore, the initial patient evaluation, regardless of the chief complaint, should include the entire arterial system in order to identify signs of other significant atherosclerotic disease that sometimes is asymptomatic and may have been previously unrecognized. This comprehensive examination usually provides a reasonably accurate impression of the patient's general cardiovascular condition, especially the cardiac status. Such an evaluation should include the following:

   A. Checking of heart rate and rhythm.
   B. Checking of bilateral arm blood pressures.
   C. Neck auscultation for carotid bruits.
   D. Cardiac auscultation for arrhythmias, gallops, and murmurs.
   E. Abdominal palpation for an aortic aneurysm.
   F. Abdominal auscultation for bruits.
   G. Palpations of peripheral pulses.
   H. Auscultation of the femoral region for bruits.
   I. Inspection of the legs and feet for ulcers, gangrene, and microembolic phenomena.

II. **Head and neck.** The vascular problems of the head and neck that are most commonly referred for evaluation are carotid bruits, transient neurologic attacks, and an enlarged carotid pulsation suggesting a possible aneurysm or carotid body tumor.

   A. **Inspection**. Normally, the carotid pulsation is not visible. However, it may become prominent at the base of the right neck in patients with long-standing hypertension. Such patients often are referred with the clinical diagnosis of carotid aneurysm, when in fact they simply have a tortuous carotid artery. Carotid artery aneurysms generally occur near the carotid bifurcation and consequently are located at the middle or upper anterior neck area. Carotid body tumors also originate at the carotid bifurcation. Unless an aneurysm or tumor is fairly large, it may not be visible on simple inspection of the neck.

   If the patient complains of transient monocular blindness (amaurosis fugax), funduscopic inspection after dilation of the pupil may reveal bright, reflective spots in the retinal arteries. These intraarterial defects are called **Hollenhorst plaques** and represent cholesterol emboli from ulcerated plaques in the carotid or innominate arteries or the aortic arch.

   B. **Palpation**. The common carotid pulse is palpable low in the neck between the midline trachea and the anterior border of the sternocleidomastoid muscle. It is difficult to distinguish separate internal and external carotid pulses in the mid-neck, where the common carotid artery bifurcates. The internal carotid artery may be totally occluded, and the carotid pulse may feel normal as long as the external carotid artery remains patent. A strong temporal artery pulse anterior to the ear usually indicates a patent external carotid artery. Simple palpation often cannot distinguish a carotid aneurysm or carotid body tumor from benign conditions such as an enlarged deep cervical lymph node or tortuous artery. This differentiation generally requires ultrasonography or arteriography.

The vertebral artery is not readily accessible to palpation since it lies deep at the posterior base of the neck and is surrounded by cervical bone for most of its course. Pulsatile masses at the base of the neck or in the supraclavicular fossa generally originate from the thyrocervical trunk or subclavian artery.

C. Auscultation. Normally, the stethoscope can detect heart sounds over the carotid artery. Pulsatile cervical bruits are an abnormal physical finding. They may originate from local carotid stenosis or be transmitted from stenotic lesions of the aortic valve or aortic arch branches. A bruit from a carotid stenosis usually is loudest at the midneck over the carotid bifurcation. Transmitted bruits tend to be loudest over the upper chest and at the base of the neck. A duplex ultrasound may help localize the source of the bruit.

The significance of a cervical bruit depends on the presence of any associated cerebrovascular symptoms and the results of other diagnostic tests. The severity of the stenosis cannot be determined by the loudness of the bruits, since a tight carotid stenosis may have minimal flow and a faint bruit. Transient ischemic attacks (TIAs) associated with a carotid bruit suggest a hemodynamically significant carotid stenosis. Of course, TIAs also may be caused by intracranial vascular disease, by emboli from the heart or aortic arch, or by an ulcerated carotid plaque. These latter causes of TIAs generally are not accompanied by any cervical bruits. If the carotid bruit is asymptomatic, noninvasive vascular testing can help the clinician determine the hemodynamic significance of the stenosis. Arteriograms generally are performed when the noninvasive vascular testing suggests a hemodynamically significant carotid stenosis or when the patient is experiencing TIAs.

III. Upper extremity. The most common symptoms suggesting upper-extremity arterial insufficiency are pain, coldness, and exertional muscle fatigue.

A. Acute arterial ischemia is characterized by the sudden onset of pain, pallor, paresthesias, and finally paralysis. The etiology usually is embolic, although occasionally the problem is thrombosis of a subclavian-axillary aneurysm or stenosis.

B. Chronic exertional muscle fatigue or arm claudication suggests a **severe occlusive lesion** of a more proximal upper-extremity artery, such as a left subclavian occlusion. Patients with thoracic outlet syndrome also may complain of arm pain or numbness with activity. These symptoms generally are initiated by elevation or hyperabduction of the arm and are more the result of brachial plexus nerve compression than of arterial occlusion. However, thoracic outlet syndrome may be associated with acute arterial ischemia from thrombosis of the subclavian artery or embolism from a clot in a poststenotic aneurysmal dilatation of the subclavian-axillary segment.

C. Intermittent hand coldness, pain, and numbness, especially associated with cold exposure, suggest **small vessel vasospasm or Raynaud's syndrome**. The etiology may be idiopathic (Raynaud's disease) or associated with other systemic collagen vascular diseases or prior frostbite (Raynaud's phenomenon).

D. **Physical examination**

1. **Inspection**. Inspection of the upper extremity provides a considerable amount of information about the arterial circulation. Pink fingertips with a capillary refill time of less than 3 seconds is a reliable sign of adequate perfusion of the arm and hand. In contrast, the acutely ischemic upper extremity generally is pallid, and its motor function may be diminished or absent. The main change in appearance of the extremity with chronic arterial ischemia is muscle atrophy, especially in the forearm and proximal hand. Recurrent microemboli or severe small-vessel disease may be recognized by fingertip lesions, such as painful mottled areas, skin ulcerations, or gangrene. Raynaud's phenomenon is associated with a triphasic color change that the fingers undergo after cold exposure or emotional stress. The fingers appear pallid (white), then cyanotic (blue), and finally hyperemic (red) as circulation is restored.

2. **Palpation**. Normally, the upper-extremity arterial pulse can be palpated at three locations: the upper medial arm just distal to the axilla and in the groove between the biceps and triceps muscles (axillary and proximal brachial); the antecubital fossa just medial to the biceps tendon (brachial); and the wrist over the distal radius (radial) or distal ulna (ulnar).

   Skin temperature also can be grossly assessed by palpation, especially using the more sensitive back of the examining hand or fingers. The level of skin temperature demarcation in the acutely ischemic arm usually is just distal to the level of occlusion. For example, if the extremity is cold to the midforearm, the occlusion is most likely in the brachial artery at the elbow.

   Aneurysms of the upper-extremity arteries generally are detectable if they occur in regions where the pulse normally is accessible to palpation. Large subclavian aneurysms may be palpable in the supraclavicular fossa. Axillary aneurysms may be detected high in the axilla. However, small aneurysms in these locations may be missed by palpation.

3. **Auscultation**. Auscultation of upper-extremity arteries should include measurement of bilateral brachial blood pressures and examination of the supraclavicular fossa for subclavian bruits. A difference of more

than 10 mm Hg between arm blood pressures indicates a hemodynamically significant innominate, subclavian, axillary, or proximal brachial stenosis on the side with the lower blood pressure. Because collateral blood flow to the arm is so extensive, a proximal subclavian stenosis may be relatively asymptomatic.

When pulses are not palpable, the Doppler unit can be used to assess arterial signals and measure arm and forearm blood pressures. If the patient has symptoms suggesting arm claudication, the arm should be exercised for 2–5 minutes and the brachial pressures rechecked. Brachial pressures should fall if significant arterial occlusive disease exists. Digital perfusion in patients with vasospastic symptoms can be assessed by digital plethysmography.

IV. Abdomen. The retroperitoneal position of the abdominal aorta and many of its branches limits the amount of information that can be obtained by physical examination. However, certain important abnormalities can be recognized by inspection, palpation, and auscultation of the major abdominal arteries. In most cases, the abdominal vascular anatomy must ultimately be defined by further tests such as ultrasonography, computed tomography (CT) scans, magnetic resonance imaging (MRI) scanning, and arteriography.

A. Symptoms. Certain distinct clinical syndromes suggest both the presence and location of significant abdominal arterial disease. The most common symptom patterns include the following:

1. Bilateral leg claudication and impotence (chronic aortoiliac occlusive disease).
2. Mottled, painful "blue toe" syndrome and abdominal bruits (atheroembolism from ulcerated aortoiliac atherosclerosis).
3. Sudden catastrophic bilateral leg pain, coldness, paresthesias, and paralysis (acute distal aortic occlusion).
4. Intestinal angina (chronic mesenteric artery disease).
5. Sudden, severe general abdominal pain with minimal abnormal physical findings (acute mesenteric artery occlusion).
6. Acute progressive back pain and pulsatile abdominal mass (aortic aneurysm rupture).
7. Severe hypertension in a child or young adult (renovascular stenosis).

Later chapters discuss the details of each of these clinical problems.

B. Physical examination

1. **Inspection** of the abdomen probably is the most limited part of the examination of the abdominal aorta and its branches. The normal aortic pulsation usually is not visible. However, a large abdominal aortic aneurysm may be seen pulsating against the anterior abdominal wall, especially in thin patients.
2. **Palpation** remains the simplest technique of detecting an abdominal aortic aneurysm and should be a part of the routine general physical examination of any adult over 40 years of age. Many aneurysms are

asymptomatic and are first recognized incidentally by palpation of the abdomen. In addition, palpation for diminished or absent femoral pulses often is the quickest way to confirm a clinical history suggesting severe aortoiliac occlusive disease.

Certain anatomic features of the normal aorta should be remembered when one palpates the abdomen. The aorta bifurcates at about the level of the umbilicus. Unless the patient is excessively obese, the aortic pulse is palpable, especially if the abdominal wall is relaxed. This relaxation can be optimized by having the patient bend his or her knees, rest his or her feet on the examining table, and consequently flex the hips and relax the anterior abdominal musculature. The normal aorta is approximately the width of the patient's thumb.

An aortic aneurysm should be suspected when the aortic pulse feels expansile and larger than 4–5 cm. Elderly patients with kyphoscoliosis of the lumbar spine may have a tortuous, anteriorly displaced aorta that is easily mistaken for an aneurysm. An incorrect diagnosis of aortic aneurysm also may be made if one palpates too low in the abdomen and mistakes the outer limits of both iliac arteries for an aortic aneurysm.

In addition to size, other characteristics of an aneurysm may be identified by palpation. If the expansile mass extends to the xiphoid and costal margins, a suprarenal or thoracoabdominal aneurysm should be suspected. Aneurysm tenderness or referred abdominal or back pain with aneurysm palpation also are important signs. These signs may indicate imminent rupture, a perianeurysmal leak, or surrounding inflammation secondary to recent aneurysm expansion or infection. In general, iliac aneurysms cannot be palpated unless they are large, since the iliac vessels travel in a deeper anatomic position than does the distal aorta. Occasionally, a large internal iliac artery aneurysm is palpable by digital rectal examination.

3. **Auscultation** with a stethoscope commonly reveals bruits when significant occlusive disease of the aorta or its branches is present. Aortoiliac disease generally causes bruits in the middle and lower abdomen and the femoral region. Bruits secondary to isolated renal artery stenosis usually are faint and localized in the upper abdominal quadrants just lateral to the midline. Mesenteric artery occlusive disease may be associated with epigastric bruits.

Asymptomatic abdominal bruits are an occasional incidental finding on routine abdominal examination of young adults, especially thin women. If the patient is not hypertensive and does not have intestinal angina or leg claudication, these bruits may be considered benign. The bruits may originate from impingement of the diaphragmatic crura on the celiac axis.

V. **Lower extremities.** Physical examination is especially helpful in the initial evaluation of arterial problems of the lower extremities. Chronic and acute arterial insufficiency produce changes that can be recognized by inspection, palpation, and auscultation. The physical examination probably is more revealing in the lower extremities than in any other body region where common arterial problems occur.

A. Symptoms. Lower-extremity arterial problems generally present in one of three main clinical patterns. The most common presentation is chronic intermittent **claudication**. If the ischemia progresses, the patient develops so-called **threatened limb loss**. The manifestations of such severe ischemia are rest pain, nonhealing ulcers, microemboli, or gangrene of the foot. The third general clinical presentation is **acute arterial ischemia**. Its classic findings often are referred to as the five Ps: pain, pallor, paresthesias, paralysis, and pulselessness. When a patient presents with any of these clinical pictures, examination of the leg is the best method to assess the severity of ischemia and to determine the urgency for further tests and treatment.

B. Physical examination

1. **Inspection** of the leg and foot will reveal most of the important signs of chronic or acute arterial insufficiency. Early chronic arterial disease may cause no appreciable change in the appearance of the lower extremity. Eventually, muscle atrophy may become apparent. Hair loss on the foot also has been associated with poor peripheral circulation but is not a consistent sign. One of the most reliable indicators of chronic severe ischemia is elevation pallor and dependent rubor of the forefoot. Finally, tissue necrosis may occur and nonhealing ulcers or frank gangrene will appear.

   Likewise, acute arterial insufficiency will produce definite changes in the appearance of the extremity. The sudden color change of marked pallor is unmistakable in such patients. With time, cyanosis or skin mottling may become predominant. In addition, muscle weakness or paralysis, especially of the foot dorsiflexors (anterior compartment), becomes obvious. After approximately 24 hours of severe ischemia, the leg usually is swollen and the skin may blister. Black gangrene of the skin is the final change in appearance but may not occur for several days.

2. **Palpation** of lower-extremity pulses remains a time-honored method of checking peripheral arterial circulation. Four lower-extremity pulses normally are palpable. The common femoral pulse is best felt just below the inguinal ligament and approximately one and a half to two fingerbreadths lateral to the pubic tubercle. In obese patients, external rotation of the hip may facilitate palpation of the artery. The popliteal pulse is more difficult to palpate because it lies deep in the popliteal space. With the patient supine and the knee slightly flexed, the examiner should hook the fingertips of both hands around the medial and lateral knee tendons and press the fingertips into the popliteal space. The popliteal pulse usually lies slightly lateral

of midline. The dorsalis pedis artery is a terminal branch of the anterior tibial artery. This pulse normally is found in the mid-dorsum of the foot, between the first and second metatarsals. The posterior tibial artery is found in the groove behind the medial malleolus of the tibia at the ankle. The peroneal pulse generally is not palpable because of its position deep in the lower leg.

Grading of pulses is somewhat subjective. The simplest classification is either presence or absence of the pulse. This simple classification may be the most objective and reproducible way to annotate pulses. However, some physicians use a graded system: 0, absent; 1+, barely palpable; 2+, palpable but diminished; 3+, normal; 4+, prominent, suggesting local aneurysm. Pedal pulses that disappear with exercise suggest arterial occlusive disease of the lower limb.

Palpation also is helpful in the assessment of the acutely ischemic leg. Extremity skin coldness and the level of temperature demarcation can be detected by palpation of the ischemic limb with the back of the examiner's hand and fingers, which are most sensitive to temperature differences. Acute ischemia also may be associated with tenderness and tenseness of the ischemic calf muscles, especially the anterior compartment. In addition, acute arterial insufficiency may cause sensory nerve damage, detectable by simple pinprick sensory examination.

3. **Auscultation** of lower-extremity arteries is most useful in the femoral area, where bruits indicate local femoral artery disease or more proximal aortoiliac disease with bruits transmitted to the groin. If the femoral bruit is questionable, walking the patient for 25–50 quick steps at the bedside often will increase lower-extremity blood flow enough to make the bruit louder and easier to auscultate. Auscultation also is important when an arteriovenous fistula is suspected, which generally has a characteristic continuous to-and-fro bruit.

Examination of
the Venous System

Venous disease usually is localized to one anatomic area, unlike atherosclerotic arterial disease, which often involves several body regions. The lower extremities most commonly are involved, although significant venous problems can impair function of the upper extremities.

I. **Upper extremities.** Acute or chronic obstruction of the axillary or subclavian veins constitutes the main serious venous disorder of the arms. The chief complaint in most cases is arm swelling. Diffuse aching pain may accompany the swelling and generally is worse with prolonged use or dependency of the extremity.

Acute axillary or subclavian vein thrombosis usually occurs in one of two clinical settings. The first setting is chronic subclavian vein catheterization for parenteral nutrition, intravenous therapy, and pacemaker therapy. The second setting is thoracic outlet syndrome, in which extrinsic compression may cause stasis and thrombosis. The term **effort thrombosis** is usually used if acute thrombosis occurs following vigorous upper extremity exercise, work, or lifting.

Chronic arm swelling may be the result of venous or lymphatic obstruction. Venous obstruction may follow acute thrombosis or result from partial extrinsic compression of the subclavian vein by a thoracic outlet syndrome. Lymphatic obstruction generally is associated with an operation (e.g., radical mastectomy), infection, or irradiation that involved the axillary lymph nodes.

A. **Inspection.** Subclavian vein thrombosis causes swelling of the entire arm and hand. Acutely, the arm may appear bluish or cyanotic. Rarely, extensive subclavian-axillary venous thrombosis results in venous gangrene. These patients often have underlying malignant disease or a coagulopathy such as heparin-induced thrombocytopenia and thrombosis. Characteristically, they have palpable arterial pulses despite cutaneous gangrene. Around the shoulder region, numerous superficial venous collateral channels may become visible, especially compared to the opposite normal arm.

The upper extremity generally does not develop the stasis dermatitis appearance that accompanies postphlebitic syndrome of the legs. However, upper-extremity chronic venous swelling, hyperpigmentation, and ulceration may occur after construction of an arteriovenous fistula for hemodialysis. Differentiation of venous obstruction from lymphedema may be difficult, although the clinical setting may suggest the most likely etiology.

B. **Palpation** offers limited information about venous problems of the arm. The axillary and subclavian veins are not palpable because they lie deep to the clavicle. In contrast, phlebitis of a superficial arm vein classically is recognized by a tender venous cord with local erythema and heat.

C. Auscultation. Normally, venous sounds are not audible with a stethoscope. If arm swelling follows a penetrating injury or operation of the arm, listening over the scar may reveal a bruit caused by an arteriovenous fistula. A continuous-wave Doppler unit can be used to listen to deep venous sounds.

II. Lower extremities. The most common venous problems of the legs are varicose veins, deep venous thrombosis, and postphlebitic syndrome. Although these conditions may be asymptomatic, they generally are associated with some degree of leg pain and swelling. Physical examination is the primary method of evaluating varicose veins and postphlebitic syndrome, since these conditions cause visible changes on the surface of the leg. In contrast, the patient history and physical examination often are unreliable in making an accurate diagnosis of deep venous thrombosis. In fact, only about 50% of patients who are initially thought to have deep venous thrombosis by history and physical examination will have an abnormal venogram. This latter finding should not be surprising, since acute leg pain and tenderness may have so many etiologies other than thrombophlebitis. Gastrocnemius musculotendinous rupture is one condition that may mimic thrombophlebitis.

Before describing the physical evaluation for the leg veins, several aspects of the history deserve mention. First, the severity of symptoms does not necessarily correlate with the appearance of varicose veins. In fact, some patients may exaggerate symptoms to convince the physician that something must be done about the unsightly appearance of the varicosities. Second, acute deep venous thrombosis may not cause typical calf pain and tenderness. The presenting sign may be nothing more than leg swelling. In some situations, the patient's first sign of lower-extremity deep venous thrombosis may be a symptomatic pulmonary embolus. Finally, postphlebitic syndrome generally does not occur until months or years after the acute thrombophlebitis. In fact, some patients with postphlebitic problems will not have a positive history of previous deep venous thrombosis. Acute deep venous thrombosis may have been silent or mistaken for some other problem such as a calf muscle strain.

A. Inspection should be done with both legs completely exposed from the groin to the feet. Important findings may be recognized by comparing the abnormal and normal extremities. When possible, the patient should stand so that superficial veins fill. We prefer that the patient stand on a short stool while the examiner sits on a chair or stool. This examining position provides a better view of the legs. If good overhead lighting or sunlight is not available for illumination of all aspects of the leg, an adjustable bedside examining lamp is useful. The entire leg should be examined as the patient turns 360 degrees.

1. Varicosities most commonly involve the greater saphenous vein on the medial side of the leg. Varicose branches of the greater saphenous vein often course around the upper calf to appear on the posteromedial aspect of the midcalf. Lesser saphenous varicosities appear on the posterior calf from the knee to the ankle. The location of the varicosities may suggest the etiology. For example, a dilated greater saphenous vein from the groin to the ankle is typical of familial valvular incompetence and vein dilatation. In contrast, varicosities that begin at or below the knee often are secondary to incompetent communicating veins from the deep venous system. These incompetent perforating veins may be acquired after thrombophlebitic damage. Two simple bedside tests may help identify whether the greater saphenous valves or the communicating (perforating) veins are incompetent.

   a. Trendelenburg's test (modified). For Trendelenburg's test, the patient lies supine and the leg is elevated to empty all varicosities. A soft rubber tourniquet is applied to the leg just below the knee, and the patient stands. If the lower leg varicosities fill slowly with the tourniquet in place but then dilate suddenly when the tourniquet is released, the greater saphenous valves are incompetent. In contrast, incompetent deep and communicating veins will immediately cause filling of the varicosities despite a tourniquet above them.

   b. Perthes' test checks the patency and competency of the communicating and deep venous system. While the patient stands, a soft tourniquet is applied around the upper calf. The patient repeatedly plantar flexes the foot, contracting the gastrocnemius and soleus muscles (musculovenous pump). Normally, this exercise causes flow from the superficial to the deep venous system and results in partial emptying of the surface veins. However, if the communicating and deep veins have incompetent valves, the varicosities remain distended.

2. Acute deep venous thrombosis usually causes a change in the appearance of the leg. Extremity swelling is the most common sign and generally is limited to the lower leg, with tibial or popliteal venous thrombosis. If the iliac vein is obstructed, swelling may extend to the groin. The amount of swelling should be documented by measurements of calf and thigh diameters of both legs. Serial examinations will be more accurate if these measurements are made at a given distance above and below a bony landmark such as the anterior tibial tuberosity. With extensive iliofemoral thrombosis, **phlegmasia cerulea dolens** may be observed: massive tight leg edema, severe leg pain, and cyanotic mottled skin that progresses to cutaneous gangrene.

Inspection also helps with the differential diagnosis of acute leg pain and swelling. Superficial thrombophlebitis often is evidenced by a localized erythematous streak along the course of the involved vein, usually the greater saphenous vein. A break in the skin with surrounding erythema and induration suggests cellulitis. A localized ecchymosis over the thigh or calf may indicate that the leg pain is caused by a muscle contusion or hematoma. Diffuse, nonpainful leg edema with a thick "pigskin" appearance (peau d'orange) is typical of lymphedema.

3. **Postphlebitic syndrome** is associated with rather specific changes in the appearance of the lower leg. Because of incompetent deep venous valves and venous hypertension, the lower leg becomes chronically swollen, mainly at the ankle. With progression, irregular thickened areas of brownish skin pigmentation (hemosiderin) appear around the ankle. This stasis dermatitis may be complicated by superficial skin ulceration. These venous ulcers classically occur on the medial ankle at the site of the lowest perforating vein. They usually are shallow ulcers with healthy-appearing granulations that bleed easily with manipulation.

4. **Chronic diffuse lower-limb swelling** without postphlebitic stasis dermatitis may be caused by either iliac vein obstruction, deep valvular incompetence, or lymphedema. Compression of the left common iliac vein by the right common iliac artery (May-Thurner syndrome) can eventually result in venous intimal fibroplasia, partial obstruction, and progressive left leg swelling. In contrast, primary or secondary lymphedema can result in chronic leg swelling that typically has a diffuse pitting "pigskin" appearance and does not resolve with bedrest at night. Venous edema, on the other hand, may resolve completely with bedrest and worsen with prolonged dependency.

B. **Palpation** provides useful information in the evaluation of varicose veins and acute venous thrombosis but does not add much data to initial evaluation of the postphlebitic limb.

1. If the varicosities on the medial leg are palpated, sites of communicating veins often can be recognized by indentations of the muscle fascia where these veins perforate to the deeper veins. It is important to identify these perforating sites when an operation to ligate the incompetent communicating veins (Linton flap procedure) is planned.

2. Deep venous thrombosis may cause tenderness of calf or thigh muscles. Such tenderness is not specific for thrombophlebitis, since muscle strain, contusion, or hematoma may cause similar tenderness. Forceful dorsiflexion of the foot contracts the gastrocnemius muscle and may cause pain when deep vein thrombophlebitis is present (Homans' sign). Again, this sign is suggestive of but not diagnostic for deep venous thrombophlebitis. In contrast, tenderness, heat, and induration over a superficial vein are the primary diagnostic criteria for superficial thrombophlebitis.

3. Palpation may help determine the possible cause of leg swelling associated with chronic venous insufficiency. Occasionally, chronic venous obstruction is secondary

to extrinsic compression by a pelvic, femoral, or popliteal mass, and so these regions should be palpated for aneurysms or tumors.

C. **Auscultation** with a stethoscope does not provide much information about superficial or deep venous flow. However, the Doppler unit is especially helpful in the examination of lower-extremity veins (see Chap. 5). It allows assessment of both deep vein patency and incompetency of valves. If leg edema or varicosities occur after a penetrating leg injury, the stethoscope or Doppler unit may detect a bruit from an arteriovenous fistula.

Noninvasive Vascular Testing

This chapter summarizes the basic principles of selecting, performing, and interpreting noninvasive hemodynamic studies for both arterial and venous problems. We emphasize that these noninvasive tests do not replace but **supplement** a thorough patient history and physical examination. In some situations, the results of noninvasive studies help the clinician determine the need for an invasive study such as an arteriogram or venogram. In addition, noninvasive tests provide a physiologic baseline before therapy and an objective assessment of outcome after treatment.

The development of clinical vascular laboratories lagged behind the introduction of angiography, synthetic grafts, and modern operative techniques for the treatment of peripheral vascular disease. However, in the past 25 years, noninvasive vascular equipment has become common in medical centers, community hospitals, and office practices. Although experienced clinicians can adequately treat many vascular problems without noninvasive testing, the vascular laboratory provides useful physiologic information that previously was not available from history, physical examination, or angiograms. Of course, such noninvasive testing must be selected carefully to avoid unnecessary studies that add considerably to the cost of patient care. Health care reform is focusing more attention on the use and abuse of the noninvasive vascular laboratory.

I. **The vascular laboratory.** The laboratory should be in a quiet area and located for convenient use by both inpatients and outpatients. Initial equipment costs obviously will vary and may range from $30,000–$300,000 depending on the installation of sophisticated duplex ultrasonography. A technician usually performs the tests, which then are reviewed by a staff physician.

In some situations, a sophisticated vascular laboratory is not feasible. Nonetheless, physicians can use a simple pocket or portable continuous-wave Doppler unit to auscultate arterial and venous sounds and measure leg blood pressures. We recommend that physicians, nurses, and other paramedical personnel who care for vascular patients learn to use a portable Doppler unit for arterial monitoring.

II. **Instrumentation**. Instruments for noninvasive vascular testing should be (1) reliable and reproducible, (2) capable of intrinsic standardization, (3) suitable for use by paramedical personnel, (4) suitable for measurements during and after exercise, and (5) adaptable to current recording devices. Our experience indicates that the following list of equipment is sufficient for most arterial and venous problems:

1. Continuous-wave bidirectional Doppler system—9 MHz for arteries, 5 MHz for veins.
2. Plethysmography (optional for various arterial and venous examinations).

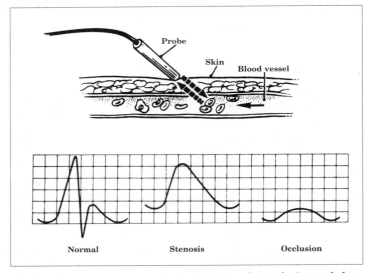

Fig. 5-1. Doppler arterial examination. The Doppler probe is coupled to the skin with acoustic gel and angled toward the direction of arterial flow. The normal Doppler arterial signal is triphasic. Stenosis and occlusion cause diminished monophasic signals.

3. A direct method of bruit analysis and imaging (e.g., duplex ultrasonography).
4. Treadmill—speeds 1.5 and 2.5 mph, 10–12.5% grade.
5. Transcutaneous oximetry (optional for documenting cutaneous perfusion).

A. Doppler ultrasound. Low-intensity ultrasound (range 1–10 MHz) can detect blood flow velocity and has been applied in monitoring arterial and venous blood flow since its introduction over 30 years ago. Simply stated, the Doppler effect shows that the average flow velocity is proportional to the frequency shift in sound waves that are transmitted toward moving blood cells and reflected back to the Doppler-receiving crystal (Fig. 5-1). A hand-held Doppler probe is placed over the course of the blood vessel being examined and is coupled to the skin with an acoustic gel. Skin lubricants other than an acoustic gel do not have the proper electrolyte content and can damage the probe crystal. Transmitted sound waves strike moving blood cells and are reflected back to the Doppler probe. An amplifier filters the sound and gives a flow signal or tracing that is proportional to the blood flow velocity.

Two types of Doppler instruments are commonly used: **continuous-wave** and **pulsed**. In practice, the continuous-wave (CW) Doppler unit is most commonly used for arterial and venous studies. The most useful Doppler instrument for examination of extremity vessels operates at 5–10 MHz. Some Doppler units are bidirectional—that is, they can detect direction as well as velocity of flow. Pulsed ultrasound was developed to provide both an image and a velocity profile of an arterial lesion. Unlike the CW Doppler, the pulsed Doppler instrument emits bursts of ultrasound waves. Between each burst, the crystal receives reflected signals. This feature allows the pulsed Doppler to sample a discrete portion of flow in a vessel being examined. Such discrete sampling provides accurate measurement of frequency (velocity) of flow through a focal stenotic lesion. The velocity patterns correlate with the degree of stenosis. Although CW Dopplers can also analyze velocity patterns, CW flow detectors may collect other signals from adjacent arteries or veins, making signal interpretation more difficult.

B. **Plethysmography**. One of the earliest means of measuring extremity blood flow was plethysmography, the measurement of volume change of an organ or body region. This principle has been applied in several forms: volume displacement (air or water), strain gauge (mercury-in-Silastic), mechanical, photoelectric, impedance, and ocular plethysmographs.

1. **The pulse volume recorder (PVR)**, developed by Raines and Darling at the Massachusetts General Hospital, is a segmental plethysmograph that has been used to monitor lower-extremity pulsatility as an indirect reflection of blood flow. The PVR uses air-filled cuffs placed at different levels around the extremity. Momentary volume changes of the limb are detected by pressure changes in the air-filled cuffs. These pulse volume changes are recorded on a strip recorder as arterial pulse contours (see Fig. 5-5). The PVR contour closely corresponds to direct intraarterial pressure waveform recordings at that level. The PVR tracings supplement Doppler segmental limb pressures and allow assessment of perfusion of the forefoot and digits where the Doppler unit cannot easily measure pressures.

2. **Ocular pneumoplethysmography (OPG)** records changes in eye volume caused by pulsatile flow in the ophthalmic artery. This vessel is the first branch of the internal carotid artery, and changes in eyeball pressure are related to significant occlusive disease of the carotid artery.

   The OPG-Gee provides direct measurement of the systolic ophthalmic artery pressure, a reflection of internal carotid pressure. An air-filled cup system is applied to the anesthetized sclera of both eyes. A vacuum draws the sclera into the cup, causing intraocular pressure to rise. When the rise in intraocular pressure exceeds systolic ophthalmic artery pressure, the eye pulse trace disappears. As the vacuum is released, pulsations return and an eyeball pressure is recorded. This pressure correlates directly with internal carotid pressure on that side.

3. **Impedance plethysmography (IPG)** measures volume changes in a limb by changes in electrical resistance. Developed by Wheeler and colleagues, IPG has become a common test for deep venous obstruction due to acute or chronic thrombosis. The rationale for the IPG is based on Ohm's law (voltage = current × resistance). Blood is a good conductor of electricity. Resistance to passage of an electrical current is lower when more blood is present in the extremity. Since deep venous obstruction increases resistance to venous outflow, the IPG can detect deep vein obstruction, although it cannot always determine whether the decreased venous outflow is caused by deep venous thrombosis, peripheral vasoconstriction, congestive heart failure, hypotension, or pulmonary hypertension.

4. **Phleborheography (PRG)** uses air-filled cuffs on the thigh, calf, and foot plus a special thoracic cuff to record volume changes of the leg with respiration. A deep venous thrombus (DVT) attenuates or eliminates the respiratory waves distal to the occlusion, with normal waves seen proximally. With extensive DVT, the respiratory waves are absent at all levels. According to a study by Cranley et al., the PRG is highly accurate (95%) for detecting acute venous occlusion. A relative drawback is that the technique requires significant time to learn and interpret.

5. **Photoplethysmography (PPG)** uses a sensor that shines light into the superficial skin layers and a photoelectric detector that measures reflected light. The intensity of reflected light correlates with venous congestion and consequently estimates venous limb pressure. A tracing is made at rest, during exercise, and through the recovery phase. The result is defined by the magnitude of the pressure drop during walking and the time required for the pressure to return to baseline. A normal recovery time is over 20 seconds. Recovery times below 20 seconds indicate venous reflux. Since the test is easy to perform and interpret, PPG provides a simple, objective means of assessing chronic venous insufficiency, especially in postphlebitic patients. Unlike the Doppler venous examination that identifies reflux at a given valve level, the PPG indicates the overall effect (recovery response) at the level studied.

C. **Duplex scanning** combines a real-time B-mode ultrasound image with a pulsed Doppler spectral analysis of flow velocity pattern. A water-soluble acoustic gel is used to couple the sound from the B-mode scan head to the skin surface. Blood vessels are identified by their characteristic B-mode images with prominent wall echoes separated by a dark, sonolucent lumen. In arteries, calcified plaques are recognized by bright intraluminal echoes and regions of posterior acoustic shadowing. The operator can place the pulsed Doppler beam in the center stream of the vessel and adjust the Doppler angle. An angle of 60

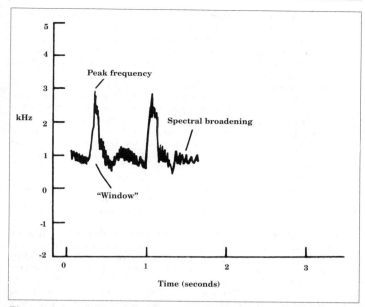

Fig. 5-2. Arterial spectrum analysis. The Doppler spectral analysis allows classification of the degree of stenosis. The most common parameters used for this classification are (1) spectral width (broadening) during systole, (2) peak systolic frequency (normal <4 kHz) or peak systolic velocity (normal <125 m/second), and (3) diastolic frequency or velocity.

degrees generally provides the best return signal for spectral analysis and velocity measurements. The Doppler sample is placed near the center stream of the vessel to avoid detection of slower velocities and eddies close to the wall. These disturbances can cause false readings of stenosis in normal arteries.

The spectral analysis allows classification of the degree of stenosis. The most common parameters used for this classification are (1) spectral width during systole, (2) peak systolic velocity, and (3) diastolic velocity. A normal Doppler spectrum of the carotid artery (Fig. 5-2) consists of a relatively low systolic peak velocity (e.g., less than 1.25 m/second in the internal carotid system) and a narrow band of frequencies during systole, resulting in a clear region beneath the systolic peak (window). With minimal stenosis, spectral changes occur as spectral broadening during the deceleration phase of systole. Further stenosis results in increased spectral broadening until the entire window beneath the systolic peak is filled, followed by an increase in peak systolic and diastolic frequencies.

Although duplex scanning was applied originally to analysis of carotid bifurcation disease, further applications have included examination of lower-extremity arteries, intestinal arteries, veins, and renal arteries. Currently, the two major disadvantages are the high cost of the equipment relative to other noninvasive techniques and the extensive operator experience required to obtain good studies.

D. Transcutaneous oximetry (TcPO$_2$) provides local measurement of skin oxygen tension and can reflect the adequacy of arterial and capillary perfusion. The principle of transcutaneous oxygen determination involves heat application (45°C) to the skin, which produces a localized hyperemia and oxygen excess. Since oxygen diffuses along a concentration gradient from the capillaries to the tissues, it can diffuse across the skin where it is electrochemically reduced and measured by a modified Clark platinum oxygen electrode. It is important to standardize vasodilation since, at skin temperatures above 43°C, the ratio of TcPO$_2$ to arterial PO$_2$ remains constant and is close to 1.

III. Lower-extremity arterial occlusive disease. Patients who are evaluated for lower-extremity arterial occlusive disease generally can be categorized into two broad groups after preliminary history and physical examination: patients with **intermittent claudication** (discomfort, tiring, or pain in lower-limb muscles with walking) or patients with severe ischemia (rest pain, nonhealing ulcers, and/or gangrene). Noninvasive vascular testing helps document the severity of claudication and provides a baseline for follow-up. Such vascular testing also may be used to confirm the degree of severe ischemia and to predict whether certain types of nonhealing skin lesions may heal without arterial revascularization.

A. Intermittent claudication. Patients with leg claudication should undergo a complete lower-extremity arterial study. This evaluation usually includes a Doppler survey of ankle and pedal arterial signals and measurement of resting ankle-brachial pressure indices (ABIs). Some laboratories also record segmental pressures and plethysmographic wave forms (PVRs) at rest and repeat these measurements after exercise.

1. Doppler survey. All major peripheral arteries can be examined by the Doppler probe. A normal arterial signal has two, and sometimes three, components (see Fig. 5-1). The first part of this crisp, high-pitched sound represents the forward blood flow during systole. The second component is reversed and brief and probably corresponds to flow reversal in early diastole. As forward flow resumes, a third low-pitched sound may be heard.

When a severe proximal arterial stenosis or occlusion is present, the Doppler signal at rest becomes lower-pitched and monophasic (see Fig. 5-1). In the case of a lesser stenosis, the resting Doppler signal may even sound normal. However, after exercise a less intense monophasic sound may be noted. This change in the Doppler sound indicates a stenosis that becomes hemodynamically significant only after exercise.

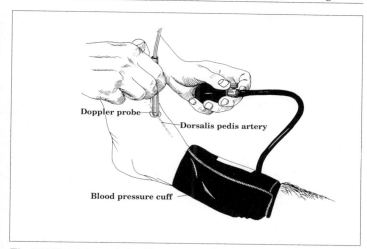

Fig. 5-3. Measurement of ankle blood pressure with a standard blood pressure cuff and a hand-held portable continuous-wave Doppler unit. This ankle pressure can be compared to the brachial (arm) blood pressure to calculate the ABI (normal = 1.0, claudication usually 0.5–0.9, rest pain or tissue necrosis usually less than 0.5).

The initial Doppler survey should note the presence or absence and the quality (biphasic or monophasic) of the femoral, popliteal, posterior tibial, and dorsalis pedis arteries.

2. **Segmental leg pressures.** The concept that segmental leg pressures (thigh, calf, and ankle) can indicate the level and significance of arterial occlusive disease was introduced more than 35 years ago but was not widely applied to clinical practice until the last 20 years. The test is performed while the patient is at rest in the supine position. Appropriately sized pneumatic cuffs (thigh, 18–20 cm in width; calf and ankle, 12 cm in width) are placed as high on the thigh as possible, on the calf immediately below the knee, and on the ankle just above the medial malleolus. A standard blood pressure manometer is used to measure the pressures. Since it is difficult to auscultate ankle pressures with a stethoscope, a Doppler probe or plethysmograph is used. We prefer the Doppler probe and place it over the ankle artery that has the loudest signal (Fig. 5-3). Next, the thigh cuff is inflated until the Doppler signal disappears. As the cuff is slowly deflated, the thigh systolic pressure is recorded when the signal reappears. In a similar fashion, calf and ankle systolic pressures are recorded. All pressures are taken by auscultating the arterial signal **at the ankle level.**

Interpretation of segmental leg pressures is based on the following principles:

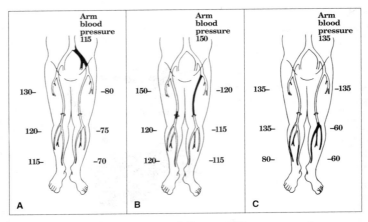

Fig. 5-4. Segmental leg pressures. A. Segmental leg pressures in a normal right lower extremity and one with isolated iliac artery occlusion (left). B. Segmental leg pressures in distal, segmental occlusions of the right superficial femoral artery (SFA) compared to proximal occlusion of the left SFA. C. Segmental leg pressures in distal (right) tibial artery occlusions and tibial disease extending into the proximal left popliteal artery. (Modified from RF Kempczinski, RB Rutherford. Current Status of the Vascular Diagnostic Laboratory. In C Rob et al [eds], *Advances in Surgery* Vol. 12. Copyright ©1978 by Year Book Medical Publishers, Inc., Chicago.)

    a. Normally, systolic ankle pressure should be equal to or greater than systolic arm pressure. In other words, the ankle-brachial pressure ratio should be 1.0 or greater. In limbs with one primary arterial occlusion, the index is usually 0.5–0.8. An ankle-arm ratio of less than 0.5 usually indicates multilevel occlusive disease.

    b. A pressure gradient of more than 20 mm Hg between cuff levels strongly suggests a hemodynamically significant occlusive lesion in the intervening arterial segment. Figure 5-4 provides several examples of arterial occlusive disease at various anatomic levels. It must be remembered that the thigh pressure may be falsely elevated if the cuff width is too narrow.

    c. Segmental leg pressures can be misleading in the following situations:

        (1) Severely calcified vessels (e.g., in dibetics) may not be compressible, so leg pressures will be falsely elevated.

        (2) Collateral blood flow may be so well developed that a 20-mm gradient is not present across a significant occlusive segment.

        (3) An extensive superficial femoral occlusion may give a thigh to arm ratio that is identical to that seen with an iliac occlusion. Of course, simple

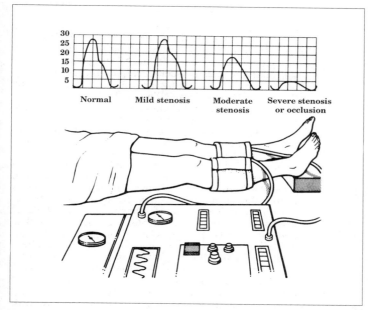

Fig. 5-5. Pulse volume recordings. The normal pulse volume recording becomes progressively flattened and prolonged with increasing arterial stenosis.

palpation for a femoral pulse should differentiate between these two situations. When the femoral pulse strength is equivocal, the hemodynamic significance of proximal aortoiliac arterial disease can be estimated. This can be accomplished by a common femoral artery Doppler blood flow velocity wave form or signal analysis.

These limitations of segmental leg pressures emphasize that results must be combined with physical findings for more accurate location of the significant occlusive lesions. Exercise testing, PVRs, and Doppler wave form analysis also add important information to the noninvasive evaluation of such patients.

3. **Pulse volume recordings** supplement the segmental leg pressures and are taken using the same pressure cuffs. Characterized by a sharp upstroke (anacrotic slope), distinct pulse peak, and rapid decline (catacrotic slope), the normal PVR tracing becomes progressively flattened and prolonged with increasing stenosis (Fig. 5-5). Segmental leg PVR tracings normally show an augmentation from thigh to calf. This augmentation is actually an artifact caused by differences in cuff

volume. In other words, the calf PVR should have greater amplitude than that of the thigh. If it does not, a superficial femoral artery occlusive lesion should be suspected. The PVR also is especially helpful in evaluating the young patient whose claudication may be due to popliteal artery entrapment by the medial head of the gastrocnemius muscle. Such patients usually have normal ankle PVR tracings at rest. With active plantar flexion or passive dorsiflexion of the foot, the gastrocnemius contracts and compresses the popliteal artery, and the ankle PVR tracing flattens.

4. **Exercise testing.** Leg exercise normally increases total limb blood flow, but systolic ankle pressures show little or no decrease. However, when significant arterial occlusive disease is present, ankle pressures drop after exercise. This pressure fall occurs for two main reasons. First, increased flow across a stenosis results in turbulence and a consequent pressure drop. Second, blood flow is diverted into higher-resistance collateral beds of the leg muscles. If actual exercise of the limb is not possible, similar pressure drops can be demonstrated by a reactive hyperemia test: inflation of a high thigh cuff to 50 mm Hg above arm pressure for 5 minutes. However, we prefer the patient to walk on a treadmill at 2 mph on a 10% incline for a maximum of 5 minutes. This walking test more accurately simulates the activity that most commonly causes claudication. Also, the cardiorespiratory reserve of the patient can be grossly evaluated.

In addition to the measurement of ankle pressures and PVRs after exercise, the recording of time of onset, location, and severity of claudication is important. This claudication profile objectively defines how much the claudication limits the patient. Serial treadmill examinations then can detect disease progression and early anastomotic stenosis after operation. Exercise testing is also helpful if there is confusion about whether the patient's leg complaints are caused by arterial occlusive disease, a musculoskeletal hip or knee disorder, or a neurologic condition such as spinal stenosis or a herniated lumbar disc.

Since patients with peripheral arterial disease often have significant heart disease, **continual electrocardiogram (ECG) monitoring** during treadmill exercise should be considered if the patient (1) has suffered previous myocardial infarction, (2) has angina pectoris requiring nitrates, (3) presents with severe chronic obstructive lung disease, (4) exhibits signs of cardiac arrhythmia as seen on the arterial PVR during initial resting examination, (5) is taking antiarrhythmic medications, (6) has undergone previous cardiac surgery, (7) has a permanent pacemaker, or (8) has suffered a recent stroke or transient ischemic attacks (TIAs). Approximately 33% of our patients undergoing lower-extremity arterial testing will have one or more of these indications for ECG monitoring. When ECG

Table 5-1. Criteria for ischemic rest pain

Noninvasive study	Unlikely	Probable	Likely
Ankle pressure (mm Hg)			
Nondiabetic	>55	35–55	<35
Diabetic	>80	55–80	<55
Ankle PVR category (mm)			
Nondiabetic	>15	5–15	<5 or flat
Diabetic	>15	5–15	<5
Transcutaneous oxygen tension (torr)	>40	10–20	0–10

PVR = pulse volume recorder.
Source: Adapted from JK Raines et al. Vascular laboratory criteria for the management of peripheral vascular disease of the lower extremities. *Surgery* 79:21, 1976.

monitoring is not available, treadmill exercise should not be performed on patients with (1) a history of angina pectoris with minimal exertion, (2) a myocardial infarction suffered in the past 6 months, or (3) unknown or untreated cardiac arrhythmia noted on initial pulse check. With or without ECG monitoring, exercise should be terminated if the patient complains of (1) chest pain or chest discomfort, (2) dyspnea, (3) dizziness, or (4) severe claudication. With ECG monitoring, additional indications for stopping exercise include (1) a heart rate greater than 120, (2) a new or increased ventricular arrhythmia, or (3) ST segment depression of more than 2 mm.

5. **Penile/brachial pressure index (PBI).** Aortoiliac occlusive disease may cause vasculogenic impotence. Distinction between vasculogenic and nonvasculogenic impotence may not be clear after urologic, endocrinologic, and psychiatric evaluations. In patients with aortoiliac disease and no other risk factors (e.g., diabetes mellitus and impotency-related drugs), a PBI less than 0.6 is highly diagnostic of vasculogenic impotence. Accuracy for borderline cases (PBI is 0.60–0.70) can be enhanced if the following criteria are used: (1) the resting PBI is less than 0.70 and stays the same or falls after standardized exercise treadmill testing (SETT); or (2) the resting PBI is greater than 0.70 but falls by greater than 0.10 and is less than 0.70 after SETT. If neither of these criteria is met, vascular occlusive disease is unlikely to be the cause of the impotence.

B. **Severe ischemia.** Patients who present with severe ischemic symptoms (rest pain, nonhealing foot lesions, or gangrene) require only resting noninvasive arterial studies. Treadmill exercise usually is not appropriate or feasible for such debilitated patients. The Doppler system and PVRs can help in the following ways:

1. **To ascertain that rest pain is ischemic and not neuropathic** (Table 5-1). Patient history and physical

Table 5-2. Criteria for healing foot lesions

Noninvasive study	Likely	Probable	Unlikely
Ankle pressure (mm Hg)			
Nondiabetic	>65	55–65	<55
Diabetic	>90	80–90	<80
Ankle PVR category (mm)			
Nondiabetic	>15	5–15	<5 or flat
Diabetic	>15	5–15	<5
Transcutaneous oxygen tension (torr)	>50	40–50	<10

PVR = pulse volume recorder.
Source: Adapted from JK Raines et al. Vascular laboratory criteria for the management of peripheral vascular disease of the lower extremities. *Surgery* 79:21, 1976.

examination usually are sufficient to diagnose ischemic rest pain. However, diabetics may have foot pain caused by both peripheral neuropathy and arterial occlusive disease. In such cases, rest pain secondary to severe ischemia should be suspected when the systolic ankle pressure is less than 55 mm Hg. In nondiabetics, rest pain is likely when ankle pressures drop below 35 mm Hg but may occur at levels between 35 and 50 mm Hg. The ankle PVR usually is flat or shows minimal deflection (less than 5 mm). The higher ankle pressure criterion for rest pain in diabetics is due to false pressure elevations secondary to decreased arterial compressibility from severe medial calcinosis of the vessel. Another method analogous to ankle pressure is measurement of systolic blood pressure in toe arteries. A small pneumatic cuff is wrapped around the toe and a photoplethysmograph, applied to the terminal phalanx, is used to sense the return of blood flow. A toe pressure less than 30 mm Hg indicates severe ischemia. In addition, we have used $TcPO_2$ of the forefoot to help differentiate ischemic pain from diabetic or alcoholic neuropathic discomfort. Forefoot $TcPO_2$ levels greater than 55 mm Hg can be considered normal at any age. Resting supine levels less than 30 mm Hg suggest arterial ischemia, especially if they drop to 0–10 mm Hg with leg elevation.

2. **To predict healing of leg or foot ulcers** (Table 5-2). Ulcers of the foot or leg have diverse etiologies that are not always clear by history and physical examination. These lesions may be the result of arterial insufficiency, venous disease, diabetic neuropathy, infection, frostbite, a variety of systemic collagen vascular illnesses, or numerous other conditions. Foot lesions are unlikely to heal if ankle pressures are less than 55 mm Hg in nondiabetics and less than 80 mm Hg in diabetics. A severely attenuated (<5 mm) or flat PVR tracing at the ankle or transmetatarsal level also correlates

with poor healing. Our experience with foot $TcPO_2$ measurements indicates that levels less than 20–30 mm Hg are generally associated with nonhealing. Chronic ischemic ulcers and gangrene are often accompanied by forefoot $TcPO_2$ levels of 0–10 mm Hg. These criteria apply only if local infection has been controlled.

3. **To predict healing at various amputation levels** (see Chap. 15). Vascular laboratory findings alone have not been sufficient to select an appropriate amputation level. Physical examination remains the best method of selecting an amputation level, although noninvasive studies may help. In general, an amputation is unlikely to succeed if the PVR tracing is nonpulsatile at the proposed amputation level. Ankle pressures have not correlated well with healing of below-knee amputations (BKAs). The outlook of a BKA has been favorably correlated with distal thigh or calf pressures of greater than 65 mm Hg. The presence of a pulsatile PVR tracing at the transmetatarsal or digital level also is encouraging for likely healing of local amputations at these levels. Our data also suggest that a $TcPO_2$ tension value of at least 40 mm Hg measured on the anterior skin flap at the proposed level of amputation is predictive of success. The conversion of absolute values to a $TcPO_2$ tension index by dividing by the corresponding anterior chest value appears to offer a slightly better discrimination, with a threshold value of 0.59.

C. **Postoperative surveillance.** Chapter 9 focuses on the importance and methods of detecting intraoperative problems with arterial reconstructions. Several authors have documented improved long-term graft patency when hemodynamically failing grafts are recognized before occlusion. Although the majority of patients with failing grafts will notice recurrent or worsening claudication, some will not become symptomatic until acute graft thrombosis. The simplest office method of detecting hemodynamic failure is the measurement of the ankle-brachial pressure index. A decline of 0.15 between office visits is considered significant enough to justify further duplex scanning or arteriography. In addition, a progressive fall in resting ankle pressure after treadmill exercise is another noninvasive means to detect a failing graft.

Duplex scanning may be a better method of detecting a problem requiring revision since resting ankle pressures may fail to detect graft problems in some patients. A decrease in peak systolic flow velocity to less than 40–45 cm/second generally identifies a femoropopliteal-tibial graft prone to failure. Real-time B-mode imaging of the graft and anastomoses should be attempted when a low velocity is noted. If scanning of the graft locates a stenosis where the ratio of the poststenotic (V_2) to prestenotic (V_1) velocities is greater than 2 **and** the peak graft velocity is less than 40 cm/second (Fig. 5-6), the graft is at higher risk of occlusion. Long-term postoperative surveillance with duplex scanning and flow velocity determina-

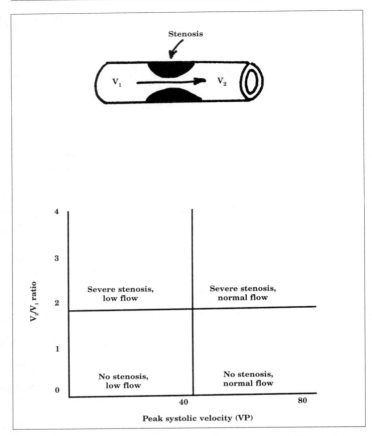

Fig. 5-6. Surveillance of lower-extremity femoropopliteal-tibial vein bypass grafts. This graph categorizes vein graft functional performance into categories based on peak systolic velocity (V_P) measured at the midpoint of the graft and the velocity ratio (V_2/V_1) across a stenosis. The grafts at greatest risk for occlusion have both low velocity (V_P <40 cm/second) and a high velocity ratio across a stenosis (V_2/V_1 >2). (Based on clinical observations by Bandyk et al.)

tion detects anatomic or hemodynamic abnormalities in at least 5–10% of vein arterial bypasses. Most experts agree that graft longevity can be enhanced by correcting such stenoses, even if they are asymptomatic. In fact, about 60% of vein grafts with a significant stenosis will not be associated with symptoms at the time of initial recognition on duplex scanning.

IV. **Extracranial cerebrovascular disease.** Noninvasive cerebrovascular testing is still under development. The search continues for a noninvasive test that can match the anatomic information and accuracy of an arteriogram.

Although the risk of angiography is low (1–2% morbidity) in experienced hands, the technique is invasive and expensive. In addition, the routine use of angiography in evaluating patients with possible extracranial vascular disease reveals many patients with no significant surgical pathology. Furthermore, the arteriogram does not provide hemodynamic information about physiologic importance of an anatomic lesion. Consequently, various noninvasive tests have been devised to assist with better selection of patients for arteriography and surgery.

A. **Indications for noninvasive cerebrovascular tests.** Before describing the common noninvasive tests for extracranial cerebrovascular disease, we must consider the appropriate indications for such testing.

1. **An asymptomatic cervical bruit** in an acceptable surgical candidate. (Obviously an asymptomatic bruit in a patient who is severely debilitated by any medical condition would be more appropriately followed without further testing or surgery.)

2. **Nonspecific neurologic symptoms** (e.g., dizziness).

3. **Follow-up** of patients after previous carotid endarterectomy to detect restenosis.

4. **Follow-up** of patients with known mild asymptomatic carotid stenosis (less than 50% diameter).

5. **Head and neck surgery** in which one carotid artery may require ligation or resection.

6. **Early postoperative neurologic deficit** after carotid endarterectomy to detect carotid thrombosis.

7. **Baseline data in symptomatic patients.** The value of noninvasive testing in patients with classic TIAs or strokes is debatable. Such patients generally need a cerebral angiogram before any cerebrovascular operation, although some surgeons are proceeding to carotid endarterectomy with only a duplex ultrasound. In our experience, an angiogram remains the best method of imaging the entire extracranial and intracranial cerebrovasculature. A good arteriogram clearly shows the intrathoracic origins of the brachiocephalic arteries, the degree and extent of carotid bifurcation lesions, ulcerative or stenotic lesions of the carotid siphon, and the smaller intracranial arteries where occlusions or aneurysms may cause neurologic symptoms. Neither noninvasive tests, intravenous digital subtraction arteriograms (IV-DSAs), or magnetic resonance angiography can provide the clarity and extent of information available on intraarterial cerebral angiograms.

Although noninvasive cerebrovascular tests may not change the need for arteriography in symptomatic patients, they can generally identify the presence of hemodynamically significant carotid stenoses that are appropriate for endarterectomy. Recently, carotid duplex scans have been used to screen patients with atypical neurologic symptoms or contrast allergies before arteriography.

Duplex sonography may also provide some useful information about the vertebral arteries in patients with nonlateralizing, posterior cerebral symptoms such as dizziness, vertigo, blurred vision, ataxia, and syncope. In most patients, the proximal vertebral arteries can be identified. Origin stenosis can be detected, and the direction of flow can be ascertained. Direction of flow may be important if proximal innominate or subclavian stenosis or occlusion is present (e.g., subclavian steal). Since the vertebral arteries are surrounded by the vertebral bodies for most of their cervical course, most of their length cannot be seen by ultrasound.

Transcranial Doppler (TCD) may also provide some useful hemodynamic information in patients with symptoms suggesting posterior circulation insufficiency. However, the utility of TCD is still debated.

B. Noninvasive carotid artery studies are generally classified as indirect or direct. Most early tests (supraorbital Doppler analysis and ocular plethysmography) provided indirect measurement by detecting changes in blood flow and pressure distal to the carotid stenosis or occlusion. Common limitations of **indirect** methods are that they only detect lesions that are sufficiently advanced to reduce mean blood flow and consequently can miss ulcerative lesions that are not associated with severe stenosis. In addition, they cannot differentiate a tight stenosis from an occlusion since the hemodynamic changes in the distal arterial bed are indistinguishable. In contrast, **direct** methods focus on imaging the extracranial carotid arteries (ultrasonic scans) and on determining the degree of stenosis (continuous or pulsed Doppler spectral analysis).

In general, the diagnostic accuracy of noninvasive cerebrovascular testing may be enhanced by performing two complementary procedures. The best combination usually includes one direct method (e.g., duplex scan) to assess the carotid bifurcation with one indirect method (e.g., OPG-Gee) to ascertain the distal hemodynamic significance of any lesion. The selection of tests depends on what equipment is available in a specific lab and on what the accuracies are for the specific techniques used in that lab. Each laboratory must learn its own limitations if accuracy is to be optimized. The following emphasizes some of the common problems we have encountered in performing and interpreting various tests.

1. Indirect methods. Our experience has been greatest with the ocular pneumoplethysmography (OPG-Gee) and transcranial Doppler.

a. Ocular pneumoplethysmography (OPG-Gee). Ophthalmic artery pressure correlates reliably with pressure in the distal internal carotid artery. The OPG-Gee can determine ophthalmic artery pressure and identify a hemodynamically significant carotid stenosis (more than 50% diameter) with 85–95% accuracy. In our experience, the OPG-Gee has been easier to perform and interpret than other OPG methods. Its main limitations are its inability to detect nonobstructive, ulcerated plaques and to distinguish between severe stenosis and occlusion of the internal carotid artery.

Since a plastic monitoring eye cup is placed on the lateral sclera after topical anesthesia, the test is not recommended in patients with (1) allergy to topical anesthesia, (2) acute or chronic conjunctivitis, (3) a history of detached retina, (4) eye surgery within the previous 6 months, (5) untreated or unstable glaucoma, (6) recent eye trauma, or (7) an intraocular lens prosthesis, or in an uncooperative or agitated patient.

Our criteria for an abnormal test include:
(1) A difference of 5 mm Hg or more between the two ophthalmic artery pressures.
(2) A ratio of ophthalmic artery to brachial artery pressure of less than 0.60 when the eye pressures are equal (i.e., severe bilateral carotid disease).
(3) A difference of 1–4 mm Hg when the ophthalmic to brachial pressure ratio is below 0.66.

One must remember that a low OPG can be caused by one or more occlusive lesions at any point along the carotid pathway, including its intrathoracic origin, carotid bifurcation, carotid siphon, or ophthalmic artery itself.

b. **Transcranial Doppler** is a relatively new noninvasive method to assess the intracranial circulation. TCD devices emit pulses of ultrasound from a 2-MHz probe. Specific bony "windows" to the intracranial arteries are used (Fig. 5-7). By placing the probe superior to the zygomatic arch, one can insonate the distal internal carotid artery siphon, anterior cerebral artery A1 segment, middle cerebral artery M1 segment, and posterior cerebral artery P1 and P2 segments. The ophthalmic artery and a portion of the internal carotid siphon may be assessed with the transorbital approach. The suboccipital window is used to insonate the distal intracranial segment of the vertebrobasilar system.

A variety of clinical applications have been established for TCD. These include (1) assessment of intracranial collateral patterns and hemodynamic reserve in occlusive carotid disease, (2) diagnosis of intracranial stenosis and occlusion, (3) diagnosis of vasospasm in the setting of subarachnoid hemorrhage, (4) monitoring the hemodynamic effects of arteriovenous malformation treatment, (5) assessment of intracranial circulation in patients with increased intracranial pressure and cerebral death, and (6) intraoperative and postoperative monitoring. However, the total impact of TCD on the current evaluation of cerebrovascular disease remains relatively small compared to the role of extracranial carotid duplex ultrasonography.

2. **Direct methods** include carotid phonoangiography, continuous-wave Doppler velocity wave form analysis, quantitative bruit analysis, various ultrasonic Doppler

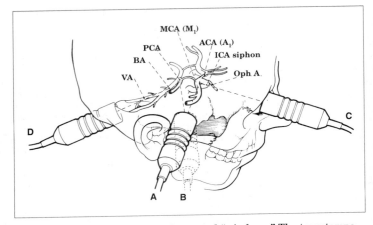

Fig. 5-7. Transcranial Doppler ultrasound "windows." The transtemporal approach (A) is used to study the middle cerebral artery (MCA), M1 segment, anterior cerebral artery (ACA), A1 segment, and the distal siphon of the internal carotid artery (ICA). By directing the probe slightly inferiorly and posteriorly (B), the posterior cerebral artery (PCA) P1 and P2 segments may be insonated. The transorbital approach (C) permits insonation of the ophthalmic artery (Oph A) and the ICA siphon in the region of the clinoid and cavernous sinus. The suboccipital window (D) allows examination of the distal intracranial segments of the verterbral arteries (VA) and the basilar artery (BA). (By permission of the Mayo Foundation.)

scans, and duplex scanning. Because it combines the benefit of real-time B-mode ultrasound imaging and pulsed Doppler velocity wave form analysis, duplex scanning has become the direct method of choice despite its relatively higher cost and dependency on operator experience.

Duplex scanning was developed by Strandness and colleagues at the University of Washington to combine the benefits of a real-time B-mode ultrasound image system with a pulsed Doppler detector. The ultrasound image not only shows the vessel and plaque anatomy but also allows precise positioning of the Doppler beam in the center stream of the vessel for optimal study of velocity patterns. The duplex scanner can study calcified lesions since the B-mode scanning allows the examiner to position the Doppler beam distal to the calcification and sample disturbed velocity patterns at this point. Based on flow signal characteristics (Table 5-3, Fig. 5-8), the degree of internal carotid disease is placed in one of six categories: (1) normal, (2) minimal disease (0–15% diameter reduction), (3) moderate stenosis (16–49%), (4) severe stenosis (50–79%), (5) critical stenosis (80–99%), and (6) occlusion.

Different investigators have demonstrated that the technique is highly accurate, with a sensitivity and

**Table 5-3. Categories of internal
carotid artery disease based on duplex scanning**

Grade	Angiogram description	Wave form criteria	Clinical impression
A	Normal	ICA: Peak systole <1.25 m/sec (or <4 kHz); clear window under peak systole; no spectral broadening	No lesions detected in the internal carotid artery
B	0–15% diameter reduction	ICA: Peak systole <1.25 m/sec (or <4kHz); clear window under peak systole; minimal or no spectral broadening in deceleration phase of systole	Minimal disease
C	16–49% diameter reduction	ICA: Peak systole <1.25 m/sec (or <4 kHz): spectral broadening throughout systole; no window	Moderate disease
D	50–79% diameter reduction	ICA: Peak systole >1.25 m/sec (or >4 kHz); increased diastolic flow; marked spectral broadening, ICA/CCA ratio >1.8:1	Severe disease hemodynamically significant
D+	80–90% diameter reduction	ICA: End diastolic peak >1.35 m/sec (or >4.5 kHz), ICA/CCA ratio 3.5:1	Severe disease hemodynamically significant
E	Occluded	CCA: Unilateral flow to zero or reversed ICA: No signal	Occluded

ICA = internal carotid artery; CCA = common carotid artery.

Fig. 5-8. Internal carotid artery Doppler spectrum patterns. The criteria for each category are summarized in Table 5-3. The percentages refer to degree of stenosis.

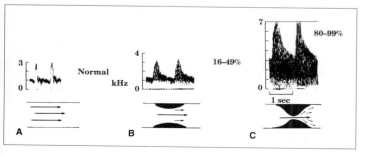

specificity over 90%. Of special importance is the high accuracy (95–97%) of separating severe stenosis from occlusion. A natural history study of asymptomatic carotid bruits categorized and followed by duplex scanning has also documented that stenoses greater than 80% are the lesions most commonly associated with subsequent TIAs, strokes, and asymptomatic internal carotid occlusions. This information makes duplex scanning a powerful tool for selecting low-risk patients for possible prophylactic carotid endarterectomy.

Since duplex scanning can provide high-quality ultrasound images of carotid lesions as well as hemodynamic information, some investigators have raised a provocative question: Can selected patients with good quality duplex scans and no signs of proximal brachiocephalic disease (normal proximal carotid pulses, normal arm pressures, and no supraclavicular bruits) and normal brain imaging (computed tomography or magnetic resonance imaging) undergo carotid endarterectomy without the risk and expense of carotid arteriography? The answer is debatable, but advances in the quality and accuracy of noninvasive cerebrovascular imaging and flow analysis does not make this provocative question seem so radical now.

V. **Deep venous thrombosis.** Patient history and physical examination are notoriously unreliable for the diagnosis of lower-extremity DVT because leg swelling and tenderness can be caused by several etiologies that physical examination cannot always differentiate. A venogram was once the definitive diagnostic study for deep venous disease but causes discomfort and sometimes serious allergic reaction or phlebitis. In our experience, about 50% of patients with suspected DVT will have a normal venogram; therefore, noninvasive venous studies (Table 5-4) have replaced venography in the initial evaluation of acute DVT.

The major noninvasive venous studies are Doppler venous auscultation, I^{125} fibrinogen scanning, radionuclide phlebography, various types of venous plethysmography, and Doppler ultrasonic imaging. Currently, we prefer duplex ultrasound for the initial evaluation of patients with a high risk or suspicion DVT. Impedence plethysmography also remains a relatively low-cost screening test for DVT in low-risk patients. The other noninvasive venous tests are not of much clinical use.

A. **Venous plethysmography.** The diagnostic accuracy of venous plethysmography makes it a reasonable screening test. Although its sensitivity for acute DVT is high, specificity is lower (60–70%), and positive predictive value is only 50% in our recent experience. Nonetheless, the equipment is portable and can be used at the bedside. The plethysmographic tracing also provides an objective recording for the patient's chart. Plethysmography is highly reliable above the knee but less sensitive for calf thrombosis.

Several types of plethysmography can be used: impedance, mercury strain gauge, and volume displacement.

Table 5-4. Noninvasive methods of assessing venous disease

Test	Measures	Detect acute DVT	Detect chronic occlusion	Detect value reflux
Duplex Doppler ultrasound	Venous flow patterns with respiration and muscle compression Valvular competence	+	+	+
Impedance plethysmography	Venous capacity Maximum venous outflow	+	+	−
Phleborrheography	Venous flow patterns with respiration and muscle compression	+	+	−
Photoplethysmography	Response of venous pressure to exercise	−	−	+

DVT = deep venous thrombosis; + = reliable in detection; − = unreliable in detection.
Source: Modified from JD Baker. The Vascular Laboratory. In WS Moore (ed), *Vascular Surgery: A Comprehensive Review.* Orlando: Grune & Stratton, 1986. Pp. 205–241.

The accuracy of each type is comparable. Thus we discuss the general principles of venous plethysmography and emphasize pitfalls in its application.

Approximately 80% of the lower-extremity blood volume is in the veins. The use of plethysmography in detecting deep venous obstruction is based on the principle that venous occlusion will change deep venous resistance and outflow. These volume changes can be recognized by a plethysmograph.

A normal venous plethysmograph of the leg shows a gradual increase after temporary occlusion of venous outflow by a thigh cuff inflated to 45–50 mm Hg for 45 seconds. With cuff release, the tracing drops rapidly toward the baseline. The plateau in calf inflation is called the **venous capacitance (VC)** (Fig. 5-9). The decrease in volume during the first second after cuff deflation is termed the **maximum venous outflow (MVO)**. By plotting VC against MVO, it can be predicted with 90% accuracy whether the deep veins are normal or obstructed.

Leg position is especially critical to an accurate examination. The leg should be slightly elevated to minimize differences in venous pooling. External rotation of the leg enhances muscle relaxation, and slight knee flexion minimizes extrinsic popliteal vein compression.

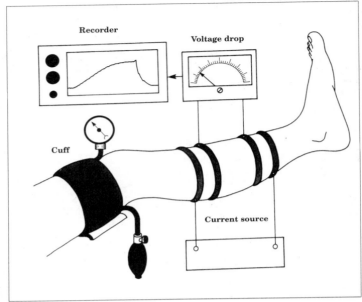

A

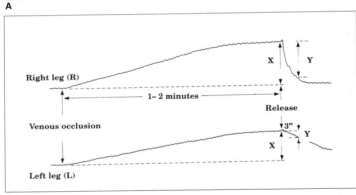

B

Fig. 5-9. A. A high-frequency, low-intensity electrical current is passed
between the two outer electrodes, and the voltage change is measured
between the two inner electrodes. An inflatable thigh cuff is used to
produce venous occlusion. B. An IPG tracing from a normal right limb
(above) and an obstructed left limb (below). When venous obstruction
is present, IPG is typically affected in two ways. (1) The rise in leg volume occurring during venous occlusion is decreased (because the deep
venous thrombosis has already occluded venous outflow and thus causes limb distension and a reduction in limb compliance). (2) The
decrease in leg volume occurring during the first 3 seconds following
cuff deflation is reduced (i.e., the rate of venous outflow is reduced).
(From Schlant et al [eds]. *The Heart* [8th ed]. New York: McGraw-Hill,
1994.)

Certain limitations should be emphasized. Plethysmography is insensitive for detection of calf vein thrombi and small nonocclusive proximal thrombi, which explains the poorer performance in postoperative patients in whom calf vein thrombi are known to occur. Also, plethysmography cannot differentiate between an acute or chronic occlusion. This limitation explains its low positive predictive value. False positive results can also occur in bedridden patients, those suffering from heart failure, and pregnant women in the second and third trimesters. It is also technically difficult to obtain reliable results in patients with altered mental status, with significant obesity, on mechanical ventilation, and after recent orthopedic procedures or trauma.

B. **Duplex venous ultrasonography** has become the predominant noninvasive test in the detection of venous thrombosis in various anatomic locations, including the vena cava and the jugular, portal, renal, and lower-extremity veins. The common femoral and popliteal veins can be visualized for the presence or absence of an intraluminal soft-tissue mass, compressibility of the veins, and response to the Valsalva maneuver. In patients in whom sonography detects a thrombus in either the common femoral or popliteal veins, the veins are generally noncompressible. When the common femoral vein is obstructed, collateral flow does not respond to the Valsalva maneuver, which normally stops femoral flow when iliofemoral valves are competent.

Venous duplex ultrasound has both a high sensitivity (95%) and specificity (98%) for proximal lower-extremity DVT. Although the success decreases for detecting clots in the calf, several authors are reporting improved accuracy.

If the noninvasive tests are normal and clinical suspicion DVT is low, we do not perform venography and pursue other reasons for leg pain or swelling. When the clinical picture strongly suggests calf vein thrombosis but noninvasive tests are equivocal, we recommend venography since it remains the best method to visualize calf veins. When calf and thigh swelling are accompanied by abnormal noninvasive tests suggesting iliofemoral venous thrombosis, anticoagulation without venography is reasonable for most patients.

Selected Reading

Bernstein EF (ed). *Vascular Diagnosis*. St. Louis: Mosby, 1993.

Fronek A. *Noninvasive Diagnostics in Vascular Disease*. New York: McGraw-Hill, 1989.

Kempczinski RE, Yao JST (eds). *Practical Noninvasive Vascular Diagnosis* (2nd ed). Chicago: Year Book, 1987.

Strandness DE Jr, van Breda A (eds). *Vascular Diseases: Surgical and Interventional Therapy*. New York: Churchill Livingstone, 1994.

Sumner DS. Vascular Diagnostics. In LJ Greenfield (ed), *Surgery: Scientific Principles and Practice*. Philadelphia: Lippincott, 1993.

Zwiebel WJ (ed). *Introduction to Vascular Ultrasonography* (3rd ed). Philadelphia: Saunders, 1992.

Vascular Radiology

The vascular radiologist has become an integral member of the medical team caring for the vascular patient. He or she provides anatomic and diagnostic information using a number of imaging techniques and performs therapeutic interventions such as percutaneous angioplasty and thrombolytic therapy. The time-honored imaging techniques of arteriography and venography have been supplemented by ultrasonography, computed tomography (CT), digital subtraction angiography (DSA), magnetic resonance imaging (MRI), positron emission tomography (PET), and angioscopy. Using the anatomic information provided by these imaging modalities, the vascular radiologist can use angiographic catheterization to deliver drugs, embolize arteries, and dilate occlusive lesions.

The responsibility for ordering either an imaging study or angiographic therapy remains with the primary physician or surgeon. Therefore, he or she must understand the indications, risks, limitations, and management of any complication associated with both the diagnostic and therapeutic activities of the vascular radiologist.

Arteriography

Most arteriograms are performed in preparation for an operation or some other therapeutic intervention. Arteriography can also help solve certain diagnostic dilemmas—for example, vasospastic disorders versus occlusive disease of the hands, ergotism, Buerger's disease, temporal arteritis, and periarteritis nodosa. The decision to order an arteriogram must be made with the patient's understanding that the study is invasive, may require hospitalization, and has definite risks. The following guidelines should assist in the preparation and selection of appropriate angiographic views.

I. Preparation. A member of the vascular radiology department should evaluate each patient before angiography. This person should explain the study and risks to the patient, record patient consent, and write appropriate premedication orders.

    A. Any **allergy to iodine** contrast material or other complications of prior angiography should be ascertained.

    B. All **peripheral pulses** should be noted.

    C. Renal function is checked by measuring serum creatinine, because contrast material can be nephrotoxic, especially in dehydrated patients and diabetics.

    D. The patient should be questioned about any **past bleeding problems.** Generally, platelet count, partial thromboplastin time, and prothrombin time are checked.

    E. Adequate urine output (0.5 ml/kg/hour) should be established in dehydrated patients and diabetics by intravenous hydration, usually with Ringer's lactated solution at 100–125 ml/hour before the study.

F. Skin preparation of the puncture site should include cleansing with an antiseptic soap such as chlorhexidine or povidone-iodine.

II. Risks. The main risks of angiography are hemorrhage from the needle puncture site, allergic reactions to the contrast material, thrombosis of the punctured vessel, and embolization of a clot from the catheter, air, or atheromatous material. In experienced hands these complications occur in about 1% of all cases. Mortality is less frequent (0.05%) but is a definite risk that the patient must understand.

III. Methods. The method of angiography must include consideration of both the puncture site for injection of contrast and some type of analgesia or anesthesia to alleviate the anxiety and pain of the procedure. We think the puncture site and anesthetic technique should be selected to meet the specific needs of each patient Thus, the angiographer should be skilled in the performance of transfemoral, translumbar, and axillary angiography.

A. The most widely used **contrast agents** are sodium or methylglucamine salts of triiodo-2,4,6-benzoic acid. Because their osmolarity is higher than that of blood, these agents cause a sensation of heat, vasodilation, and pain during injection. Excreted by the kidneys, these angiographic contrast agents can also produce a transient decrease in renal blood flow and induce acute renal dysfunction in patients with or without a past history of renal disease. However, individuals with preexisting renal failure, proteinuria, diabetes mellitus, and dehydration are at higher risk. Postangiographic renal dysfunction can be minimized by intravenous hydration, limited contrast loads, and mannitol infusion in patients with poor renal function. Contrast-induced renal insufficiency is generally transient, improving within a week.

In addition, contrast agents can cause allergic reactions in 2–5% of patients. These reactions are usually mild, with itching or urticaria. Rarely, more severe anaphylactoid reactions occur and are manifested by hypotension, bradyarrhythmias, wheezing, and collapse. Patients with allergies or prior contrast reactions seem to be at higher risk for recurrent allergic complications with repeat angiography. Although the benefits of some type of pretreatment in this high-risk group are controversial, we recommend that steroids and diphenhydramine be administered prior to the arteriogram. One previously studied regimen includes prednisone, 50 mg PO q6h for three doses ending 1 hour before the arteriogram, and diphenhydramine, 50 mg PO, 1 hour before the study.

Newer, less toxic contrast media are available but are considerably more expensive. Some of these newer agents (Iopamidol and Iohexol) are nonionic monomers that have a lower osmolality and consequently cause less pain with injection. Both of these agents, plus an ionized monoacidic dimer (iothalamate methylglucamine [Hexabrix]), have a

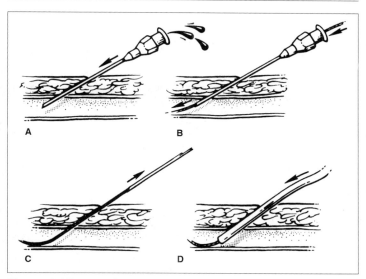

Fig. 6-1. Seldinger technique for percutaneous catheter angiography.
A. Introductory needle is passed into femoral or axillary artery.
B. Smaller flexible guidewire is passed through the introductory nee-
dle into the artery. C. Introductory needle is withdrawn over the
guidewire, which is left in the artery. D. Larger flexible angiographic
catheter, passed over the smaller guidewire, then is manipulated
through the arterial system until the desired level of study is reached.
Angiographic dye is injected through this catheter.

relatively low osmolality because of the higher number of
iodine atoms per number of dissolved particles.

B. The **pain of angiography** is related to the local puncture site and the contrast material. Angiographic contrast
has a direct irritating effect on vascular endothelium.
This pain accompanying contrast injection is described as
an intense hot or burning pain that lasts only seconds but
is remarkably uncomfortable for some patients. In general, pain can be sufficiently managed by premedication
with a sedative (e.g., diazepam), a narcotic, and local
anesthesia at the puncture site. Additional diazepam or
narcotics can be administered just before contrast injection. Some institutions prefer general anesthesia for all
cases, but we generally reserve this technique for children. We have found local anesthesia and intravenous
sedation to be sufficient and safe for most studies.

C. We prefer **transfemoral catheterization** by the
Seldinger technique (Fig. 6-1). Our main exception to this
approach has been to avoid puncturing grafts in the groin
when possible. The introductory needle could cause local
graft complications such as local infection, suture line
injury, graft thrombosis, or distal thromboembolism.
Several reports, however, have documented a low compli-

cation rate following prosthetic graft punctures for angiography. Although the incidence of problems from direct graft puncture is usually higher than that associated with puncture of native vessels, alternative approaches (e.g., transaxillary) are also associated with higher complication rates. In some cases, a translumbar aortogram can provide the needed information but not when renal, visceral, or thoracic aortic views are critical. The Seldinger technique allows:

1. Placement of a catheter that can be moved to various positions in the arterial tree.
2. Measurement of pressures across an iliac stenosis to determine its hemodynamic significance.
3. Safe movement of the patient into various oblique positions to evaluate the origin of various vessels (e.g., the profunda femoris artery).

D. One alternative is **translumbar aortography.** Its proponents claim that it is simpler and more rapid than transfemoral studies. They also claim that improvements in translumbar technique have made it safe and have improved the quality of the study.

E. **Transaxillary or transbrachial angiography** provides the third main access to the arterial system. It has been the least preferred method because of possible brachial plexus injury, axillary hematomas, and emboli to the cerebral circulation. However, the transaxillary route provides excellent access in situations where transfemoral puncture is not feasible. By the transaxillary approach, the cervical and intracranial circulation can be studied as well as the abdominal aorta and its major branches.

F. Regardless of the approach selected, angiographic studies should be designed to maximize anatomic information but minimize pain, contrast load, and the time the catheter remains in the arterial system. To attain these goals, the physician ordering the arteriogram should discuss them with the vascular radiologist **before the study.**

IV. **Angiographic series.** The following views are suggested for the evaluations of peripheral arterial occlusive disease, renovascular hypertension, intestinal angina, and aneurysmal disease.

A. **Symptomatic cerebrovascular disease (transient ischemic attacks [TIAs]).** Angiographic study of symptomatic cerebrovascular disease begins with an aortic arch injection to visualize the origins of the innominate, both common carotid, vertebral, and subclavian arteries. In addition, selective images of both carotid arteries with intracerebral views are done to show both the anteriorposterior (AP) and lateral projections. The carotid bifurcation usually is visualized better on the lateral view. The AP view of the intracranial vasculature demonstrates any cross-circulation to the opposite hemisphere. In the symptomatic patient, the intracranial images are essential to identify any central pathology such as an aneurysm, an arteriovenous malformation, a mass (e.g., tumor), or small-vessel occlusions. We also have found that 105-mm camera spot images enhance the details of the carotid bifurcation and may reveal ulcerative plaques that other views do not clearly demonstrate. In our experience, intravenous DSA has not been as accurate as conventional selective carotid angiography for visualizing the intracranial vessels in symptomatic patients. At the Mayo Clinic, 8% of the intravenous DSA images have missed intracranial lesions found on standard arteriography. Likewise, magnetic resonance angiography lacks the clarity necessary to make therapeutic decisions in some patients.

B. **Asymptomatic carotid disease.** Patients with asymptomatic carotid disease usually have asymptomatic neck bruits and positive noninvasive carotid studies that suggest a hemodynamically significant stenosis at the carotid bifurcation, where the majority of extracranial occlusive lesions occur. Thus, aortic arch injections in each oblique projection usually reveal a significant stenosis of either carotid bifurcation. If an arch injection does not clearly show the carotid bifurcations, selective carotid injections can be performed. Limiting the study to arch injection reduces the risk of additional contrast and selective catheterizations.

Intravenous carotid DSA is another method of studying asymptomatic cervical bruits. However, good to excellent carotid images are obtained in only 60–75% of patients. The most frequent causes of an inadequate study are the superimposition of the origins of the internal and external carotid arteries and patient breathing or motion that cause poor clarity of the images. Such poor intravenous DSAs lead to additional contrast loads and costs for at least 20% of patients. Consequently, we are less enthusiastic about carotid intravenous DSAs and prefer a combination of intraarterial DSA and selective conventional arteriography.

An increasing number of surgeons are advocating **only duplex ultrasound** to define extracranial carotid lesions before endarterectomy. This approach may be safe when the ultrasound study is performed by a laboratory with a proven record of accuracy.

C. **Aortoiliac disease.** When occlusive disease appears to be limited to the terminal aorta and iliac arteries, we request an abdominal aortogram with lower-extremity runoff. This study can be biplanar, giving a lateral aortic view that includes the origins of the mesenteric blood supply (celiac, superior mesenteric, and inferior mesenteric). Since the inferior mesenteric artery may be ligated during aortic grafting, knowledge of celiac and superior mesenteric artery patency is critical to prevent acute or chronic intestinal ischemia. Oblique views of the iliac system also may reveal significant posterior plaques that may be missed on the AP view.

D. **Multilevel occlusive disease.** Patients with multilevel occlusive disease have clinical findings of combined disease of the aortoiliac, femoropopliteal, and tibial segments. In addition to a biplanar aortogram with runoff, oblique views of the femoral artery may help delineate any profunda origin stenosis, which is difficult to visualize on the AP projection.

One of the perplexing problems with multilevel occlusive disease is determining whether the patient needs aortoiliac or femoropopliteal reconstruction or bypasses at both levels. A **femoral artery pressure (FAP) study** helps make this determination. A transfemoral angiographic catheter can measure a distal aortic pressure and then be pulled back across an iliac stenosis into the femoral artery for a femoral pressure. In our experience, the iliac stenosis is significant when the resting pressure gradient across the iliac segment is greater than 5 mm Hg or falls more than 15% after reactive hyperemia.

E. **Femoropopliteal and tibial disease.** Patients with femoropopliteal and tibial disease, who often present with a severely ischemic foot, usually have multiple medical problems, including poor renal function. Thus, the amount of angiographic contrast **must be limited** if further renal damage is to be avoided. An appropriate approach to such patients is a transfemoral arteriogram of the ischemic leg and an FAP study to detect any proximal significant iliac stenosis. If the FAP study indicates poor iliac flow, extra contrast is injected to delineate the distal aorta and iliac system. In some patients, a focal iliac stenosis can be dilated by a balloon catheter, and the distal superficial femoral artery occlusion can be treated later by femoropopliteal bypass grafting. Some of these patients also have severe tibial occlusive disease and require visualization of the distal leg and arterial arches of the foot. These views can be obtained by proper timing for x-ray exposure, intraarterial injection of vasodilators (e.g., papaverine), or balloon-occlusion arteriography. In most cases, proper exposure times will be sufficient to show the runoff. When conventional runoff views are inadequate, intraarterial DSA images may yield further delineation of distal tibial and foot arteries.

F. **Renovascular hypertension.** The specific angiographic views needed before renal artery reconstruction is attempted depend on what particular surgical procedure is planned. In general, an abdominal aortogram will demonstrate both proximal and distal renal arteries in addition to the infrarenal aorta, which is commonly used as the origin for an aortorenal bypass graft. Selective renal artery injections, especially in oblique views, may be needed to further delineate the renal artery anatomy. A biplane celiac artery view is needed when use of the splenic artery for a splenorenal anastomosis or the hepatic artery for a hepatorenal bypass graft is planned. Selective inferior vena cava and renal vein renins may be sampled after the patient has been volume restricted or given captopril, 25 mg PO, to enhance renin ratios. When renal function is poor (creatinine >2 mg/100 ml or creatinine clearance <30 ml/minute), the total angiographic contrast load should be limited to less than 125 ml, since larger volumes may deteriorate renal function. Although some physicians use intravenous digital subtraction angiograms to screen patients with suspected renovascular hypertension, recent advances in duplex scanning may allow adequate and safer noninvasive imaging and velocity pattern analysis. Since intravenous DSA can involve a substantial contrast load (100–200 ml) with unclear renal artery views, a conventional renal arteriogram with selective injections remains the optimum method to obtain good images and minimize contrast-related nephrotoxicity. The role of magnetic resonance renal angiography is still being assessed in many centers.

G. Chronic intestinal angina. The angiographic evaluation for chronic intestinal angina should include biplanar aortography, since the origins of the mesenteric arteries are best visualized on the lateral view. Selective catheterizations may help if the aortogram does not clearly define the distal distribution and venous return of the mesenteric vessels.

H. Aneurysmal disease

1. Abdominal aortic aneurysm. Unless the patient has poor leg pulses, a biplane abdominal aortogram and a pelvic view alone are sufficient to show the extent of any abdominal aortic aneurysm and any associated lesions of the iliac, renal, or mesenteric vessels. Lower-extremity runoff requires additional contrast and is unnecessary if leg pulses are normal. A thoracic aortogram should be performed when a thoracoabdominal aneurysm is suspected by chest x-ray, physical examination, CT scan, or sonogram. Again, contrast load should be restricted to defining only essential anatomic information.

2. Femoral aneurysms. Since patients with femoral aneurysms often have diffuse aneurysmal disease, an abdominal aortogram with runoff is appropriate.

3. Popliteal aneurysms. These patients frequently have diffuse aneurysmal disease. If the physical examination and ultrasonography or CT have ruled out proximal femoral or aortic aneurysms, a transfemoral arteriogram with runoff is adequate to define local anatomy before popliteal aneurysm repair is undertaken.

V. Postangiogram care. Any patient who has undergone angiography should be monitored hourly for at least 6 hours. Most early complications become evident during this time. Nursing personnel can perform these routine checks, but a physician also should examine the patient sometime during this recuperative period. The routine examination should include (1) evaluation of the patient's general appearance and mental status (especially after cerebral studies), (2) heart rate, (3) blood pressure, (4) inspection of puncture sites, (5) palpation of extremity pulses, and (6) hematocrit if any signs of hemorrhage exist.

In addition, adequate hydration must be maintained for 12–24 hours, since the angiographic contrast causes a diuresis and can lead to dehydration. The combination of diuresis and the nephrotoxicity of the contrast material can cause renal deterioration. Patients with diabetes mellitus or chronic renal insufficiency are most susceptible to this complication. We maintain an intravenous infusion for 4–6 hours after the angiogram, because it is during this period that diuresis and other early complications are most likely to occur.

VI. Complications

A. Neurologic deficits.

Aortic arch and selective cervical artery injections can result in transient or permanent neurologic deficits. These changes may be delayed, occurring several minutes to hours after the angiogram is completed. Neurologic deficits that happen during the angiogram study probably are embolic from dislodged atheroma or catheter clots. Delayed neurologic damage may be secondary to hypoperfusion or thrombosis associated with angiograpic contrast material–induced diuresis and dehydration. Emergency carotid endarterectomy should be considered in the event of an immediate neurologic deficit on the appropriate side of a tight carotid stenosis, especially if a previous carotid bruit suddenly disappears.

Sometimes the neurologic change is subtle, such as confusion, mild facial paresis, dysarthria, or dysphagia. If the neurologic deficit is not recognized for several hours and is persistent, the patient probably has suffered a stroke. Emergency endarterectomy is not advised in such cases, since it can worsen neurologic deficits by changing an ischemic infarct to a hemorrhagic infarct. A CT or MRI scan should be done in 12–24 hours to define any infarct areas and the amount of cerebral edema.

If a cerebral vascular accident has occurred, several measures can help minimize cerebral edema and stroke progression. Intravenous fluids should be limited to maintenance levels (1 ml/kg/hour) so that cerebral edema is not worsened by excessive hydration. Steroids also may be useful during the period of maximum cerebral edema (3–7 days). We avoid systemic anticoagulation as it may cause intracerebral bleeding.

B. Hemorrhage.

Small hematomas and ecchymosis at the puncture site are not uncommon. Expanding hematomas indicate continued bleeding from the arterial puncture site into perivascular spaces. This complication can be prevented by application of direct pressure over the puncture site for 15–30 minutes after the arterial catheter is removed and bed rest of the extremity for 6–12 hours. Sandbags and ice packs are of dubious value since they provide diffuse rather than point pressure and may hide an underlying expanding hematoma. They also may provide a false sense of adequate hemostasis.

Expanding or pulsatile hematomas should be evaluated immediately by ultrasound. Often, an active pseudoaneurysm can be closed by ultrasound-guided compression. In some patients an acute arteriovenous fistula may also resolve with ultrasound-guided compression. After axillary puncture, any hematoma that compresses the brachial plexus, causing pain or other neurologic change, should be decompressed in the operating room.

Significant retroperitoneal hemorrhage can occur after translumbar aortography. The only early indications of such bleeding may be persistent back pain, tachycardia, falling blood pressure, and a falling hematocrit. Flank ecchymosis is a late physical finding. An abdominal CT scan will demonstrate a periaortic or psoas muscle hematoma.

C. **Diminished pulses.** Postangiogram pulses that are diminished or absent when compared to baseline pulses suggest partial or complete arterial obstruction. Although arterial spasm may occur, it is rarely the cause of diminished pulses that persist beyond 30–60 minutes. The most common causes of diminished extremity blood flow after angiography are (1) arterial injury (intimal flap), (2) a clot stripped off the catheter, and (3) compression by a hematoma in the arterial wall or extrinsic to it.

The acutely ischemic extremity that is painful, pallid, and pulseless obviously needs emergency revascularization. In contrast, a small intimal flap may diminish but not obstruct arterial flow. The extremity will be asymptomatic, but pulses and Doppler pressures will be diminished compared to preangiogram findings. Such asymptomatic cases with mild pressure reduction (10–20 mm Hg) can initially be managed nonoperatively. Small intimal flaps usually will adhere to the arterial wall and heal in several days to a few weeks. Systemic heparinization for 24–48 hours followed by antiplatelet drugs for 4–6 weeks has been a successful regimen in our experience. Noninvasive Doppler ankle pressures at rest and after treadmill exercise can be followed to document improvement or deterioration. However, we emphasize that the presence of any ischemic symptoms and the absence of previously palpable pulses require emergency surgical intervention to restore normal extremity circulation.

D. **Pulsatile mass.** It can be difficult to ascertain whether a pulsatile mass at the angiogram puncture site is a hematoma or a false aneurysm. An aneurysm is not only pulsatile but also expansile on palpation. Ultrasonography is diagnostic.

Any postarteriogram hematoma that suddenly causes pain and local subcutaneous hemorrhage is a ruptured pseudoaneurysm and usually requires urgent surgical evacuation of the clot and repair of the artery. Pseudoaneurysm rupture is most likely to occur within 7–10 days of the initial angiogram. For this reason, we suggest that all patients with local hematomas remain close to a surgical facility during this time. In some situations, smaller (<3–4 cm) acute pulsatile hematomas can be eliminated by compression under ultrasonic control. It may take more than an hour to obliterate them, but the success rate is over 90%. Pseudoaneurysms that are initially missed and then noted at a later examination should be repaired about 6–8 weeks after the arteriogram. By this time, local inflammation generally has resolved and dissection and repair may be easier. Chronic pseudoaneurysms have a developed capsule that is generally not likely to resolve with ultrasound-guided compression.

E. Infection. Local infection at arteriogram puncture sites is unusual with meticulous surgical technique. Such technique should include (1) cleansing the site with a surgical scrub soap before the study, (2) standard surgical operative preparation at the time of the study, and (3) standard surgical attire for members of the angiogram team.

Local superficial pustules at the skin puncture site should be incised, drained, and cultured. If cellulitis extends around this site, oral or parenteral antibiotics should be started. Most local infections will be secondary to hospital-acquired *Staphylococcus aureus* or *Streptococcus*. Abscesses should be incised and drained in the operating room, since hemorrhage from an infected artery may occur and require repair or ligation. **Any elective synthetic bypass, especially aortofemoral grafting, should be postponed until local groin infections are completely resolved.**

Venography

 I. Indications. The use of contrast venography to diagnose deep venous thrombosis (DVT) of the lower extremity has decreased recently. Duplex ultrasound has assumed the primary role in DVT diagnosis at and above the knee. Nonetheless, venography remains useful in defining lower-extremity venous anatomy in patients undergoing deep venous valve reconstructions or venous bypasses. With increasing use of chronic subclavian vein catheters for parenteral nutrition and chemotherapy, venography also has been the most accurate method of defining subclavian vein thrombosis when acute arm pain and swelling occur.
 II. Patient preparation. Minimal preparation is required prior to venography. Past allergy to contrast material must be ascertained. The extremity must also be examined for a suitable puncture site.
III. Risks. About 3% of venographic studies will be complicated by minor allergic reactions, contrast-induced thrombophlebitis, or contrast extravasation at the puncture site. Major allergic reactions of hypotension and bronchospasm occur in less than 1% of cases.
 IV. Methods. The quality and safety of contrast leg venography can be optimized by paying attention to several aspects of the technique.
    A. The patient should be positioned at 30–45 degrees on a tilt table, with no weightbearing on the affected limb. Weightbearing tends to contract the gastrocnemius and soleus muscles, thus preventing adequate filling of some deep veins.
    B. Generally, a vein on the dorsum of the foot is punctured with a 21-gauge needle. Rarely, a cutdown exposure of the greater saphenous vein at the ankle is necessary.
    C. Dilute contrast material, ionic or nonionic, is suitable. The usual volume is 60–90 ml per extremity.
    D. Views of both the superficial and deep veins can be obtained **without** a tourniquet unless leg swelling

appears severe and causes markedly increased compartmental pressures. Then an ankle tourniquet is used to promote better filling of the deep veins.

E. Exposures of the leg are made with external and internal foot rotation.

F. Next, the same views are obtained over the knee and thigh.

G. Finally, the pelvic film is exposed after the table is returned to the horizonal position and the leg is elevated.

H. The venous system of the lower limb is flushed with 60 ml of normal saline.

V. Interpretation

A. The **normal venogram** will opacify the deep and superficial veins except for the profunda femoris vein, which is rarely filled with contrast material. Deep venous trunks in the calf are paired and have smooth, straight walls except at valve sites, which have a beadlike appearance. The anterior tibial veins are the smallest. Deep muscle venous plexuses are large and fusiform in young people but appear smaller with advancing age. The femoral vein usually is single but may be paired for a variable length. Normally, contrast material should flow quickly up the deep system after leg elevation.

B. **Acute deep venous thrombosis** is confirmed by filling defects in the deep veins on more than one view. The contrast column will end abruptly when the thrombosis completely obstructs the vein. Deep veins also may be nonopacified because of external compression from muscle swelling in the fascial compartments. Mixing defects can be seen at major junction sites such as the femoral triangle and iliac bifurcation.

VI. Postvenographic care. Complete drainage of the leg is performed immediately after filming by the examiner. The filming should proceed rapidly to minimize the amount of contact time between the contrast material and the venous endothelium. This process will reduce the risk of postvenographic phlebitis to near zero. Patients with positive studies should remain at bed rest with the leg elevated, and systemic heparinization should be continued.

Ultrasound and Computed Tomography

The search continues for noninvasive methods of imaging the vascular system. So far, ultrasonography and CT scanning have proved useful in defining arterial aneurysms in certain locations and also in detecting various graft complications. These methods, however, have been considered inferior to arteriography for clear identification of stenotic lesions and ulcerated plaques. This limitation is already being overcome by newer duplex scanners with high-resolution imaging capabilities. The entire field of noninvasive vascular diagnosis is also being changed by MRI, spectroscopy, and blood flow measurements. For example, MRI has proved to be excellent in depicting the anatomic rela-

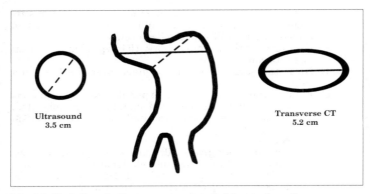

Fig. 6-2. Variations in the measurement of abdominal aortic aneurysm diameter from ultrasound versus computed tomography (CT). Anterior-posterior measurements on ultrasound are accurate to within 3–5 mm of actual size measured at operation. CT measurements are also accurate but may over-estimate size if they are made at an oblique angle. This problem arises since CT scans make measurements perpendicular to the body axis while aneurysms are often tortuous and consequently may appear distorted on CT scanning.

tionships of hemangiomas, arteriovenous malformations, and aortic arch anomalies. Until these new techniques receive more extensive clinical evaluation, ultrasonography and CT scanning will remain safe, cost-effective methods of vascular imaging for most common vascular problems.

I. **Risks.** Present ultrasound techniques do not appear to produce any harmful effects on humans. CT does involve contrast administration in most cases and a radiation exposure, although the dose usually is no greater than that of an intravenous pyelogram. Likewise, MRI does not appear to have an identifiable risk at present field strengths.

II. **Indications**

   A. **Abdominal aortic aneurysm** size can be accurately measured by gray-scale ultrasound to ± 3–5 mm (Fig. 6-2). In addition to size measurement, sonography can identify an intraluminal thrombus and reveal a periaortic hematoma from aneurysm leakage. The most common problem in obtaining an accurate abdominal aortic sonogram is interference by overlying bowel gas, which degrades the image. Past limitations of sonography were its inaccuracy in defining whether the aneurysm was infrarenal or suprarenal and its inability to show iliac aneurysms. Current ultrasound equipment, however, can image the mesenteric, renal, and iliac arteries in most patients. If ultrasound does not clarify suprarenal or iliac aneurysm involvement, a CT scan should be performed. CT is also useful in defining other abdominal or retroperitoneal pathology in patients with unexplained symptoms (e.g., retroperitoneal fibrosis, tumors). In the acute setting, CT can quickly evaluate hemodynamically stable patients with a high suspicion of a leaking aortic aneurysm. Angiography should be done when ultrasound or CT reveal a horseshoe kidney. This renal anomaly can be associated with multiple renal arteries that may complicate repair.

B. Peripheral aneurysms of the common femoral and popliteal arteries can be accurately defined by ultrasound.

C. Graft complications such as abscesses, a perigraft hematoma, graft dilation, and false aneurysms can be delineated by ultrasound or CT. Ultrasound is especially useful in the groin and lower limb, while CT is preferable in the abdomen or chest. Nonetheless, high-resolution ultrasound can currently provide excellent images of most abdominal grafts, including the common iliac areas. Arteriography is necessary to define detailed arterial anatomy before most arterial reconstructions for graft complications. Also, indium[111]-labeled leukocyte scans can help document and localize prosthetic vascular graft infections.

Digital Subtraction Angiography

Intravenous arteriography by computerized fluoroscopy allows direct visualization of the arterial system by injection of a contrast medium into a peripheral vein rather than a peripheral artery. A bolus of contrast is power-injected into a catheter passed through an antecubital vein into the superior vena cava. Immediately, a fluoroscope images the area under study, and a computer subtracts these early images from subsequent images taken at only a few-second intervals. Images of bone and other soft tissues are eliminated, and the only image recorded is the contrast-filled artery. The images can be enhanced by a factor of eight, displayed on a video monitor, and stored on videotape. A standard multiformat camera can convert the video images to hard-copy arteriograms. Radiation exposure is comparable to that of standard arteriography: 50 mR per image for extremities and 300 mR for abdominal images. The technique avoids direct arterial puncture and its attendant complications, and DSA is less expensive than conventional arteriography. Intravenous DSA is also an important alternative to imaging arteries in patients who do not have suitable arterial access sites for catheterization due to occlusive disease or prosthetic grafts. Since its revival in the early 1980s, intravenous DSA has been used to detect arterial disease in every body region. These anatomic regions include the aortic arch, brachiocephalic branches, abdominal aorta, renal and mesenteric vessels, and peripheral arteries. Experience has demonstrated several disadvantages of this intravenous technique: (1) simultaneous opacification of all vessels, precluding selective views unless intraarterial DSA is used; (2) superimposition of paired arteries, making true lateral views not feasible; (3) inferior resolution due to misregistration artifacts caused by breathing or motion; and (4) a significant contrast load if several views are taken (usually 40–50 ml per injection).

Consequently, these disadvantages of intravenous DSA have prevented it from replacing conventional arteriography. Currently, the trend with DSA appears to be the increasing use of intraarterial catheters that deliver small volumes of contrast media for **intraarterial digital subtraction arteriography** (IA-DSA). Current DSA equipment offers larger film formats, less soft-tissue motion artifact by hybrid subtraction (combined temporal and energy subtraction), and improved image quality with postprocessing computer programs.

Magnetic Resonance Imaging

MRI relies on the principle that hydrogen nuclei (protons), when subjected to a magnetic field, tend to align themselves in the direction of the field's poles. However, bursts of radio waves of appropriate frequency will alter this alignment (excitation). Following each radio frequency (RF) burst, the protons realign themselves with the magnetic field. This realignment (relaxation) is associated with the emission of a faint radio signal of their own. A computer translates these faint signals into an image of the scanned area. The image reveals varying densities of protons that correlate with different tissues (e.g., soft tissue and bone).

The physics of MRI are well suited for imaging vascular disease. In rapidly moving blood, the hydrogen nuclei do not line up in the applied magnetic field and thus produce little or no signal when stimulated by an RF burst. The result is a natural contrast between the blood and the vessel wall.

MRI can study several nuclei of biologic significance, including hydrogen, sodium, phosphorus, calcium, oxygen, carbon, chlorine, and potassium. Hydrogen is ideally suited for MRI because it has the greatest sensitivity of the stable nuclei and is the most abundant atomic nucleus in the body. Phosphorus **MR spectroscopy** can analyze the tissue content of adenosine triphosphate (ATP), adenosine diphosphate (ADP), and phosphocreatine, making ^{31}P MR spectra a powerful research tool to study the effects of ischemia on the depletion and recovery of high-energy phosphates. Techniques for blood flow measurement by MRI are also in various developmental stages.

Although its long-term place in vascular imaging remains unclear, MRI has been used to assess several aspects of peripheral vascular disease. Visualization of the aorta is the area where MRI has shown its greatest promise. Mesenteric and renal arteries can also be readily seen in patients with occlusive disease. Attempts to image extra- or intracranial vessels have achieved lesser success because of the complex three-dimensional anatomy of these systems. On the other hand, MRI is superior to CT scanning in evaluating cerebral edema and has the potential to accurately stage strokes and to determine the optimal time for any cerebrovascular operation in such patients.

Obviously, MRI offers several advantages in evaluating cardiovascular disease: (1) noninvasive imaging, (2) blood flow velocity estimation, (3) avoidance of any contrast medium, and (4) multidimensional images (transverse, sagittal, and coronal planes). Despite these advantages, several significant limitations currently exist. Present MRI resolution is limited to 1.0–1.5 mm. Other major limitations are cost ($800,000–$2,000,000) and a special room completely insulated from external radio frequencies. In addition to these equipment limitations, patients dependent on metallic life-support systems (e.g., pacemakers) are excluded since the magnet creates problems with their operation. Intracranial magnetic arterial aneurysm clips also preclude MRI scanning. Patients with joint prostheses or intraabdominal clips have been evaluated by MRI without problems. Some authors also caution that less expensive but effective methods of vascular imaging must not be abandoned during the current rapid proliferation of this new diagnostic modality.

Positron Emission Tomography

CT and MRI have improved our ability to visualize three-dimensional structures. In contrast, MR spectroscopy and PET allow us to analyze cellular function in vivo. PET is a noninvasive technique to quantify regional physiologic and biochemical function in vivo. Biochemically active substances, labeled with positron-emitting isotopes, are administered and the subsequent distribution of radioactivity measured. Although images are produced, they are of secondary importance to the ability to measure cellular metabolic function. The capability of PET to measure regional blood flow, oxygen consumption, and substrate (e.g., glucose) utilization make it particularly useful in conditions of ischemia. Brain and heart have been studied extensively during normal function and while ischemic. PET can distinguish ischemic from normal tissue and reversibly from irreversibly injured tissue. PET has been used to document the metabolic response to revascularization operations. Although it is complex and expensive, PET may offer a means for establishing a more metabolic basis for the management of vascular disease.

Balloon Angioplasty

One of the most active topics in the treatment of vascular disease remains nonoperative dilatation of arterial stenoses by inflatable balloon-tip catheters. This procedure has most commonly been called **percutaneous transluminal angioplasty (PTA)** and usually is performed by vascular radiologists. Some surgeons and cardiologists have also applied the technique in the peripheral vascular system. PTA generally uses polyethylene catheters that have an inflatable balloon

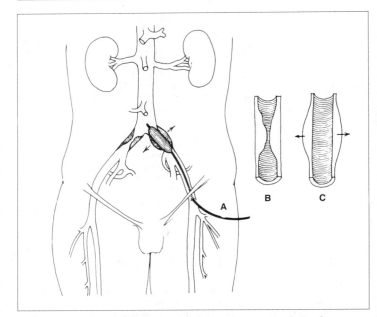

Fig. 6-3. Percutaneous transluminal angioplasty (PTA). A. By the Seldinger technique, a catheter with an internal flexible guidewire is passed to and gently insinuated through the area of arterial stenosis. B–C. The balloon is inflated to several atmospheres of pressure. When the PTA is complete, the arterial lumen is larger and the local artery is stretched.

near the tip. The balloon angioplasty represents a variation of the transluminal arterial dilatation described originally by Dotter and Judkins. The older Dotter technique used a relatively large No. 12 French Teflon catheter introduced over an inner No. 8 French catheter and passed through the stenosis to dilate it. No balloon was involved. Gruntzig popularized balloon catheters in the late 1970s, and their use is increasing. Larger balloon catheters usually are only No. 5–7 French, but the balloon tip inflates to a predetermined diameter (4–25 mm) at 3–20 atm pressure. Even smaller catheters (2.5–3.3 French) are available for small tibial lesions. The smaller catheter size obviously reduces local complications at the arterial puncture site, and the rigidity and pressure characteristics of the balloon allow for greater force to be exerted in dilating the stenosis.

I. Mechanisms of balloon angioplasty (Fig. 6-3). The mechanisms by which percutaneous balloon angioplasty can dilate a stenotic artery are complex. Pathologic studies demonstrate several changes in the atherosclerotic plaque and the vessel itself. First, balloon dilatation disrupts both the plaque and the artery wall, with separation of the plaque from the media, rupture of the plaque and possibly the media, and stretching

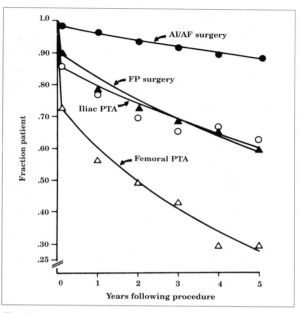

Fig. 6-4. Limb patency rate among survivors of surgical procedures or percutaneous transluminal angioplasty (PTA) during a 5-year period. (AI/AF = aorto-iliac or aortofemoral; FP = femoropopliteal.) These primary results of PTA and surgery have not changed significantly since this graph was compiled in 1984. (Modified from P Doubliet, HL Abrams. The cost of under-utilization: Percutaneous transluminal angioplasty for peripheral vascular disease. Reprinted by permission of the *New England Journal of Medicine* [310:95, 1984].)

of the adventitia to increase the lumen cross-sectional area. Second, the intimal plaque protrudes into the lumen, accounting for the angiographic appearance of local flaps and dissection channels. Third, remodeling occurs by readherence of the intimal flaps with little change in plaque volume. Thus, long-term patency depends on sufficient stretching of the vessel and an adequately remodeled lumen. Finally, restenosis may occur because of insufficient dilatation (compliance), from extension of dissection channels into nondilated segments of the artery, and from intimal hyperplasia.

II. **Indications.** Since its revival in the late 1970s, PTA has been used successfully to dilate or recanalize arteries or grafts in every anatomic region. Generally, PTA has been relatively safer than surgery and less expensive since hospitalization is shorter. However, controversy continues over whether PTA is as durable as operative revascularization (Fig. 6-4). Regardless of one's opinion, PTA is a reasonable therapeutic option for selected patients. Based on our reported experience and other studies, we suggest that the following indications are justified based on long-term follow-up. We agree with others that success must be documented by significant improvement of both clinical symptoms **and** hemodynamic measurements (ankle/brachial indices, Doppler wave forms, pulse volume recordings, exercise distance, or transcutaneous oxygen measurements).

A. **Iliac stenosis.** A focal mid-common iliac artery stenosis (1–3 cm in length) is considered an ideal lesion for dilation, especially in a patient with unilateral claudication and good femoropopliteal runoff. The best results are achieved when PTA is limited to lesions that appear hemodynamically significant by either a 10-mm gradient at rest or a 15% pressure drop after either intraarterial injection of a vasodilator agent or after reactive hyperemia following tourniquet occlusion for 5 minutes. Initial clinical and hemodynamic improvement is achieved in 80–90%, but long-term functional success falls to 60% at 4–5 years. These results can be enhanced in selected patients with balloon angioplasty plus metallic stenting of the lesion (e.g., Palmaz stent). Generally, patients with diffuse bilateral aortoiliac disease or common iliac artery occlusion should be treated by surgery and not by PTA.

B. **Femoral, popliteal, and tibial lesions.** Balloon angioplasty of infrainguinal arterial lesions is less successful than PTA for iliac artery stenosis. Success is more likely if the lesions are more proximal in the leg, are a focal stenoses less than 3 cm in length, and are associated with good distal runoff. Initial clinical and hemodynamic improvement ranges from 50–75% but diminishes to as low as 30% at 5 years. Smokers and diabetics have particularly poor results.

Despite these disappointing results, PTA represents a reasonable option for younger claudicants with focal superficial femoral stenosis or high-risk patients whose rest pain may be relieved more safely by PTA of one or more sequential short femoropopliteal stenoses. More aggressive angiographers are also attempting more distal popliteal and tibial angioplasties using smaller balloon catheters. This approach cannot be judged until long-term results are clearly documented. Recanalization of noncalcified superficial femoral occlusions less than 10 cm long has been possible, but recurrent stenosis or occlusion is common. Thus, saphenous vein femoropopliteal bypass remains the most durable treatment for most superficial femoral, poplitial, and tibial artery occlusions.

C. **Combined disease.** In a high-risk patient with a focal iliac stenosis and a superficial femoral artery occlusion, we have dilated the iliac stenosis to improve inflow and then performed a distal femoropopliteal bypass to achieve limb salvage. This approach avoids an abdominal or retroperitoneal procedure such as aortofemoral or ileofemoral bypass, which is often difficult for an elderly, debilitated patient. In other cases of combined femoropopliteal and tibial disease, a standard femoropopliteal bypass can be performed and a tibial stenosis can be dilated in the operating room through the popliteal arteriotomy under fluoroscopic control.

D. Renal artery disease. Renal balloon angioplasty has achieved distinctly different results for fibromuscular disease compared to atherosclerosis.

PTA is probably the treatment of choice for renovascular hypertension due to fibromuscular dysplasia (FMD). The mechanism of dilation in dysplastic stenosis is presumably stretching, shearing, and rupture of the fibrous septa. PTA is particularly attractive when the FMD extends into intrarenal branches that are difficult to repair surgically. Since FMD tends to be a disease of younger women, PTA may delay the need for surgical revascularization until the patient is older. Initial technical success is possible in 80–90% of lesions, and blood pressure becomes normal or improves in slightly more than 90% of patients who have had a successful renal PTA. In short-term follow-up to 3 years, success with PTA is comparable to surgical bypass for FMD. In some patients, PTA can be repeated successfully.

Focal unilateral atherosclerotic stenosis beyond the renal aortic orifice can be adequately dilated in 50–60% of patients, but dilation of bilateral atheromatous stenoses, especially ostial lesions, succeeds in less than 50% of patients. Such ostial lesions are extensions of more extensive aortic plaques that cannot be effectively dilated by a balloon in the renal artery orifice. Currently, renal balloon angioplasty plus stenting appears to be achieving better early results. The durability of renal artery stenting, however, has not been proved. Nonetheless, blood pressure is improved in 80–85% of atherosclerotic patients who have good renal dilation with significant improvement in the pressure gradient across the lesion. Although some radiologists have successfully dilated solitary renal arteries and have improved failing renal function by PTA of high-grade stenoses, we have generally avoided PTA in solitary kidneys and have not found PTA to be a durable method of preserving renal function in patients with atherosclerosis.

Since the complications of renal PTA can include renal artery perforation, thrombosis, or dissection, a vascular surgeon should be available to handle such problems when they occur. In addition, close monitoring of blood pressure is essential for at least 6–12 hours since significant hypotension can occur after successful PTA of high-grade renin-stimulating stenoses.

E. Other applications. Additional uses for PTA are evolving. Success has been achieved in relieving atherosclerotic stenoses of the axillary, subclavian, and mesenteric arteries. The dilatation of atherosclerotic carotid bifurcation lesions has been performed in a few centers. Cerebral microembolism presents a small but real danger, and no long-term results of carotid PTA are available. In contrast, high intimal-carotid fibromuscular lesions may be more suitable for either percutaneous or intraoperative balloon dilatation. In addition, the following types of anastomotic stenoses may be relieved by balloon dilatation: splenorenal or mesocaval shunts, saphenous vein grafts, renal transplants, renal dialysis angio-access, and synthetic grafts. Again, the durability of such angioplasties is often limited, but even temporary successes may be important in severely ill patients.

III. **Complications.** The complications of PTA occur in 3–5% of patients. Thrombosis is the main problem that requires urgent surgical intervention. Any angioplasty should be planned so that a vascular surgeon is available to manage any significant complications.

IV. **Use of antiplatelets and anticoagulants.** There is no consensus regarding the administration of antiplatelet and anticoagulant agents for angioplasty. A general regimen that is followed by many angiographers is as follows:

A. **Antiplatelet therapy** is begun 24–48 hours before angioplasty. Aspirin, 81–325 mg (i.e., one children's aspirin or one adult aspirin) daily are common doses and are generally continued for 2–3 months after the procedure.

B. **Systemic heparin** (2,500–5,000 units) is administered intraarterially during the procedure.

C. **Warfarin sodium (Coumadin) therapy** has been used for 1–3 months for angioplasties at low-flow sites such as the popliteal and tibial arteries, as well as a variety of venous sites. However, such therapy places the patient at increased risk for serious bleeding complications, and no prospective, randomized data to date support its long-term use after angioplasty.

Thrombolytic Therapy

Despite recent widespread interest in thrombolytic drugs, their role in clinical practice remains debatable. Enthusiastic reports of the early 1980s have been balanced by more critical analyses. Although we have used streptokinase and urokinase in a variety of clinical settings, thrombolytic drugs play a very selective role in our practice. Their use must be undertaken after careful consideration of the pharmacokinetics, contraindications, indications, and complications of these powerful agents. They are not a substitute for the safe, proved record of standard medical or surgical therapy for most arterial and venous problems.

I. **Pharmacokinetics.** The most widely available thrombolytic agents are streptokinase, urokinase, and tissue plasminogen activator (t-PA). These drugs are plasminogen activators that lead to clot lysis by enhancing the fibrinolytic system via conversion of plasminogen to its active form, plasmin. **Urokinase**, currently produced by renal tubular cells in tissue culture, acts directly on plasminogen to form plasmin. In contrast, **streptokinase**, manufactured by beta-hemolytic streptococci, must first form an activated complex with plasminogen. The activated complex completes the conversion of excess plasminogen to plasmin. These fibrinolytic agents not only act on plasminogen within a clot but also on plasminogen throughout the circulation. A systemic fibrinolysis results. **t-PA** acts primarily on plasminogen bound to fibrin clot. Although systemic fibrinogenolysis occurs with t-PA, it happens to a less degree than that observed with streptokinase. This advantage reduces bleeding complications.

Each drug has unique disadvantages. The main side effect of streptokinase is an allergic reaction in about 10% of patients who have past exposure to streptococci and therefore antibodies. Urokinase and t-PA have the disadvantage of being considerably more expensive than streptokinase.

These agents can be administered intravenously or intraarterially in full systemic doses or lower regional infusions. Typical systemic dose regimens of streptokinase are a loading dose of 250,000 units followed by a continuous IV infusion of 100,000 units/hour. Urokinase is given IV at a loading dose of 2,000 units **per pound** followed by a continuous hourly rate of 2,000 units/lb. For peripheral arterial occlusions, an intraarterial high-dose urokinase (4,000 IU/minute) infusion directly into the thrombus has been recommended, followed by 1,000–2,000 IU/minute after the thrombus has been recanalized and until it resolves completely. Investigational regimens for arterial infusions for t-PA (0.5 mg/ml) have been 0.1 mg/kg/hour through an angiographic catheter embedded in the thrombus. Two common laboratory tests to document a lytic state are measurement of thrombin time and fibrinogen level. When clot lysis occurs, fibrin split products generally rise, too. However, changes in the constituents of the fibrinolytic system do not correlate with bleeding complications. Hemorrhagic problems usually occur at the arterial puncture site and are related to catheter size and manipulation.

The half-life for each drug is short: streptokinase, 10–12 minutes; urokinase, 11–16 minutes; and t-PA, 6 minutes. Consequently, the effects of the drugs dissipate rapidly, although depleted fibrinogen levels may take at least 24 hours to normalize. In our experience, the need to use aminocaproic acid or fibrinogen concentrates to reverse the thrombolysis rarely occurs.

So-called **low-dose regional** thrombolytic therapy was popularized to achieve clot lysis without causing systemic fibrinolysis. Streptokinase can be administered at 5,000–10,000 units/hour and urokinase at 10,000–20,000 units/hour into a regional thrombus. Generally, however, regional therapy has to be continued for 12–72 hours, and systemic effects are evident by a falling fibrinogen level within 24 hours.

Whether the thrombolytic drug should be administered concomitantly with heparin is debatable. Those who favor concomitant heparin state that it prevents clot accumulation around the infusion catheters. On the contrary, heparin may increase the risk of hemorrhage at the catheter infusion site. We generally start heparin (1,000 units/hour IV without a loading dose) at the onset of regional lytic therapy to avoid pericatheter thrombus formation.

II. **Contraindications.** Since thrombolytic drugs can lyse recent clots anywhere in the body and result in serious bleeding, they generally should **not** be used in the presence of (1) an active bleeding site, (2) a recent stroke, (3) operation or organ biopsy within the past 10 days, and (4) a coagulopathy. In addition, patients with severe acute ischemic and neuromotor impairment should undergo emergency surgical revascularization. They are **not** good candidates for thrombolytic therapy that takes several hours and may delay reperfusion until irreversible neuromuscular damage has occurred.

III. **Indications.** Definite indications for lytic therapy are difficult to define. Prospective, randomized studies have confirmed benefit in selected patients with acute DVT of the lower limbs and for pulmonary embolism (see Chap. 21). Thrombolytic infusions can alleviate acute subclavian vein thrombosis associated with central venous catheters, effort thrombosis, or thoracic outlet syndrome. Urokinase is also commonly used to clear fresh thrombus in central venous lines (e.g., urokinase, 5,000 units in 1 ml).

The benefits of thrombolytic therapy for arterial thrombosis are more controversial than those for venous thrombosis. The recently completed STILE study (*S*urgery versus *T*hrombolysis for *I*schemia of the *L*ower *E*xtremity) concluded that patients with acute ischemia (0–14 days) who were treated with thrombolysis had improved amputation-free survival and shorter hospital stays. There were no differences in efficacy and safety between urokinase and rt-PA. Of practical note, failure of catheter placement occurred in 28% of patients who were randomized to lysis. In contrast, surgical revascularization was more effective and safer than thrombolysis for patients with chronic ischemia (>14 days). Currently, a multicenter clinical trial (TOPAS: *T*hrombolysis *O*r *P*eripheral *A*rterial *S*urgery) is in progress for patients with acute arterial occlusions of less than 14 days' duration. In the meantime, the best results with peripheral arterial occlusions are achieved in patients with clots of less than six weeks' duration. Acute thrombosis associated with balloon angioplasty has been a good indication for thrombolytic therapy. Likewise, lysis of a recent thrombosis secondary to a focal iliac or superficial femoral artery stenosis has allowed subsequent PTA of the causative stenosis. Results of thrombolytic therapy for thrombosed aortic or femoropopliteal grafts have been mixed.

Other uses of thrombolytic drugs for arterial occlusions are focused on clinical situations for which surgery has traditionally given poor results or in which an anticipated operative mortality makes a nonoperative approach a particularly attractive alternative. Examples of such situations include acutely thrombosed popliteal aneurysms with extensive tibial artery thrombosis, thrombosis of autogenous vein grafts, and lower-extremity arterial embolism associated with acute myocardial infarction. These are examples reported in the literature, although our experience with them has not been uniformly successful.

IV. **Complications.** Systemic or regional thrombolytic therapy is complicated by bleeding, thrombosis, or embolism in 15–50% of patients. In our experience, bleeding at the angiographic catheter site has been the most common problem. Distal emboli are often small and sometimes can be resolved with continued thrombolytic administration. Nonetheless, about 10% of patients will require surgical intervention to manage these complications. Unfortunately, regional low-dose infusions have not eliminated these problems.

Laser Angioplasty

Lasers were introduced in the late 1980s as another tool to debulk atherosclerotic lesions. For several years, research in this area was intense. The general public became enamored with the idea of laser therapy for vascular disease. Hot-tipped laser-assisted angioplasty proliferated, but relatively poor results eventually tempered the initial enthusiasm.

If there is a future for lasers in vascular interventional therapy, the primary focus remains on developing fiberoptic catheters that can be introduced percutaneously and guided to the lesion. Laser energy must then be directed at the target plaque, which is to be vaporized. The products of this process are oxygen, nitrogen, and hydrocarbons that are absorbed by the surrounding fluid medium. Although the concept is simple, several factors make clinical application more complex. First, only certain types of lasers (e.g., argon and eximer) can be easily delivered by fiberoptic catheters. Second, soft atheroma can be vaporized, but the calcific matrix of the plaque can be more difficult to eliminate. Third, normal vessel wall can be damaged just as easily as the plaque. Consequently, perforation of the vessel is a real risk. Finally, a major consideration will be the high costs of any laser system. Nonetheless, laser angioplasty, either percutaneously or by surgical arteriotomy, is likely to play some role in the future treatment of atherosclerosis.

Selected Reading

Ahn SA. Atherectomy Devices. In FJ Veith, RW Hobson, RA Williams, SE Wilson (eds), *Vascular Surgery*. New York: McGraw-Hill, 1994.

Bettmann MA. Principles of Angiography. In J Loscalzo, MA Creager, VJ Dzau (eds), *Vascular Medicine*. Boston: Little, Brown, 1992.

Graor RA. Interventional Treatment of Peripheral Vascular Disease. In JR Young, RA Graor, JW Olin, JR Bartholomew (eds), *Peripheral Vascular Diseases*. St. Louis: Mosby-Year Book, 1991.

Polak, JF. Magnetic Resonance Imaging of Vascular Disease. In J Loscalzo, MA Creager, VJ Dzau (eds), *Vascular Medicine*. Boston: Little, Brown, 1992.

The STILE Investigators. Results of a prospective randomized trial evaluating surgery versus thrombolysis for ischemia of the lower extremity: The STILE trial. *Ann Surg* 220:251, 1994.

Strandness DE Jr, van Breda A (eds). *Vascular Diseases: Surgical and Interventional Therapy*. New York: Churchill Livingstone, 1994.

Tumeh SS, Seltzer SE, Wang A. Computed Tomography in Vascular Disorders. In J Loscalzo, MA Creager, VJ Dzau (eds), *Vascular Medicine*. Boston: Little, Brown, 1992.

White RA. Application of Laser Technology to Vascular Disease. In FJ Veith, RW Hobson, RA Williams, SE Wilson (eds), *Vascular Surgery*. New York: McGraw-Hill, 1994.

White GH, Yu W. Vascular Stents. In FJ Veith, RW Hobson, RA Williams, SE Wilson (eds), *Vascular Surgery*. New York: McGraw-Hill, 1994.

Zimmerman JJ, Fogarty TJ. Adjunctive Intraoperative Dilatation (Angioplasty). In FJ Veith, RW Hobson, RA Williams, SE Wilson (eds), *Vascular Surgery*. New York: McGraw-Hill, 1994.

Preoperative Preparation

Many patients who undergo major vascular surgery have multiple medical problems that increase operative risk. Hypertensive cardiovascular disease, chronic obstructive pulmonary disorders, and diabetes mellitus are common among vascular surgery patients. Preoperative preparation must include accurate assessment of anesthetic risk and stabilization of these chronic or acute medical problems. This chapter focuses on the general topics of assessing anesthetic risk, managing cardiovascular medications, optimizing pulmonary function, and controlling diabetes mellitus. Subsequent chapters discuss the preoperative evaluation of specific vascular problems.

I. **Anesthetic risk.** One of the key factors in achieving excellent results from elective vascular surgery is accurate assessment of anesthetic risk. Identifying patients with low versus high anesthetic risks may be difficult, since many vascular patients have various combinations of chronic heart, lung, or renal dysfunction. Some patients have varying degrees of diabetes mellitus. Although common clinical sense and experience provide a great deal of the surgeon's initial impression of anesthetic risk, more objective data also can assist with final assessment of operative risk.

One common approach to correlating a patient's preoperative condition with postoperative mortality is the Dripps-American Society of Anesthesiologists (ASA) classification (Table 7-1). The ASA grading system refers only to a patient's **general physical condition** and does not consider the type of anesthesia, extent of operation, or experience of the surgeon. Another multifactorial index by Goldman et al. focuses on cardiac risk in noncardiac surgery and has been suggested as a useful method of evaluating patients with vascular disease. However, a prospective study using Goldman's criteria in patients undergoing elective aortic reconstruction found that cardiac complications were more common in **all** risk groups than Goldman's scale would predict (Table 7-2). The New York Heart Association (NYHA) classification of angina pectoris is also commonly used for anesthetic risk assessment (Table 7-3). Of note is the observation that stable angina pectoris alone, in the absence of marked ventricular dysfunction, generally does **not** increase operative risk.

A. **Cardiac problems** are the leading cause of death after major vascular surgery. Perioperative fatal myocardial infarction (MI), arrhythmias, or heart failure occur in approximately 3–6% of major vascular operations. Patients with the following risk factors are considered to be at high risk of life-threatening or fatal cardiac complications: (1) MI in the past 6 months, (2) progressive or unstable angina pectoris, (3) symptomatic aortic valve stenosis, (4) symptomatic congestive heart failure, and (5) chronic atrial or ventricular arrhythmias.

Table 7-1. Dripps-American Society of Anesthesiologists classification and postoperative mortality correlation[a]

Class	Description	Mortality (%)[b]
1	Normal healthy	0.08
2	Mild systemic disease	0.27
3	Severe systemic disease with limited activity but not incapacitated	1.8
4	Incapacitating, constantly life-threatening systemic disease	7.8
5	Moribund, not expected to survive 24 hours with or without operation	9.4

[a]Modified from ER Jewell, AV Persson. Preoperative evaluation of high-risk patients. *Surg Clin North Am* 65:3, 1985.
[b]Modified from CJ Vacanti, RJ Van Houten, RC Hill. A statistical analysis of the relationship of physical status to post-operative mortality in 68,388 cases. *Anesth Analg* 49:565, 1970.

Table 7-2. A multifactorial cardiac risk index

Criteria	Points
History	
Age >70 yrs	5
Myocardial infarction in past 6 mos	10
Physical examination	
S_3 gallop or JVD	11
Important aortic valve stenosis	3
Electrocardiogram	
Rhythm other than sinus	7
5 PVCs/min anytime before surgery	7
General status	
PO_2 <60 mm Hg or PCO_2 >50 mm Hg, K less than 3 mEq/liter or HCO_3 less than 20 mEq/liter, BUN >50 or Cr >3 mg/dl, elevated SGOT or signs of chronic liver disease, bedridden or malnourished	3
Operation	
Intraperitoneal, intrathoracic, aortic surgery	3
Emergency operation	4
Total possible	53

JVD = jugular venous distention; PVC = premature ventricular contractions; K = potassium; BUN = blood urea nitrogen; Cr = creatinine; SGOT = serum glutamic oxaloacetic transaminase.
Source: Modified from L Goldman et al. Multifactorial index of cardiac risk in noncardiac surgical procedures. *N Engl J Med* 297:845, 1977.

Table 7-3. New York Heart Association angina classification

Class	Description
1	Angina with strenuous exercise
2	Angina with moderate exercise
3	Angina after one flight of stairs or walking 1–2 blocks
4	Angina with any activity

Source: Modified from ER Jewell, AV Persson. Preoperative evaluation of high-risk patients. *Surg Clin North Am* 65:3, 1985.

Table 7-4. Cardiac risk index: Categories of increasing risk

Class	Points	Abdominal aortic surgery		Noncardiac surgical procedures (Goldman et al.)		
		No. of patients	Cardiac complications[a]	No. of patients	Cardiac complications[a]	P[b]
1	0–5	56	4 (7%)	537	5 (1%)	0.01
2	6–12	35	4 (11%)	316	21 (7%)	NS
3	13–25	8	3 (38%)	130	18 (14%)	NS
4	>26			18	14 (78%)	c
Total		99	11 (12%)		44 (4%)	0.01

NS = not significant.
[a]Documented intraoperative or postoperative myocardial infarction, pulmonary edema, or ventricular tachycardia without progression to cardiac death.
[b]Pearson's chi-square and likelihood ratio chi-square of abdominal aortic patients vs. Goldman's group.
[c]In this highest risk group, life-threatening cardiac problems affected 22% and cardiac-related mortality was 56%.
Source: Modified from CC Jeffrey, J Kunsman, DJ Cullen, DC Brewster. A prospective evaluation of cardiac risk index. *Anesthesiology* 58:462, 1983.

1. Table 7-2 shows one method of tabulating a **multifactorial index** of cardiac risk. A **cumulative point system** allows for placement of a patient into one of four categories of increasing risk (Table 7-4). We believe patients in categories 1 and 2 (cardiac mortality less than 2%) are acceptable risks for elective major vascular procedures. Elective surgery should be carefully considered in class 3 patients, and class 4 individuals generally are unacceptable risks for elective procedures. In some cases, risk can be improved by medical or surgical therapy, allowing for an elective vascular procedure at a later date. Obviously, increased risks must be taken for life- or limb-threatening problems such as symptomatic aneurysms or ischemic extremities.

2. Hertzer and colleagues at the Cleveland Clinic have emphasized the high prevalence and mortality of coronary artery disease (CAD) in their study of 1,000

Table 7-5. Preoperative evaluation of coronary heart disease before abdominal aortic aneurysm (AAA) repair

Class I: No evident coronary heart disease and normal exercise tolerance
   30–40% of AAA patients
   No special cardiac testing
   Proceed with AAA repair with good cardiovascular monitoring and anesthesia

Class II: Clinically evident or probable coronary heart disease
   50% of AAA patients
   Angina pectoris, prior MI, history of heart failure, long-standing diabetes mellitus, premature AAA disease (<60 yrs of age)
   Assess ventricular function (e.g., echocardiography)
   Assess cardiac perfusion (e.g., thallium scan)
   Coronary angiography and revascularization for high-risk patients

Class III: Severely symptomatic or unstable heart disease
   5–10% of AAA patients
   Assess ventricular function (e.g., echocardiography)
   Cardiac catheterization
   Coronary revascularization (CABG or PTCA) ± valve replacement(s)

MI = myocardial infarction; CABG = coronary artery bypass grafting; PTCA = percutaneous transluminal coronary angioplasty.

patients with peripheral vascular disease who underwent preoperative coronary angiography. Severe but correctable CAD was documented in 25% of patients presenting for surgical management of peripheral vascular disease (abdominal aortic aneurysm, 31%; cerebrovascular disease, 26%; arteriosclerosis obliterans of the lower limbs, 21%). Severe, correctable CAD was present in approximately 50% of all patients with angina pectoris, as well as in one of every three patients with a previous MI or with ischemia on routine electrocardiogram (ECG). These data have stirred controversy over whether patients with severe, correctable CAD should undergo myocardial revascularization before elective peripheral vascular operations, especially before aortic reconstruction. Several large series have documented reduced perioperative myocardial ischemia and death in patients who have had coronary artery bypass grafting or percutaneous coronary angioplasty before peripheral vascular operations.

3. We perform **noninvasive cardiac testing** in patients who have coronary or valvular heart disease by history, physical examination, or preliminary ECG (Table 7-5). In addition, we pursue further cardiac evaluation in patients who develop angina, dyspnea, arrhythmias, or ischemic ECG changes during treadmill exercise testing for claudication. Current methods used to assess the heart include **ECG-monitored treadmill exercise, two-dimensional echocardiography (stress-exercise or dobutamine-stimulated),**

**radio-nuclide angiography, thallium or ses-
tamibi myocardial perfusion scans, 24-hour
ambulatory ECG monitoring,** and **coronary arteriography.**

a. An exercise radionuclide angiogram (**MUGA
scan**—*m*ultiple *g*ated *a*cquisition) was once a common noninvasive cardiac test but recently has been
replaced with thallium scanning and stress
echocardiography in many centers. Two-dimensional echocardiography (2-D echo) is an excellent technique for evaluating global left ventricular size and
function, segmental wall motion abnormalities, and
valve characteristics, including anatomic defects,
motion, and area. For claudicating patients who
cannot be exercised adequately on a treadmill,
dobutamine can be used to stress the heart phar-
macologically.

b. We have also relied on **dipyridamole thallium-
201 imaging** to evaluate suspected CAD in
patients with peripheral vascular disease. Dipyridamole thallium scans are especially helpful in
patients who cannot be stressed by exercise. In this
test, intravenous dipyridamole is administered, followed by an intravenous bolus of thallium radioisotope. Intravenous dipyridamole is as potent as exercise in causing coronary vasodilatation but does not
increase myocardial oxygen consumption. The
rationale for the test is that atherosclerotic vessels
have a fixed stenosis and cannot dilate in response
to dipyridamole. Thus, normally perfused
myocardium absorbs the thallium-201 promptly
and is visualized on the initial scan. Ischemic
myocardium, beyond a fixed stenosis and at risk of
infarction, takes up thallium-201 more slowly ("cold
spot") but does visualize on a delayed scan done 3–4
hours later (redistribution). Previously infarcted
myocardium fails to absorb thallium-201 on either
the initial or late scan. Dipyridamole thallium-201
imaging has a sensitivity of 85–90% and a specificity of 65–80% in detecting hemodynamically important coronary stenosis, which is seen subsequently
on coronary arteriography. Patients on theophylline
should have this medication withdrawn for 72
hours before dipyridamole testing, since dipyridamole will not increase coronary blood flow effectively in the presence of theophylline.

In using thallium stress testing, one must factor
**clinically evident signs of coronary heart dis-
ease** into any clinical decision. In analyzing the
experience at the Massachusetts General Hospital,
Eagle and colleagues have stressed the importance
of combining clinical risk factors for ischemic coronary events with the need and results of thallium
scanning. **The most important clinical risk factors are angina pectoris, past MI, congestive
heart failure, diabetes mellitus, and Q waves**

on the ECG. If none of these factors is present and the patient performs normal daily activities, the risk of a ischemic coronary event following peripheral vascular surgery is low (3%). Such patients do not need any special preoperative cardiac stress testing. Most patients, however, will have one or two cardiac risk factors. When their thallium scan is normal, they also face a low perioperative cardiac risk (3%) and can proceed to vascular surgery without cardiac catheterization. In contrast, a positive thallium scan (redistribution) in this subset of patients is predictive of an approximate risk of 30% for a postoperative cardiac event. If the patient has three or more clinical risk factors, the risk of serious postoperative myocardial ischemia escalates to 50%. Likewise, two or three coronary areas of redistribution should heighten concern for operative cardiac event risk (50%). Consequently, patients with **clinical cardiac risk factors plus thallium redistribution** should be considered for coronary angiography and revascularization of left main lesions or three-vessel disease with compromised ventricular function.

4. At the Massachusetts General Hospital and at the Mayo Clinic, we have **selectively** evaluated and treated patients for coronary artery or valvular heart disease. We consider valve replacement or coronary revascularization for individuals with unstable angina, critical valvular disease, asymptomatic three-vessel coronary disease associated with decompensated post-stress ventricular function (ejection fraction falling to less than 35%), and left-main coronary artery stenosis. For example, 5–10% of our patients undergoing abdominal aortic aneurysm repair have significant heart pathology needing preoperative revascularization (85% by coronary bypass grafting and 15% by percutaneous coronary angioplasty). With this selective approach, operative mortality for abdominal aortic aneurysm repair has been about 1–2% for patients with a negative history of CAD and 3–5% for those with a positive history of CAD.

5. **Cardiac conduction abnormalities** must be clearly defined before operation. First-degree atrioventricular (AV) block, right bundle branch block (RBBB), left bundle branch block (LBBB), and bifascicular or trifascicular block are usually chronic abnormalities that seldom progress to complete heart block (CHB), except in the setting of acute MI, aortic valve endocarditis, or surgical trauma. Thus, temporary pacing is usually not required for these conduction disturbances. In contrast, patients with Mobitz II AV block, third-degree AV block, or significant impairment of AV-nodal function should have temporary perioperative pacing support, regardless of whether a history of syncope or near-syncope is obtained. Permanent pacemakers are required for CHB or intermittent CHB.

Placement of a Swan-Ganz pulmonary artery catheter places a patient with LBBB at risk for induced RBBB and can precipitate CHB. Due to this occasional occurrence, a multipurpose pacing Swan-Ganz catheter should be used in patients with LBBB and placed by physicians familiar with pacing equipment.

Patients with **implanted permanent cardiac pacemakers** may present a special problem during operation. The electrocautery may inhibit or rapidly stimulate the pulse generator, especially if the cautery is used within 12–18 inches of the generator. To prevent an inadequate pacemaker-dependent cardiac rate, the rate of the pacer can be easily converted to a fixed-rate mode by placing a special magnet supplied by the manufacturer over the pulse generator. Rapidly evolving technologies and complex operational characteristics of newer pacemakers mandate that the surgeon and anesthesiologist consult preoperatively with a patient's cardiologist to ascertain how a particular pacemaker is to be managed during operation.

B. **Carotid occlusive disease** is present in 10–20% of patients presenting with aortic or femoropopliteal atherosclerosis and abdominal aortic aneurysms. Often the carotid disease is asymptomatic and detected initially by cervical bruits. Controversy continues over whether asymptomatic carotid disease should be ignored or whether carotid bruits should be evaluated by noninvasive testing and selective arteriography to ascertain the exact nature of the lesions. Most studies suggest that there is no significant increase in risk of perioperative stroke in patients with asymptomatic bruits. These studies, however, do not define the anatomy of the carotid lesions and leave doubt about whether high-grade (greater than 80%) bilateral carotid lesions may increase stroke risk.

Our approach to asymptomatic cervical bruits in patients facing elective aortic or coronary reconstruction is noninvasive classification of the degree of stenosis by ocular pneumoplethysmography (OPG) or duplex scanning. High-grade lesions (greater than 80%) with poorly compensated distal cerebral pressures (positive OPG result) are generally evaluated by arteriography and corrected by carotid endarterectomy before elective aortic or coronary surgery. Obviously, patients with large or symptomatic aneurysms, unstable angina pectoris, or threatening leg ischemia must have these more pressing problems operated urgently, taking the risk of the occasional stroke. After these more critical operations, asymptomatic hemodynamically significant carotid disease can be repaired electively later.

C. **Pulmonary complications** remain another leading cause of postoperative morbidity and mortality. Most patients undergoing vascular operation have some degree of chronic lung disease since they generally are longtime smokers.

1. The initial **history and physical examination** will identify the patients at highest risk of pulmonary

problems. They often are dyspneic at rest or report dyspnea with minimal exertion, exhibit chronic cough and sputum production, or previously have suffered from pneumonia. Other typical findings include a hyperinflated chest with distant breath sounds and obvious use of accessory neck and abdominal muscles to assist with breathing. Asthmatics may have wheezing. A simple bedside assessment of the degree of airway obstructive disease can be made by having the patient take a deep inspiration and then expire as quickly as possible while the examiner listens with a stethoscope. Normal complete expiratory time is less than 3 seconds. For patients with obstructive lung disease, this time is often 4–8 seconds. This simple bedside test also can be used to monitor clinical improvement during bronchodilator therapy.

2. A **chest x-ray** may reveal important anatomic information such as an occult lung cancer, cardiomegaly, interstitial fibrosis, or giant lung blebs.

3. **Spirometry** and measurement of **arterial blood gases** need not be routine but are indicated for patients with obvious chronic lung disease. One of the most reliable predictors of high pulmonary risk is the forced expiratory volume at one second (FEV_1). Significant postoperative pulmonary complications can be expected in patients with an FEV_1 of less than 15 ml/kg or less than 1,000 ml. If the FEV_1 is less than 70% of that predicted, the spirometry should be repeated after attempted bronchodilatation with inhaled isoproterenol. An increase of at least 15% in FEV_1 generally indicates that preoperative bronchodilator therapy may enhance pulmonary function. This improvement may be significant for the patient who has marginal lung function and requires elective surgery. Although measurement of arterial blood gases need not be routine, baseline values may help in patients with severe chronic obstructive pulmonary disease (COPD). For example, an elevated PCO_2 should caution against administration of high oxygen concentrations that may suppress respiratory drive.

D. **Renal function** should be routinely checked by urinalysis and measurement of the serum creatinine level. Many vascular patients take diuretics chronically, which causes intravascular volume depletion. This chronic dehydration places them at increased risk for acute renal failure after angiography or operation. Consequently, rehydration appears to be the single most important factor in reducing postoperative renal failure.

E. **Diabetes mellitus,** a common metabolic disease of many vascular patients, often becomes difficult to control when patients are hospitalized for diagnostic tests, treatment, and surgery. When diabetics enter the hospital, their activity level decreases and diet usually changes. Consequently, the insulin administered should be adjusted. Wide swings in blood sugar levels may result, especially when patients receive insulin but miss meals because of diagnostic tests or other preoperative preparations.

F. **Poor nutritional status** has been correlated with increased postoperative complications, sepsis, and mortality. Few physicians think of vascular patients as being poorly nourished. Nonetheless, certain vascular patients tend to be malnourished and need repletion of nutritional deficits.

1. **Chronic intestinal angina** from mesenteric ischemia leads to fear of eating and therefore weight loss. This weight loss usually occurs over several months and may amount to 20–50 lb in some patients.

2. **Severe lung disease** requires extra expenditure of energy because accessory neck and abdominal muscles are used to assist with breathing. Pulmonary cachexia often is obvious on examination. Because the weight loss usually is insidious, the severe degree of malnutrition may not be appreciated.

3. **Multiple complicated vascular procedures or serious postoperative infections** also place increased caloric demands on the body. Again, the weight loss may be gradual and the severity of the malnutrition may be missed.

4. **Chronic alcoholism** and associated liver disease may result not only in poor nutrition but also in altered clotting function. If hypersplenism is present, the platelet count may be low. Liver-dependent clotting factor deficiency and thrombocytopenia can be life-threatening problems in patients who require preclotting of porous knitted grafts. Patients with chronic liver disease also become more hypoalbuminemic in the postoperative period and may develop peripheral edema, ascites, or anasarca.

5. Patients in the clinical categories above must be nutritionally assessed and may need parenteral or enteral supplemental feedings before or after surgery. A clinical "eyeball" evaluation of nutritional status is unreliable in assessing high- versus low-risk patients. Several objective **criteria for supplemental nutrition** are:

   a. **Weight loss** of 10% in the past 30 days.

   b. **Failure to reestablish** adequate nutrition (35 calories/kg/day) within 5–10 days after surgery.

   c. **Compromised immune response** indicated by anergy to common skin tests or total lymphocyte count less than 800.

   d. Preoperative **serum albumin** less than 3 mg/100 ml.

II. **Cardiovascular medications.** Vascular patients often are on various combinations of antihypertensives, diuretics, digitalis, beta-blockers, calcium channel blockers, antiarrhythmics, and nitrates. In general, most of these medications are continued until the time of operation. There are, however, a few exceptions.

A. Patients on **antihypertensive therapy** have decreased intravascular volume and consequently are prone to hypotension during the perioperative period. In the past, efforts were made to restore sympathetic activity by discontinuing drugs such as reserpine, guanethidine, and methyldopa. These drugs do not totally suppress sympathetic activity; therefore, they should be continued until the time of operation. Abrupt stoppage of clonidine, which decreases sympathetic outflow from the brain, can be accompanied by severe rebound hypertension. Because monoamine oxidase inhibitors prevent metabolic degradation of endogenous amines and have been associated with difficult control of blood pressure when a vasopressor is used, they should be discontinued or replaced by other antihypertensive medications. Otherwise, most antihypertensives should be continued until the time of operation, although bed rest and hospital diet may permit some reduction in dosage.

B. Chronic diuretic therapy depletes both intravascular volume and total body potassium stores. Diuretics generally should be reduced or discontinued 24–48 hours preoperatively and potassium replacement should be initiated.

C. Cardiac glycosides, such as digoxin, usually are continued until operation.

D. Propranolol or other **beta blockers** being administered for hypertension or ischemic heart disease should not be abruptly discontinued. Acute withdrawal has been associated with exacerbation of coronary events such as increased angina, ventricular tachycardia, and fatal MI.

E. Antiarrhythmic drugs should be continued until the operation. Their suppressing effect on the myocardium may require alteration in doses of other drugs given during anesthesia.

III. Optimizing pulmonary function. In patients with chronic lung disease, optimizing pulmonary function before the operation can decrease the incidence of postoperative respiratory complications at least twofold. Preoperative preparation may require that the patient stop smoking, that antibiotics for bronchitis and bronchodilators be administered, and that the patient be instructed in deep breathing.

A. Ideally, **smoking** should be stopped several weeks before surgery so that cilia regeneration can occur and any bronchorrhea can be resolved. However, this goal is difficult to attain in many patients who are anxious before hospitalization. Consequently, we generally enforce nonsmoking on admission, treat any anxiety with sedatives, and begin intensive pulmonary care before surgery in patients with severe lung disease.

B. Bronchitis in COPD patients usually is caused by *Streptococcus pneumoniae* or *Haemophilus influenzae*. Ampicillin, amoxicillin, or tetracycline, 250–500 mg PO tid–qid, are considered first-line antibiotics for treating bronchitis.

C. Bronchodilators remain the cornerstone of drug treatment for patients with COPD. However, we often find that COPD patients are not on optimum doses of bronchodilators when they enter the hospital for elective surgery. Simple chest auscultation may reveal a prolonged expiratory phase (>3 seconds) or wheezing.

Spirometry may show that the FEV_1 is less than 70% of that predicted and is improved after inhalation of a bronchodilator.

Initial bronchodilator therapy is usually an inhaled beta-agonist delivered by a metered-dose inhaler or nebulization three or four times daily. If bronchospasm is severe, oral or intravenous aminophylline is added. Another benefit of theophylline is its potent and long-lasting effect in improving diaphragmatic strength and suppressing fatigue in patients with fixed airway obstruction. The optimum method to maximize bronchodilatation is oral theophylline (3–5 mg/kg qid) or intravenous aminophylline (loading dose of 6 mg/kg; maintenance dose of 0.2–0.5 mg/kg/hour). This therapy should be titrated to bring plasma concentrations of theophylline to 10–20 µg/ml. Higher drug levels may cause bothersome tachycardia, restlessness, nausea, vomiting, extrasystoles, or seizures. We generally recommend that therapy continue until surgery, be withheld during the operation, and be resumed postoperatively at the first sign of bronchospasm. Newer adrenergic agents appear to achieve bronchodilatation with fewer cardiac effects than those accompanying theophylline or aminophylline administration. The main new agents are terbutaline (2.5–5.0 mg PO q6–8h or 0.25–0.50 SQ q4–6h) and metaproterenol (10–20 mg PO qid). However, blood levels cannot be monitored as easily as they can be with theophylline administration. Inhaled adrenergic agents such as isoproterenol or metaproterenol also are useful for prn postoperative bronchodilatation.

D. Deep breathing after surgery decreases postoperative atelectasis. Preoperative instruction is more effective than waiting to teach the proper method until the early postoperative period, when the patient is having incisional pain. Different types of incentive spirometers are popular methods of achieving deep breathing, but the key to deep inspiration is patient motivation, nursing instruction, and continuous encouragement after operation.

IV. Controlling diabetes mellitus can be difficult in the perioperative period, when glucose intake may be erratic and physiologic stress is so variable. In general, stress results in a state of insulin resistance due to increased levels of contrainsulin hormones such as glucagon, epinephrine, cortisol, and growth hormone. To avoid hypo- or hyperglycemia, the clinician should attempt to maintain the patient's blood glucose level in the range of 150–250 mg/100 ml.

A. The **best method to monitor** therapy remains measurement of blood glucose levels. Testing urine glucose **without** correlation with blood sugars is an inaccurate means of determining insulin requirements, since the incidence of falsely high and falsely low tests is so great. Control of diabetes with the sliding scale method of urine glucose levels and regular insulin coverage may result in wide swings of blood sugar levels and is mentioned only to discourage its use.

Table 7-6. Onset and duration of action for insulin

Type of insulin	Peak action (hrs)	Duration (hrs)
Regular	2–4	6–8
Intermediate (NPH, Lente)	8–12	18–24

B. The **perioperative drug management** of the diabetic depends on whether the patient's usual therapy has been insulin or oral hypoglycemics (Table 7-6).

1. **Insulin-taking patients** who are scheduled for surgery early in the morning (before 9 AM) should not take their insulin the morning of surgery. They may be asked to bring their insulin with them if they are a morning admission. The blood sugar level is checked on arrival at the operating room. If the blood sugar is more than 100 mg/dl, the patient should receive one-half the usual intermediate-acting insulin. If the blood sugar is less than 100 mg/dl, the patient should receive 15 g of carbohydrates (i.e., fruit juice or an intravenous infusion containing dextrose) and one-half the usual dose of intermediate-acting insulin(no regular insulin) at that time.

2. **Insulin-taking patients who are NPO** after breakfast and scheduled for a procedure later in the day should be asked to take one-half the usual dose of intermediate-acting insulin instead of the full dose (**no regular insulin**) at breakfast.

3. Patients taking oral hypoglycemic agents should be advised **not** to take the oral agents on the morning of surgery.

4. The so-called **brittle diabetic** can have wide variations in blood sugar levels despite frequent blood glucose monitoring and little change in insulin dose. In our experience, this type of patient's blood glucose is optimally controlled with continuous low-dose insulin intravenous infusion. A continuous infusion of 1–4 units of regular insulin per hour generally results in smooth control. To avoid an accidental rapid insulin infusion, we recommend mixing only 10 units of regular insulin in 250 ml of D5W or D5NS and infusing at a rate of 25–100 ml/hour (1–4 units) with **control by an infusion pump.**

V. **Preoperative weight reduction.** Obesity makes operative dissection more difficult than usual, especially in the abdomen and retroperitoneum. In our experience, it also increases wound complications in the groin. Consequently, we insist that obese candidates for **elective** major vascular surgery lose excess weight. Obviously, obese patients who require urgent treatment for symptomatic aneurysms or limb salvage cannot wait to lose excess weight before an operation. However, moderately obese patients who require elective operation for claudication or asymptomatic aneurysms generally may be followed until excess weight is lost.

Patients who are 15–40 lb above their ideal weight are considered moderately obese. Morbidly obese patients (100 lb overweight) seldom can be expected to lose substantial weight before elective surgery. Therefore, the benefits of elective abdominal or extremity vascular reconstruction in excessively obese patients must be weighed carefully against the increased risks of perioperative complications.

Occasionally, some physicians remark that weight reduction in preoperative patients is extremely difficult to achieve and may be unsafe. They are concerned that insistence on weight loss may discourage the patient from returning to them for further treatment. The added cost of dietary consultation often is mentioned. Finally, the danger of excess weight loss and protein catabolism before major surgery also is raised as an objection to preoperative weight reduction.

In our experience, safe preoperative weight reduction can be accomplished in approximately 8 of 10 moderately obese patients who require an elective operation. Ideally, we strive to bring the patient's weight to within 10% of ideal weight. The following guidelines for preoperative weight reduction are usually effective:

A. The **importance of preoperative weight reduction** as a means to facilitate operative dissection and to decrease postoperative complications must be explained to the patient. We emphasize that elective surgery can be safely postponed until excess weight is lost. Faced with major vascular surgery, most patients can be motivated to lose weight.

B. A **definite time period** for the diet is proposed and a tentative surgery date is selected. Most moderately obese patients will need to lose 10–30 lb. To ensure safe, gradual weight reduction, we recommend a weight loss of 1–2 lb/week. Thus, elective surgery is postponed for 6–8 weeks for most patients. Obviously, some patients will need 3–6 months of dieting. We also have found it important to recheck patients every 6–8 weeks to ensure that they are losing weight and not having any problems with the diet.

C. The diet should be low-calorie (800–1,200 calories/day) but **balanced.** We routinely use a relatively low-fat, low-cholesterol **1,000-calorie diet.** Strict starvation or diets that do not have a balance of carbohydrates, protein, and fat are not safe for older patients with vascular disease. Adherence to such diets may result in severe catabolism and deficiencies in vitamins, minerals, and trace elements.

D. Although consultation with a dietician may be helpful in selected cases, a simple **explanation of the diet** by the physician and office nurse generally will suffice and saves the patient the extra time and cost of a dietary consultation. In our experience, patients seem to respond best to the firm insistence on and explanation of a diet by the primary surgeon.

E. **A specified amount of weight** to lose is marked on the front page of the diet. Patients are instructed to take a baseline reading of their weight on a home scale and then to lose the specified weight.

F. **Alcoholic beverages** are commonly an overlooked source of calories. This fact should be emphasized to patients who drink regularly, as they usually must reduce alcohol intake to lose weight.

G. It is extremely difficult to lose weight and stop **smoking** at the same time. Consequently, we allow chronic smokers to continue some smoking while they diet. We make an agreement with the patient that smoking will stop when the patient is hospitalized for elective surgery. Some physicians criticize this relatively late discontinuance of smoking; however, this approach usually results in successful weight reduction and has not led to increased pulmonary morbidity in our experience.

Selected Reading

Cambria RP et al. The impact of selective use of dipyridamole-thallium scans and surgical factors on the current morbidity of aortic surgery. *J Vasc Surg* 15:43, 1992.

Coley CM et al. Usefulness of dipyridamole-thallium in preoperative evaluation of cardiac risk for nonvascular surgery. A*m J Cardiol* 69:1280, 1992.

Cutler BS, Hendel RC, Leppo JA. Dipyridamole-thallium scintigraphy predicts perioperative and long-term survival after major vascular surgery. *J Vasc Surg* 15:972, 1992.

Elmore JR et al. Myocardial revascularization before abdominal aortic aneurysmorrhaphy: Effect of coronary angioplasty. *Mayo Clin Proc* 68:1, 1993.

Gersh BJ et al. Evaluation and management of patients with both peripheral and coronary artery disease. *J Am Coll Cardiol* 18:203, 1991.

Hertzer NR et al. Coronary artery disease in peripheral vascular patients: A classification of 1000 coronary angiograms and results of surgical management. *Ann Surg* 199:223, 1984.

Lalka SG et al. Dobutamine stress echocardiography as a predictor of cardiac events associated with aortic surgery. *J Vasc Surg* 15:831, 1992.

Taylor LM et al. The incidence of perioperative myocardial infarction in general vascular surgery. *J Vasc Surg* 15:52, 1991.

Woodley M, Whelan A. (eds). *Manual of Medical Therapeutics* (27th ed). Boston: Little, Brown, 1992.

Perioperative Management

After the initial patient evaluation and preoperative preparation, the next phase of patient care may involve an operation. Perioperative management encompasses not only anesthesia but also vascular monitoring and early postoperative care. A carefully administered anesthetic is just as important as an appropriate and technically successful operation. The informed vascular surgeon should understand at least the basic concepts of anesthesia for vascular patients. To avoid early postoperative failures and reoperation, the surgeon must also develop techniques of vascular monitoring that will detect perioperative problems. Finally, he or she must have an understanding of postoperative cardiorespiratory support and common multiorgan dysfunctions that may threaten patient survival.

This section emphasizes principles of perioperative management that we have found successful. This section should be especially valuable to surgical house staff and nurses, who often are the first to recognize and treat perioperative problems.

Anesthesia

Improved anesthetic management has been a key factor in the progressive reduction of operative mortality and morbidity for major vascular surgery. Optimum anesthetic management requires that the vascular surgeon understand the principles of anesthesia involved in intraoperative care of vascular patients. The preoperative assessment of the patient and the suspected underlying disease states form the basis for selecting a successful anesthetic. The anesthesiologist must also be aware of certain parts of the operative technique that are most stressful to cardiac, cerebral, and renal function in order to treat the effects of such stresses. Good communication between the surgeon and the anesthesiologist must be maintained for smooth conduct of any major vascular operation.

Although this chapter is brief, we provide a list of selected reading for those interested in more detail. This chapter focuses on carotid and aortic operations, since these arterial reconstructions represent the most difficult challenges in anesthetic management. Appropriate anesthesia for other arterial and venous operations is discussed briefly.

I. **Perioperative physiologic monitoring.** Perioperative physiologic monitoring provides objective data that are critical to assessment and maintenance of multiorgan function. The magnitude of the operation and the patient's medical condition determine the extent of such monitoring. It should be recognized that information gathered from monitoring may be misleading, inaccurate, or imprecise. It is essential to realize the limitations of such monitoring.

A. **All patients** should have at least one large-caliber (14- or 16-gauge) intravenous line and electrocardiographic (leads II and V_5), temperature, and blood pressure monitoring. A urinary catheter and collection system to measure hourly urine output is needed for operations that last longer than 2–3 hours.

B. **Major vascular cases** usually require the addition of an indwelling radial artery line and a central venous catheter. The arterial line allows easier blood sampling for measurements of arterial blood gases, hematocrit, sodium, potassium, and glucose in addition to continuous observation of the systemic blood pressure. The central venous line allows measurements of central venous pressure and central infusion of medications, especially potassium.

C. It is unclear which patients require or benefit from monitoring of the pulmonary artery with a **Swan-Ganz pulmonary artery catheter (PAC)**. Pulmonary capillary wedge pressure or pulmonary diastolic pressure is a more reliable guide to left ventricular function and intravascular volume than is right-sided central venous pressure. The PAC also allows the assessment of cardiac index. Special PACs will also measure the mixed venous oxygen saturation (SvO_2), which is another indication of overall multior-

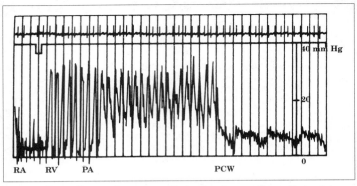

Fig. 8-1. Swan-Ganz pulmonary catheter tracings as the catheter is advanced from the right atrium (RA) through the right ventricle (RV) and pulmonary artery (PA) to a wedged position in a pulmonary artery (PCW). The pressures shown are within normal limits. Abnormal values are discussed in the text.

gan well-being. Patients with coronary artery disease and left ventricular dysfunction may be at further risk for the development of rhythm disturbances such as heart block. The PAC will allow rapid initiation of ventricular pacing. **Consequently, patients with past or present heart failure, unstable angina pectoris, or recent myocardial infarction generally require a PAC.** Some anesthesiologists prefer a PAC in all major aortic reconstructions where aortic cross-clamping is necessary and blood loss may be large. If there is a question about the need for a PAC, the surgeon and anesthesiologist should discuss both the indications for such monitoring and the surgeon's operative plan. When it is unclear whether a Swan-Ganz catheter will be needed, a No. 7.5 French catheter introducer can be placed in a central vein at the start of the operation. A PAC can then be introduced any time during or after the procedure, although doing so makes the sterile field more difficult to maintain. Figure 8-1 illustrates the various pressure tracings as the Swan-Ganz catheter is floated through the right heart to a wedge position in a pulmonary artery. The use of pulmonary artery pressures in managing cardiac function is discussed in Chap. 10. Although there are complications related to the use of a PAC, most of the risks are incurred with the process of obtaining central venous access. Therefore, once the decision to place a central venous catheter has been made, the decision to use a PAC is less difficult.

Special **oximetric pulmonary artery catheters** allow continuous monitoring and display of **SvO_2.** Decreases in SvO_2 are an indication of lowered cardiac output and oxygen delivery. SvO_2 values less than 60% are considered critically low and mandate immediate cardiorespiratory manipulations to enhance cardiac output and oxygen delivery.

D. Pulse oximeters, which attach easily to a finger or toe, are also used to continuously determine arterial oxygen saturation of hemoglobin. Pulse oximetry functions by positioning any pulsating arterial vascular bed between a two-wavelength light source and a detector. A familiar plethysmograph wave form results. Because the detected pulsatile wave form is produced safely from arterial blood, the amplitude of each wavelength related to reduced versus oxyhemoglobin allows continuous beat-to-beat calculation of arterial hemoglobin oxygen saturation. The instrument's ability to accurately calculate saturation can be impaired by (1) hypothermia, (2) hypotension (mean blood pressure <50 mm Hg), and (3) vasoconstriction by drugs. The placement of an additional pulse oximeter probe on another site is recommended (alternate extremity or more central location such as ear or nose).

E. Transesophageal two-dimensional echocardiography (TEE) is rapidly becoming an important part of monitoring in the operating room. It is the most sensitive method to detect myocardial ischemia in the operating room as evidenced by the development of myocardial wall motion abnormalities. TEE is also able to more accurately assess ventricular filling. This method requires additional expertise and training to gain a working knowledge. However, the PAC is adequate for most patients.

II. Patient positioning. Positioning of the patient on the operating table is critical if pressure-related injuries of the skin are to be avoided. The most common pressure problems in our experience have been heel ulcers. These pressure sores generally occur on the lateral heel. They usually affect patients with impaired lower-extremity arterial perfusion or with prolonged ischemic time when proximal arteries are clamped. Pressure-related heel ulcers can be prevented by one of two methods. Simply elevating the calf on soft towels can lift the heel so that it does not rest on the operating table, or a soft pad can be placed under the heel.

Another potential pressure problem occurs when the upper extremities are tucked along the side of the patient, and pressure from the edge of the operating table causes an ulnar neuropathy. This bothersome problem can be prevented by gently wrapping the elbow region with a soft pad to keep pressure off the ulnar nerve.

Another concern involves the positioning of the head, eyes, ears, and neck. Patients with carotid disease or musculoskeletal conditions such as arthritis may be particularly susceptible to serious injury secondary to poor positioning. Gentle positioning of the neck in the neutral position is best when possible. The eyes should always be taped to avoid abrasions.

Any limitations of range of motion involving the neck or extremities should be known. Positioning after induction of anesthesia should not involve any motion that goes beyond what the patient can achieve while conscious. The risk of injury to the skin should be minimized by carefully accounting for the electrocardiogram (ECG) leads, catheter connectors, and jewelry that may be in contact with the skin of the patient. The patient's skin should not be directly exposed to **metal.**

III. **Aortic surgery.** The main determinants of safe anesthesia for aortic surgery are careful control of the patient's blood pressure, intravascular volume, and myocardial performance within the context of the preoperative baseline of the patient. Since the majority of these patients have coronary artery disease, hypotension or hypertension can result in serious myocardial ischemia. The anesthesiologist must be aware of the various stages of the operation and the hemodynamic consequences with respect to the potential impact on the various organ systems. However, good anesthetic management is not simply maintaining a certain blood pressure. Moreover, it is the assessment and **maintenance of physiologic integrity** involving multiple physiologic parameters such as urine output, mean arterial pressure, pulmonary artery pressure, cardiac index, and pH. All these physiologic parameters must be considered together to treat the patient appropriately. Certain parameters may have increased significance in the context of certain disease states, such as coronary artery disease. It is important to avoid assigning too much importance to one particular value or parameter. The surgeon must understand how the anesthesiologist manages the patient at these critical points and be willing to contribute information he or she deems important.

Anesthesia may consist of a regional technique, **a mixed regional and general technique,** or a general anesthetic technique. Some centers have satisfactorily used continuous epidural anesthesia with a mixture of local anesthetics (e.g., bupivacaine) and narcotics supplemented with general anesthesia and endotracheal intubation. Epidural catheters appear to be safe in vascular patients who will be heparinized after the catheter insertion for their vascular operation. Epidural or subdural hematomas are a very rare complication, provided an atraumatic puncture is made. We have also found that a continuous epidural narcotic (e.g., fentanyl) infusion is a safe and highly effective method of controlling early postoperative pain for 48–72 hours after abdominal or lower-extremity operations. General endotracheal anesthesia may offer the greatest control of the hemodynamics and respiratory system for patients with significant pulmonary and cardiac disease. Although balanced general anesthesia with nitrous oxide, narcotics, relaxants, and barbiturates provides excellent operative conditions, a small amount of an inhalation agent or an intravenous vasodilator frequently is required to manage hypertension. Fluid requirements may also vary significantly with epidural anesthesia. Persistent hypotension may result with the occurrence of severe blood loss if an epidural technique is used.

A. **Causes of hypotension**

   1. After satisfactory induction of anesthesia, the first point of significant hypotension may occur when the intestines are withdrawn from the abdomen for exposure of the retroperitoneum. Although this response is thought to be vagally induced, atropine may not correct the problem. Vasodilating peptides that reside in the gas-

trointestinal tract may cause the fall in blood pressure. This pressure drop usually can be corrected with an intravenous dose of 5–10 mg of ephedrine or a phenylephrine drip plus increased fluid administration.

2. When a right lumbar sympathectomy is performed in conjunction with an aortic bypass, blood pressure may fall when the inferior vena cava is compressed and retracted for exposure of the lumbar sympathetic chain. This caval retraction results in decreased venous return from the lower extremities to the right side of the heart. The surgeon should inform the anesthetist whenever the vena cava is being compressed.

B. One of the most stressful steps of the operation for the myocardium is **aortic cross-clamping,** which acutely increases afterload to the myocardium. The healthy heart can tolerate this change with no evidence of myocardial failure or ischemia. However, the impaired heart is stressed. Blood pressure and pulmonary capillary wedge pressure rise. The ECG often shows ST segment changes and ventricular irritability. In the case of a severely impaired heart, the blood pressure and cardiac output may fall. Afterload must be immediately decreased by judicious titration of peripheral vasodilator drugs such as sodium nitroprusside or nitroglycerin, and inotropic support should be started or increased as required to stabilize hemodynamics. The use of vasodilating agents will require maintenance of adequate filling pressure. Sodium nitroprusside will give a more rapid and effective response on the blood pressure than nitroglycerin.

With aortic cross-clamping, **renal cortical blood flow** and urine output may decrease in spite of clamping below the renal arteries. This effect can usually be prevented by establishing an adequate urine diuresis before clamping. This diuresis is accomplished by adequate hydration and intravenous administration of 12.5–25.0 g mannitol. The preoperative pulmonary wedge pressure and left ventricular function must be considered when determining whether the patient is adequately volume-loaded. If this treatment is not effective, 10–20 mg of furosemide (Lasix) is given. During this diuresis, potassium must be carefully monitored and supplemented. Otherwise, serious arrhythmias may occur from hypokalemia. Hypokalemia during the cross-clamping period must be very cautiously treated because decreased renal function after cross-clamping may impair potassium excretion. Once again, the surgeon should inform the anesthetist several minutes before cross-clamping.

C. **Blood loss**

1. The next point of significant blood loss may occur when the **aortic clamp is released to check the proximal anastomosis.** At this time, additional blood (50–150 ml) may be taken to complete preclotting of a knitted graft.

2. Blood loss is usually substantial enough in aortic cases to require transfusion. The alternative to bank blood transfusions is **autotransfusion.** When more than

2,500 ml is autotransfused, clotting factors and platelets must be checked and administered as necessary. The use of the thromboelastogram (TEG) can also provide a qualitative analysis of the ability of the blood to clot, which can be used to guide platelet and factor replacement. Empirical transfusion of blood products may be necessary but should be carefully considered. Fresh plasma and platelets may be especially important initially when the graft is opened. Failure to replenish these factors can result in life-threatening leakage through the graft wall. The hemoglobin used to initiate transfusion of red blood cells should be determined on an individual basis for each patient based on the severity of underlying diseases, age, and surgery. The surgeon and anesthesiologist should communicate openly about the transfusion of blood and blood products.

D. Fluid replacement. Throughout the procedure, adequate amounts of fluid must be given continuously. Fluid replacement should be guided by indices of ventricular filling and maintenance of a good cardiac index. The large incision, prolonged exposure of the abdominal contents, and the usual blood loss create large fluid shifts. Lactated Ringer's solution is administered at 750–1,000 ml/hour, in addition to blood and colloid as needed. Patients can become hypothermic (T <34°C) during long operations; therefore, blood and fluids should be warmed. In addition, we prevent hypothermia by using an upper-body heating tent (Bair Hugger) during the operation. (This special heating blanket can also be used in the early postoperative period to rewarm the trunk and lower extremities.)

E. One of the most critical times of the entire operation is at **aortic unclamping.** Profound hypotension can occur. The surgeon should warn the anesthetist several minutes before unclamping. Hypotension can be minimized by adequate intravascular volume replacement. The anesthetist also can avoid additional myocardial depressants and decrease vasodilator therapy and inhalation agents prior to release of the cross-clamp. Opening the graft slowly also may minimize sudden changes in blood pressure. Occasionally, small amounts of sodium bicarbonate will be necessary, but acid metabolites from ischemic limbs are not the primary cause of "declamping shock." Generally, we also administer intravenous calcium chloride, which rapidly increases myocardial contractility, cardiac output, and blood pressure. If one reverses heparin with protamine at the end of the operation, the protamine must be administered slowly since it can cause hypotension or bradycardia. In rare cases, the administration of protamine may lead to severe bronchospasm and hemodynamic instability.

IV. Carotid artery surgery. Anesthesia for carotid artery surgery must be administered skillfully to avoid dangerous swings in blood pressure and cerebral perfusion. The surgeon must understand basic control mechanisms for cerebral blood flow, methods of monitoring cerebral perfusion, and the effects of different anesthetic agents on cerebral metabolism. The surgeon must keep the anesthetist informed of operative steps that affect blood pressure or interrupt carotid blood flow.

A. Cerebral blood flow. The major determinants of cerebral blood flow in the normal brain are:

   1. Local metabolic factors. Accumulation of local metabolic products causes vasodilatation of adjacent blood vessels and increased local flow.

   2. Arterial oxygen tension (PaO$_2$). Within wide limits, PaO$_2$ does not significantly influence cerebral blood flow.

   3. Arterial carbon dioxide tension (PaCO$_2$) affects cerebral blood flow throughout its physiologic range. As PaCO$_2$ falls, cerebral blood flow also decreases, and vice versa.

   4. Cerebral perfusion pressure (arterial pressure minus intracranial pressure or venous pressure). Within wide ranges of perfusion pressure, cerebral blood flow does not change because of autoregulation.

In diseased states, these control mechanisms are altered. Autoregulation is altered so that the acceptable mean arterial pressure is different and the point at which autoregulation becomes lost is also altered. Blood vessels in ischemic brain are maximally vasodilated, and therefore blood flow becomes a direct function of perfusion pressure. During carotid clamping, normotension to slight hypertension should optimize cerebral perfusion. In addition, normocarbia to slight hypocarbia seems preferable. Raising the PaCO$_2$ may dilate normal brain arterioles and increase intracranial pressure so that flow is diverted from ischemic to normal areas (intracranial steal).

B. Monitoring. In our experience, the best method to assess adequate cerebral perfusion during carotid cross-clamping has been a continuous electroencephalogram (EEG). Carotid artery stump pressures may not correlate with the EEG changes. Chapter 11 describes indications for use of an intraluminal shunt.

C. Anesthetic agents. The goals of anesthesia for carotid surgery include (1) consistent blood pressure control, (2) regulation of PaCO$_2$ to maximize blood flow to ischemic areas, and (3) rapid emergence from anesthesia for a postoperative neurologic examination in the operating room when possible.

   We routinely use general anesthesia because blood pressure, arterial blood gases, and the patient's airway are best controlled by this technique. General anesthesia may also be most suitable for a teaching center.

   Some surgeons prefer local or regional cervical block anesthesia because they think it is safer than general anesthesia and allows them to detect neurologic change when the carotid artery is clamped. We think a local anesthetic has no major advantage over carefully conducted general endotracheal anesthesia. Neurologic deficits can be minimized in the sleeping patient by EEG monitoring with selective or routine shunting.

   One of the most common anesthetic techniques for carotid surgery is **balanced anesthesia** of barbiturates, nitrous oxide, narcotics, and muscle relaxants. Volatile agents and barbiturates may offer some protection against ischemia because cerebral oxygen demand is reduced. Beyond the level of an isoelectric EEG, which reflects an absence of functioning neurons, barbiturates have no cerebral metabolic effect or protection.

All volatile anesthetics are considered cerebral vasodilators, with halothane being the most potent and isoflurane the least. Most of the intravenous agents for anesthesia are cerebral vasoconstrictors. The effects these agents have on the abnormal cerebral vasculature is variable. As a result, the impact of one anesthetic choice versus another may be less important as long as the hemodynamics are kept adequate. The ability of either volatile or intravenous agents to suppress metabolism and provide cerebral protection occurs only at anesthetic depths that could impair hemodynamic stability. Halothane can cause hypotension and myocardial depression. Deep anesthesia with a volatile agent such as halothane may also increase intracranial pressure and promote intracerebral blood flow steal from ischemic areas. Prevention of ischemia may be more beneficial than any attempt with anesthetics to prolong the brain's tolerance to ischemia. Light levels of anesthesia with any combination of volatile or intravenous agents with EEG monitoring can be successful. Postoperative neurologic evaluation usually is delayed because the patient is slower to awaken when deeper anesthetic techniques are used or longer-acting intravenous agents are administered.

V. **Lower-extremity arterial reconstructions.** Lower-extremity arterial reconstructions can be performed under a general or regional anesthetic. In our experience, continuous catheter epidural anesthesia is an excellent method for femoropopliteal bypass grafting. In the early postoperative period, the epidural catheter may be left in place for additional pain relief or for reoperation if early graft thrombosis occurs.

The indication and appropriateness of a regional technique should ultimately be decided by the anesthesiologist. The surgeon should give appropriate input on the choice of a regional anesthetic and any potential ramifications. Patient acceptance of a regional anesthetic as well as its safety must be considered. Many factors may reduce the advisability of a regional technique, such as dementia, risk of pulmonary aspiration, or previous neurologic injury. Prolonged sedation is often required in many of these lower-extremity arterial reconstructions. In addition, some patients may have cardiovascular conditions that may disqualify them for regional anesthesia because of venous and arterial dilation (hypertrophic cardiomyopathy or severe aortic stenosis).

The use of regional anesthesia in patients undergoing intraoperative anticoagulation is still controversial. Most studies reveal a low complication rate. The risk for patients taking aspirin or mini-dose heparin also appears very small. The use of a preoperative bleeding time or activated partial thromboplastin time (aPTT) has been advocated by some in these circumstances.

VI. Arterial embolism. Arterial embolism often occurs in critically ill patients who are poor risks for general anesthesia. In such cases, femoral thromboembolectomy may be accomplished under local anesthesia. However, general or regional anesthesia is preferred for most thromboembolectomies, especially when operative arteriograms or an associated arterial bypass or patch angioplasty is planned.

VII. Lower-extremity venous procedures. Lower-extremity venous procedures require general or regional anesthesia. A spinal or epidural anesthetic is adequate for most varicose vein operations, which generally last 1–2 hours.

Selected Reading

Brewster DC, O'Hara PJ, Darling RC, Hallett JW Jr. Relationship of intraoperative EEG monitoring and stump pressure measurements during carotid endarterectomy. *Circulation* 62(Suppl 1):1, 1980.

Brown DL (ed). *Risk and Outcome in Anesthesia*. Philadelphia: Lippincott, 1988.

Cullen ML et al. Continuous epidural infusion for analgesia after major abdominal operations: A randomized, prospective, double blind study. *Surgery* 98:718, 1985.

Hallett JW Jr, Popovsky M, Ilstrup D. Minimizing blood transfusions during abdominal aortic surgery: recent advances in rapid autotransfusion. *J Vasc Surg* 5:601, 1987.

Roizen MF et al. Monitoring with two-dimensional transesophageal echocardiography. *J Vasc Surg* 1:300, 1984.

Roizen MF (ed). *Anesthesia For Vascular Surgery*. New York: Churchill Livingstone, 1990.

9

Vascular Monitoring

The success or failure of a vascular operation often can be recognized by simple examination of the patient in the operating or recovery room. However, pulses sometimes are difficult to palpate, or distal disease may not have been corrected. In some cases, the surgeon may want some physiologic means to monitor cerebral perfusion during carotid endarterectomy or to ascertain carotid patency in the early postoperative period if a neurologic deficit is present. Numerous techniques are available for intraoperative and postoperative vascular monitoring, and this chapter describes the methods we currently use. Although the ideal methods of vascular monitoring can be debated, few surgeons would argue against some type of objective assessment of immediate technical results. **The best time to detect and correct a technical problem is in the operating room, before the patient departs for the recovery area.**

Instrumentation

Our vascular monitoring is accomplished by the following techniques.

I. **Pulse volume recorder (PVR) or other air plethysmograph.** The PVR is a segmental plethysmograph that provides a pulse volume tracing that correlates directly with arterial pressure (Fig. 9-1). The tracing can be made by application of a blood pressure cuff to the distal extremity at the calf or ankle level. A baseline tracing is made before the operation begins (see Fig. 9-1). For aortic reconstructions (e.g., aortic aneurysms), the calf cuffs can be left in place if the lower limbs are only prepped to the thighs. Sterilized cuffs can be used in the operative field following femoropopliteal bypass grafting. Tracings are recorded when the arterial reconstruction is completed.

   Interpretation of PVR tracings is fairly simple. If normal PVR tracings existed before operation, they should show no worsening after the procedure. A flat or diminished pulse contour (<5 mm) suggests significant obstruction. This obstruction may be the result of an anastomotic stenosis, a distal intimal flap, or distal thromboemboli. Corrective measures should be undertaken and the PVR tracing should be repeated when the obstruction has been relieved (see Fig. 9-1).

II. **Doppler velocity detector and duplex scanning.** The continuous-wave Doppler system represents one of the simplest methods to evaluate arterial perfusion before and after arterial reconstructions. The Doppler unit allows evaluation of the quality of the arterial signal and measurement of limb blood pressures. It is particularly useful when pulses are not palpable. Also, it is a good method to assess arterial flow sig-

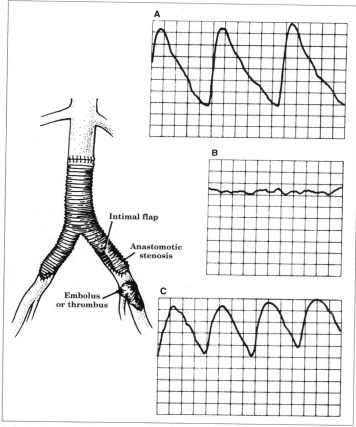

Fig. 9-1.   Pulse volume recordings during intraoperative monitoring of arterial reconstructions. A. Baseline tracings at the calf document normal preoperative pulse volume recording. B. When arterial reconstruction is completed, a flat or severely attenuated pulse volume recording (<5 mm) indicates an obstructive problem. Usual intraoperative problems are intimal flap, anastomotic stenosis, twisted or kinked graft, or distal thromboembolus. C. After the problem is corrected, pulse volume recording should return to a more normal-appearing tracing.

nal quality after carotid endarterectomy and renal reconstruction.

A. A triphasic or biphasic signal with a crisp upstroke is **normal.** Significant arterial obstruction is associated with a monophasic, dampened signal. These Doppler patterns are illustrated in Fig. 5-1.

B. Ankle blood pressures can be obtained by application of a routine blood pressure cuff at the ankle and auscultation of the dorsalis pedis or posterior tibial arteries with the Doppler unit.

C. The **primary advantages** of the Doppler system are its ability to provide an audible arterial signal and accurate distal limb blood pressures. In addition, most Doppler units are small, easily transported by one person, and relatively inexpensive. With limited training, most paramedical personnel can detect arterial signals and measure blood pressures with a Doppler unit. Some Doppler probes may be sterilized and used in the operative field to examine abdominal or extremity vessels.

D. Several **disadvantages** of the Doppler system for perioperative vascular monitoring must also be emphasized. Unless the Doppler unit is attached to some type of strip recorder, no permanent paper copy of the signal is recorded. Also, some experience is necessary for interpretation of the biphasic, triphasic, and monophasic quality of Doppler arterial signals. This experience is especially critical in examination of severely ischemic limbs in which monophasic arterial signals may be confused with low-intensity venous sounds. Finally, Doppler arterial signals and ankle blood pressures may be depressed in the immediate operative and postoperative period, when the patient is often cold and vasoconstricted.

E. The combination of B-mode ultrasound imaging and continuous-wave or pulsed Doppler flow velocity analysis **(duplex scanning)** can be used for intraoperative assessment of carotid endarterectomy, infrainguinal bypass grafts, and renal and visceral artery reconstructions. Our experience with intraoperative duplex ultrasound after carotid endarterectomy and renal revascularizations has enhanced detection and correction of technical problems. These technical defects can generally be corrected immediately and thus the risk of early postoperative arterial thrombosis at the operative site can be reduced. We have detected significant defects after 5% of carotid endarterectomies and after 10% of renal reconstructions. When major defects (>50% luminal compromise on gray-scale image and >three times normal peak systolic velocity) were corrected, the postoperative outcome was uncomplicated. Failure to correct major defects resulted in a 50% occlusion rate at the operative site in the early postoperative period.

III. **Electroencephalogram (EEG).** The EEG probably represents one of the most sensitive detectors of cerebral ischemia during carotid artery clamping for endarterectomy. Excellent correlation has been established between ischemic EEG changes and reduction of regional cerebral blood flow (rCBF) to a critical level of 17–18 ml/100 g/minute. In patients under general anesthesia, severe EEG ischemic changes have been associated with postoperative neurologic deficit.

Despite evidence of its reliability for cerebrovascular monitoring, the continuous EEG has not gained widespread use during carotid endarterectomy, and some authors have recently questioned its net benefit. It probably is not necessary if routine intraluminal shunting is used, although it can detect shunt malfunction. For surgeons who shunt selectively, internal carotid stump pressures have been a common technique to assess adequate cerebral collateral flow during carotid clamping (stump pressure >50 mm Hg). In our experience, internal carotid stump pressures may not correlate with ischemic EEG changes. Consequently, we prefer EEG monitoring if selective shunting is used.

IV. **Ocular pneumoplethysmography (OPG).** The ocular pneumoplethysmograph is abnormal when a hemodynamically significant carotid stenosis or occlusion is present. After successful carotid endarterectomy, the OPG should revert to normal. Thus, the OPG may be used to ascertain carotid patency after endarterectomy. However, neither the OPG nor the Doppler system will detect intimal flaps or thromboemboli that may be related to postoperative neurologic deficits. These lesions may not cause significant stenosis or occlusion of internal carotid flow and so may be missed by an OPG. In most practices, duplex ultrasound has become the preferred method to check the endarterectomy site in the operating room or recovery area. For patients with profound, early neurologic deficit contralateral to the operated side, we return to the operating room for an examination of the endarterectomy site, ultrasound or arteriography, and any indicated surgical correction.

V. **Arteriography.** Intraoperative arteriography remains the primary method to check the distal anastomosis of a newly placed graft and visualize the distal runoff. A PVR, continuous-wave Doppler unit, or duplex ultrasound machine also can assess graft function. An arteriogram is essential when the noninvasive tests suggest inadequate distal flow or any disturbance in flow along the graft or at the distal anastomosis. For example, an operative arteriogram may be necessary to better define lower leg and foot runoff when a distal femorotibial bypass is undertaken and preoperative arteriograms have not clearly shown the distal anatomy. Likewise, a retrograde arteriogram may be useful to ensure that thrombectomy of an occluded aortofemoral limb is complete.

If operative arteriography is anticipated, the following guidelines may ensure an adequate study.

A. An x-ray technician should be notified at least 20–30 minutes before the need for the arteriogram.

B. Any electric coil heating pads or blankets, metal instruments, retractors, or sponges with radiopaque markers should be removed from the arteriogram field as they may obstruct the detail of the angiogram.

C. The graft **proximal to the angiogram injection site** should be clamped temporarily while the contrast material is being injected. This clamping prevents the inflow of blood that may dilute the contrast material and diminish the quality of the arteriogram.

D. Usually 20–50 ml of full-strength contrast is administered: one-half of the volume over 5 seconds and one-half of the volume over the next 10 seconds, with x-ray exposure as the final milliliter is injected.

E. The needle or catheter that was used for contrast injection should then be flushed with heparinized saline while the proximal occluding clamp is removed.

F. During each exposure, a surgeon standing 1 ft from the x-ray tube receives an absorbed dose equivalent to

0.24–1.40 mrem, which is about one-half an operative cholangiogram. With a maximum yearly permissible dose of 5,000 mrem, one could safely perform 3,500 operative arteriograms per year! Fluoroscopy, however, increases radiation exposure more than four times that of nonfluoroscopic x-rays.

VI. **Electromagnetic and ultrasonic transit flowmeters.** Blood flow through arteries and grafts can be measured by an electromagnetic flow probe. Various sizes are available to fit different diameters of vessels and grafts. Common sources of error include inaccuracies due to distortion of the velocity profile by vessel bifurcations or angulations, poor probe fit, interference from adjacent metal instruments, and lack of calibration. Ultrasonic transit time flowmeters may even be more reliable and easy to use than electromagnetic flowmeters.

Selection of Monitoring

Table 9-1 outlines the purpose, data, and techniques of appropriate vascular monitoring in the preoperative, intraoperative, and early postoperative periods.

I. **Carotid endarterectomy.** The preoperative assessment of the patient who undergoes carotid surgery must begin with a complete baseline neurologic examination. All patients have a baseline preoperative carotid duplex ultrasound and/or OPG. During operation, continuous EEG monitoring is used. If carotid clamping causes severe focal ischemic EEG changes, an intraluminal shunt is inserted immediately. When the carotid endarterectomy is completed and blood flow is restored, a continuous-wave or pulsed Doppler with or without an ultrasound image can be used to assess flow velocity and any residual obstructing lesions. Although we do not routinely perform operative arteriograms, other surgeons advocate them. About 5% of endarterectomy sites need immediate revision for stenosis, occlusion, or intimal flap. However, neither duplex imaging nor angiography detect all abnormalities. The best method to ensure a good result remains a careful endarterectomy with adequate direct visualization of the internal carotid artery endpoint of the plaque.

In the early postoperative period, the neurologic examination remains the best single indicator of success. If a focal neurologic deficit complicates the operation, immediate duplex ultrasound or intraoperative arteriography are the best methods to ensure that a technical mishap has not occurred. If the postoperative neurologic deficit is not focal and one wants to ascertain whether the endarterectomy site is patent and not severely narrowed, an OPG or duplex scan is a reasonable emergent test to detect carotid occlusion.

II. **Aortic grafting.** Preoperative baseline data should include complete pulse examination. Doppler signal analysis and ankle pressures or PVRs are also useful, especially when pulses are already decreased or absent. These data should be rechecked in the operating room before beginning the proce-

Table 9-1. Techniques of perioperative vascular monitoring

Time	Purpose	Data	Technique
Preoperative monitoring	Establish baseline data	1. Appearance of patient 2. Pulses 3. Quality of arterial signal 4. Limb pressures 5. PVR tracing 6. Hemodynamic significance of carotid lesion	1, 2. Physical examination 3, 4. Doppler ultrasound 5. Plethysmograph (PVR) 6. Ocular pneumoplethysmograph, duplex scanning
Intraoperative monitoring	Ensure successful reconstruction Detect any vascular accidents	1. PVR tracings 2. Quality of arterial signal 3. Pulses, appearance 4. Adequate cerebral perfusion 5. Anatomy 6. Flow	1. PVR 2. Doppler ultrasound (duplex scan) 3. Physical examination 4. EEG 5. Arteriogram, duplex scan 6. Electromagnetic flowmeter
Postoperative (recovery room) monitoring	Recognize early failures	1. Appearance 2. Pulses 3. PVR tracings 4. Quality of arterial signal 5. Limb pressures (ankle) 6. Carotid patency	1, 2. Physical examination 3. PVR 4, 5. Doppler ultrasound 6. Ocular pneumoplethysmograph, duplex scan

PVR = pulse volume recorder; EEG = electroencephalogram.

dure. When the aortic graft is open, pulses, PVR tracings, or Doppler signals should be rechecked. We also use an electromagnetic flowmeter to measure graft flow, which normally ranges from 500 ml/minute to over 1,000 ml/minute. Flows less than 250 ml/minute combined with diminished calf PVRs (<5 mm) and monophasic or absent ankle Doppler signals usually suggest a problem with the reconstruction, uncorrected distal disease, or a distal thromboembolus. If easily palpable pedal pulses are present, their palpation is adequate for continued postoperative monitoring. If pedal pulses are not palpable because of uncorrected femoropopliteal disease, ankle or calf PVRs or Doppler ankle pressures will be necessary to ensure adequate arterial perfusion. A recently developed impedance pulse monitor (IPM, Electrodiagnostics, Burbank, CA) can also be used for continuous postoperative monitoring of lower-limb perfusion. The impedance wave

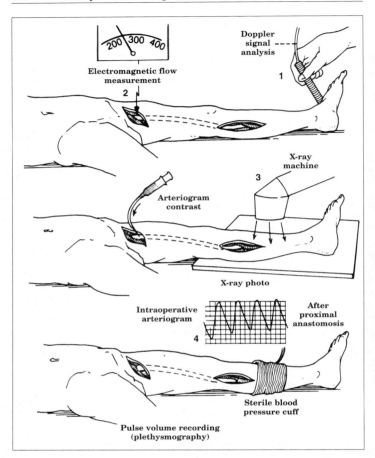

Fig. 9-2. Methods of intraoperative assessment of femorodistal bypass. Doppler signal analysis (1) with a sterile probe is the simplest method after pulse check to ensure distal flow. Electromagnetic flow measurement (2) is useful for vein grafts but cannot be done over polytetrafluoroethylene (PTFE) synthetic conduits since PTFE is an electrical insulator. An operative arteriogram (3) is the "gold standard" way to check the anatomy of the distal anastomosis and runoff. Finally, we use a sterile blood pressure cuff to check a distal pulse volume recording (4).

form can be displayed on the same bedside monitor as the electrocardiogram (ECG) and blood pressure.

III. **Lower- and upper-extremity revascularization.** Revascularization of upper and lower extremities includes bypass grafting and thromboembolectomies. In general, distal pulses are not palpable before operation. Therefore, ankle PVRs or Doppler signal analysis and distal extremity (e.g., ankle) pressures are needed as baseline measurements. Figure 9-2 demonstrates the intraoperative value of the PVR in construction of femoropopliteal bypasses. During operation, the success of revascularization may be judged by return of palpable pulses, an improved PVR tracing, or a better Doppler signal. Doppler pressures are generally 20–30 mm lower than they will be once the patient rewarms and vasoconstriction resolves. With in situ saphenous vein bypass grafts of the lower limb, we generally measure flow rates proximally and distally with an electromagnetic flowmeter. A high proximal flow rate (200–300 ml/minute) with a lower distal vein flow rate (e.g., 80 ml/minute) suggests an intervening arteriovenous fistula via a side branch that needs ligation. Generally, femoropopliteal grafts have a flow rate of at least 100–150 ml/minute, while femorodistal grafts may remain patent with flow rates less than 100 ml/minute. Because polytetrafluoroethylene (PTFE) is an electrical insulator, flow rates cannot be measured over PTFE grafts by an electromagnetic flowmeter. Duplex ultrasound is another alternative monitoring method for femoropopliteal and tibial bypasses.

IV. **Renal and visceral reconstructions.** Adequate flow through renal and visceral revascularization can be assessed by continuous-wave Doppler, an electromagnetic flowmeter, or duplex scanner. A sterile continuous-wave Doppler probe is a simple and accurate method to ascertain the presence of flow and quality of the arterial signal. In addition, we generally measure flow, which is usually 150–350 ml/minute for renal arteries and 350–1,000 ml/minute for visceral vessels such as the celiac or superior mesenteric arteries. Duplex ultrasound has also become an accurate method to assess renal and visceral reconstructions.

Selected Reading

Bandyk DF. Monitoring During and After Distal Arterial Reconstruction. In EF Bernstein (ed), *Vascular Diagnosis* (4th ed). St. Louis: Mosby, 1993.

Brewster DC, O'Hara PJ, Darling RC, Hallett JW Jr. Relationship of intraoperative EEG monitoring and stump pressure measurements during carotid endarterectomy. *Circulation* 62(Suppl I):1, 1980.

Courbier R et al. Routine intraoperative carotid angiography: Its impact on operative morbidity and carotid restenosis. *J Vasc Surg* 3:343, 1986.

Dilley RB, Bernstein EF. A comparison of B-mode real-time imaging and arteriography in the intraoperative assessment of carotid endarterectomy. *J Vasc Surg* 4:457, 1986.

Dougherty MJ et al. Optimizing technical success of renal revascularization: The impact of intraoperative color-flow duplex ultrasonography. *J Vasc Surg* 17:849, 1993.

Gee W, Lucke JF, Madden AE. Reappraisal of ocular pneumoplethysmography after carotid endarterectomy. *J Vasc Surg* 4:517, 1986.

Healy DA, Zierler RE. Intraoperative Assessment of Carotid Endarterectomy and Recurrent Carotid Stenosis. In FJ Veith,

RW Hobson, RA Williams, SE Wilson (eds), *Vascular Surgery* (2nd ed). New York: McGraw-Hill, 1994. Pp. 699–710.

Miller A et al. Comparison of angioscopy and angiography for monitoring infrainguinal bypass grafts: Results of a prospective randomized trial. *J Vasc Surg* 17:382, 1993.

O'Hara PJ, Brewster DC, Darling RC, Hallett JW Jr. The value of intraoperative monitoring using the pulse volume recorder during peripheral vascular reconstructive operations. *Surg Gynecol Obstet* 152:275, 1981.

Ramalanjaona GR, Pearce WH, Ritenour ER. Radiation exposure risk to the surgeon during operative angiography. *J Vasc Surg* 4:224, 1986.

Sundt TM Jr et al. Correlation of cerebral blood flow and electroencephalographic changes during carotid endarterectomy. *Mayo Clin Proc* 56:533, 1981.

Early Postoperative Care

Most life-threatening complications of major vascular surgery occur in the early postoperative period (24–48 hours). Fortunately, early recognition and treatment can resolve most of these problems. In this chapter we focus on methods of recognizing these problems and discuss principles of treatment that have been most successful in our experience. The management of specific complications of each type of operation is outlined in other chapters.

I. **Equipment.** The intensive care unit or recovery room for vascular patients should be equipped with volume ventilators and monitors for continuous heart rhythm, arterial blood pressure and gases, central venous pressure (CVP), and pulmonary artery pressure. The unit also should have facilities for rapid determination of arterial blood gases and pH, hemoglobin and hematocrit, serum sodium, serum potassium, and blood sugar. An urgent coagulation profile should be available for patients with bleeding problems. Other chemical parameters, such as liver and renal function tests, usually can be done by the routine laboratory.

II. **Respiratory support.** Respiratory support by a volume ventilator is often necessary for several hours after many major vascular operations, especially after prolonged abdominal procedures. In nonbreathing patients, controlled mechanical ventilation provides a preset tidal volume at a controlled respiratory frequency. For the patient with respiratory drive but inadequate blood gases or ventilatory mechanics for extubation (Table 10-1), an assist-control technique allows spontaneous breathing supplemented by assisted ventilations to prevent hypoventilation and respiratory acidosis. The best method of assist-control appears to be intermittent mandatory ventilation (IMV). With IMV, the ventilator delivers a preset gas volume at selected intervals—for example, 6–8 breaths per minute. Between these mandatory ventilations, the patient breathes spontaneously. The IMV rate can be progressively decreased to 1–2 breaths per minute as the patient improves his or her own respiratory mechanics. When the criteria for extubation outlined in Table 10-1 are met, the patient is extubated.

Some patients with reduced functional residual capacity and increased airway closure will require continuous positive airway pressure (CPAP) or positive end-expiratory pressure (PEEP) in conjunction with assisted ventilation. Although PEEP can maintain better alveolar expansion and, consequently, better arterial oxygenation, high pressures (>15 cm H_2O) can decrease cardiac output. The mechanism of this reduced cardiac output is complex but involves increased intrathoracic pressure, decreased venous return, leftward displacement of the interventricular septum, and restricted left ventricular filling before ejection.

When the patient is extubated and breathing without assistance, pulmonary complications are preventable by fair-

Table 10-1. Guidelines for ventilatory support in adults

Ventilatory parameters	Normal range	Tracheal intubation and ventilation indicated
Mechanics		
Respiratory rate/min	12–20/min	>35/min
Vital capacity (ml/kg body weight[a])	65–75	<15
FEV_1 (ml/kg body weight[a])	50–60	<10
Inspiratory force (cm water)	75–100	<25
Oxygenation		
PaO_2 (mm Hg)	75–100 mm Hg (room air)	<70 mm Hg (on mask O_2)
$P[(A-a)O_2]1.0$[b]	25–65	>450
Ventilation		
$PaCO_2$ (mm Hg)[c]	35–45 mm Hg	>55 mm Hg
Vd/Vt	0.25–0.40	>0.60

[a]Ideal weight is used if weight appears grossly abnormal.
[b]After 10 minutes of 100% oxygen.
[c]Except in patients with chronic hypercapnia.
Note: The trend of values is of utmost importance. The numerical guidelines obviously should not be adopted to the exclusion of clinical judgment. For example, a vital capacity below 15 ml/kg may be sufficient if the patient can cough "effectively," if hypoxia is prevented, and if hypercapnia is not progressive. However, such a patient needs frequent blood gas analyses and must be closely observed in a well-equipped, adequately staffed recovery room or intensive care unit.
Source: Modified from H Pontoppidan, B Geffin, E Lowenstein. Acute respiratory failure in the adult. *N Engl J Med* 287:743, 1972.

ly simple methods. Frequent deep breathing and coughing remain the best means of preventing atelectasis. A variety of incentive spirometers are available to assist the patient. Elevating the patient's head and chest 30–45 degrees in bed increases functional residual capacity. Administration of inhaled bronchodilators or mucolytic agents can assist patients with chronic obstructive lung disease. Chest percussions and postural drainage are helpful for patients with copious or thick pulmonary secretions but need not be routine for all patients. Occasionally, endotracheal stimulation and suctioning will be necessary to help the patient with deep breathing and secretion clearance. We caution that this endotracheal suctioning should be done after the patient is adequately oxygenated, and the pulse should be monitored since arrhythmias can occur. Of course, ambulation assists with deep breathing, but some vascular patients are not hemodynamically stable for several days and so require bed rest.

III. **Cardiac problems.** Since the majority of peripheral vascular patients also have coronary artery disease or chronic hypertension, postoperative cardiac problems are common.

  A. **Hypertension** is one of the most common early postoperative problems. The causes may be multiple: increased sympathetic tone, incisional pain, or elevated renin-angiotensin activity. The danger of severe hypertension is excessive cardiac work (cardiac work = stroke volume × heart rate × systolic blood pressure). Myocardial ischemia, cardiac failure, or stroke may occur if severe hypertension is not controlled promptly.

For practical purposes, we suggest maintaining the patient's systolic blood pressure at ±15% of its preoperative level. Systolic blood pressure readings from a radial arterial monitor tend to be higher than the true auscultated values. Before administering antihypertensives, a brachial blood pressure measurement taken with a sphygmomanometer and stethoscope should be compared to elevated monitor readings.

1. **Pain control** with a small intravenous dose of a narcotic (e.g., morphine, 2–5 mg) may alleviate moderate hypertension. If continuous epidural analgesia is used, the catheter position, patency, and dosage should be checked to ascertain that adequate narcotic is being delivered.

2. Otherwise, intravenous **sodium nitroprusside** (Nipride), a potent direct vasodilator, lowers blood pressure immediately and has a short duration of action (1–10 minutes). Initially, we mix 50 mg nitroprusside in 250 ml of 5% dextrose in water (D/W) (200 µg/ml) and begin administration at 0.5–1.0 µg/kg/minute, increasing to a maximum of 10 µg/kg/minute. Table 10-2 shows doses at various microdrops per minute. **Nitroprusside should be administered in an intensive care setting, where blood pressure can be monitored continuously.** The administration should be controlled by an infusion pump. In addition, care must be taken not to flush the IV line containing nitroprusside, since such a bolus can drop the blood pressure to extremely low levels instantaneously. If this mishap does occur, the nitroprusside infusion should be stopped, the patient's legs should be elevated, and phenylephrine (Neo-Synephrine), 1 mg intravenously (1 ml of a 10-mg vial in 9 ml saline) should be administered. Since nitroprusside is metabolized to thiocyanate in the liver before renal excretion, it must be used with caution in patients with hepatic or renal insufficiency. Prolonged infusion (3–4 days) or high doses (>10 µg/kg/minute) can lead to cyanide intoxication. We normally begin other antihypertensives if nitroprusside is needed for more than 6–12 hours. Other choices for immediate control of hypertension and tachycardia are esmolol or a calcium channel blocker (nifedipine).

3. Occasionally severe hypertension occurs during transport to the recovery room. If a nitroprusside infusion is not immediately available, **labetalol** can be given intravenously over a 2-minute period in doses of **20 mg** (or up to 40–80 mg for subsequent injections) and repeated at 10- to 15-minute intervals to a maximum dose of 320 mg. Labetalol possesses alpha$_1$-, beta$_1$-, and beta$_2$-blocking activity. Consequently, it should be used

Table 10-2. Infusion rates of commonly used cardiovascular drugs

	Nitroprusside: 50 mg in 250 ml 5% D/W (µg/kg/min)	Dopamine: 200 mg in 250 ml 5% D/W (µg/kg/min)	Lidocaine: 1 g in 250 ml 5% D/W (mg/min)	Nitroglycerin: 50 mg in 250 ml 5% D/W (µg/min)	Dobutamine: 250 mg in 250 ml 5% D/W (µg/min)	Esmolol: 2.5 g in 250 ml 5% D/W (10 mg/ml)	Diltiazem: 250 mg in 250 ml 5% D/W
Usual starting dose	0.5–1.0 µg/kg/min	1–2 µg/kg/min	50–100 mg IV bolus followed by 1 mg/min	5–50 µg/min*	2.5–10.0 µg/kg/min	0.5 mg/kg/min over 1 min	0.25 mg/kg; if no effect, repeat in 15 min at 0.35 mg/kg
Maintenance	2.0–4.0 µg/kg/min	2–3 µg/kg/min		50–200 µg/min	5–15 µg/kg/min	0.05–0.20 mg/kg/min	5–10 mg/hr
Maximum dose	10 µg/kg/min	50 µg/kg/min	1–4 mg/min	500 µg/min*	20 µg/kg/min	0.20 mg/kg/min	15 mg/hr

*Note that the starting and maximum doses for nitroglycerin are µg/min and not µg/kg/min.

Note: If the patient is on multiple drips, consider normal saline as diluent to prevent free water excess and hyponatremia.

cautiously in the setting of congestive heart failure because of its $beta_1$-antagonism and carefully in the setting of bronchospasm because of its $beta_2$-antagonism.

4. A variety of **chronic antihypertensives** are available, and the selection of certain agents in the early postoperative period will depend on the individual patient. If the patient has been on specific antihypertensives, they generally can be resumed orally, even if the patient has not resumed feedings. In patients who are fluid overloaded, a diuretic (e.g., furosemide, 20 mg qid or bid) may help reduce high blood pressure. A variety of beta blockers, calcium channel blockers, and angiotensin-converting enzyme inhibitors can be used as oral intake resumes (see Appendix of drugs commonly used in adults).

B. **Tachycardia** is another common early postoperative cardiac problem and adds to cardiac work, especially if the patient also is hypertensive. An analgesic may help if the patient is having pain. Hypovolemia often is the cause of tachycardia. Decreasing urine output, falling blood pressure with deep inspiration, and low heart filling pressures are good indicators that more fluids are needed. When intravascular volume appears adequate, persistent tachycardia may be caused by cardiac failure or increased sympathetic tone. An elevated pulmonary capillary wedge pressure (PCWP) (>18 mm Hg) suggests left ventricular failure. Digoxin usually is the drug of choice for heart failure and tachycardia. If cardiac failure is not evident, a beta blocker can control heart rate effectively. Careful intravenous administration of small doses of propranolol (0.1–1.0 mg) under continuous electrocardiogram (ECG) and blood pressure monitoring can rapidly slow the heart rate. These small doses can be repeated. Generally, only a few (a total of 1–3 mg) doses are necessary, and the patient can be started on an oral beta blocker. Recently continuous intravenous infusions of esmolol have been used effectively. In patients with chronic obstructive airway disease, nonselective beta blockers may cause bronchospasm. If an oral beta blocker is needed, metoprolol (Lopressor, 50 mg PO bid) may cause less bronchospasm than propranolol because it is a cardioselective beta-adrenergic agent. Since the beta blockade may mask the sympathetic signs (e.g., tachycardia) of hypoglycemia, propranolol must be administered carefully in insulin-dependent diabetics.

C. **Low cardiac output (CO)** with hypotension in the early postoperative period of major vascular surgery generally results from hypovolemia. Pump failure or cardiogenic shock is the other main cause of low CO and is more likely if the patient has severe chronic heart failure or has sustained an intraoperative myocardial infarction. Sometimes both etiologies are present. Arrhythmias also may lower cardiac output. Septic shock usually is not an early postoperative problem but must be considered if the later postoperative course is complicated by infection,

**Table 10-3. Low cardiac output states
in the immediate postoperative period**

Etiology	Recognition	Treatment
Hypovolemia	Low CVP (0–5 cm saline) Low PCWP (<8–10 mm Hg) Falling blood pressure with each deep inspiration	Volume replacement: Balanced salt solution (Ringer's lactate bolus, 5–10 ml/kg body weight) Packed red blood cell transfusion for hematocrit <25, Hb <8g
Heart pump failure	High CVP (>15 cm saline)\High PCWP (>18 mm Hg) Low cardiac index (<2.2 liters/m^2)	Afterload reduction: Nitroprusside 0.5–5.0 µg/kg/min Nitroglycerin 1.0–5.0 µg/kg/min Inotropic support: Dobutamine 2.5–15.0 µg/kg/min Dopamine 2.0–10.0 µg/kg/min
Arrhythmia	12-lead ECG Continuous ECG monitoring	See Table 10-4

CVP = central venous pressure; PCWP = pulmonary capillary wedge pressure;
ECG = electrocardiogram; Hb = hemoglobin.

fever, and hypotension. Table 10-3 summarizes low CO
states in the early postoperative period.

1. The recognition and treatment of low perfusion states
   are facilitated by the application of the **basic mechanisms of CO and blood pressure control**. CO is the
   product of heart rate (HR) and stroke volume (SV):

   $$CO = HR \times SV$$

   The main determinants of SV are preload, afterload,
   and myocardial contractility:

   $$SV = preload \times contractility/afterload$$

   Preload may be described by the end-diastolic filling pressures on the right and left hearts. SV is directly related to preload and is described by the Frank-
   Starling mechanism (Fig. 10-1). **Afterload** represents
   the resistance against which the left ventricle contracts. It is the force resisting fiber contraction and is
   inversely related to SV.

   Contractility describes factors such as beta-adrenergic agonists and antagonists that modify the force of
   contraction independent of preload and afterload.

   Systemic blood pressure (BP) depends directly
   on CO and peripheral vascular resistance (PR):

   $$BP = CO \times PR$$

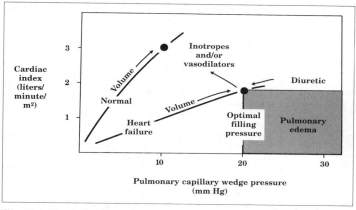

Fig. 10-1. Frank-Starling left ventricular function curve relating ventricular filling pressure (pulmonary capillary wedge pressure) to stroke volume (cardiac index). In patients with heart failure and pulmonary edema, cardiac performance can be improved by a combination of inotropes (e.g., dobutamine), vasodilators (e.g., nitroprusside), and diuretics (e.g., furosemide). (Adapted from PL Marino. *The ICU Book*. Philadelphia: Lea & Febiger, 1991.)

Although regulation of CO, blood pressure, and local tissue perfusion is a complex physiologic process, clinical recognition and treatment of low-output states can be achieved by application of these simple relationships.

2. **Recognition** of a low-perfusion state usually is made when blood pressure, urine output, or both drop. In stressful situations, heart rate may already be elevated and thus may not change. If fluid resuscitation (5–10 ml/kg bolus) does not improve perfusion, more intensive monitoring should be considered if it is not already in place. A low CVP (0–5 cm saline) suggests hypovolemia but is not reliable in assessing left ventricular function or CO. A Swan-Ganz thermistor-tipped pulmonary artery catheter allows measurement of central venous and pulmonary arterial wedge pressures (preload) and CO by thermodilation. Afterload of the left ventricle is the peripheral arterial resistance.

3. Knowledge of the PCWP and cardiac index allows categorization of patients into subsets that respond to different modes of **treatment**. Vascular congestion begins when PCWP exceeds 18–20 mm Hg. Pulmonary edema occurs when PCWP rises above 30 mm Hg. The normal cardiac index is 2.7–4.3 liters/m². Clinical hypoperfusion becomes evident when the cardiac index drops to the 1.8–2.2 liters/m² range. Below 1.8 liters/m², cardiogenic shock becomes a problem.

a. **Low filling pressures** (PCWP, CVP) are the hallmark of hypovolemia. If blood pressure and urine output are low (<90 mm Hg and <0.5 ml/kg/hour, respectively), CO usually can be optimized by fluid administration to bring PCWP to the 10–12 mm Hg level. If hemoglobin is less than 8–9 g or hematocrit is less than 25–30, we administer 1–2 units of packed red cells. Otherwise, an intravenous bolus of 5–10 ml/kg of a crystalloid solution (Ringer's lactated solution or normal saline) is given. Colloid solutions generally are not necessary unless serum albumin and protein are excessively low, as in chronic liver disease. Not uncommonly, patients after aortic surgery are both hypovolemic and hypertensive. As volume is repleted, nitroprusside can be used to control hypertension and vasodilate the patient, who is often cold and vasoconstricted. After hypovolemia is corrected, persistent tachycardia can be treated with a beta blocker or a calcium channel blocker. It must be remembered that intubated patients on PEEP may have decreased venous return and ventricular filling. PEEP, which increases intrathoracic pressure, may falsely elevate central venous and pulmonary artery pressures. These falsely elevated filling pressures may lead the clinician to conclude that hypovolemia is not a problem. In fact, CO may not increase until PEEP levels are lowered and more volume is infused.

b. Elevated left ventricular filling pressures and low CO suggest impaired heart contractility. Such patients usually have a PCWP in excess of 18 mm Hg—generally in the 25–30 mm Hg range. Their peripheral vascular resistance is usually high (>1,500–1,800 dynes/second/cm^{-5}). If an oximetric Swan-Ganz catheter is in place, a decreasing mixed venous oxygen saturation (SvO_2) (<60%) is another indication of low CO. Likewise, an arterial-mixed venous saturation difference greater than 30% indicates that tissue oxygen delivery is inadequate. These patients need both afterload reduction and inotropic support.

(1) Afterload reduction can be accomplished by vasodilation with intravenous infusion of nitroprusside or nitroglycerin. Sodium nitroprusside relaxes vascular smooth muscle in both the arterial and venous systems. When ventricular function is severely impaired, the cardiac response to reduced arterial impedance and venous pooling is a rise in CO. The dose required for a therapeutic response varies from 15–400 μg/minute (average about 50 μg/minute). Nitroglycerin acts primarily on the venous system. The net effect is a sharp fall in heart filling pressures and pulmonary artery pressures. In severe heart failure, CO is augmented. Afterload reduction can be maintained in the remaining postoperative period with other nonparenteral vasodilators: nitrates, hydralazine, prazosin, minoxidil, and captopril.

(2) Although several **inotropic drugs** are available to enhance myocardial contractility, the most useful agents are dobutamine (Dobutrex), dopamine (Intropin), and digitalis (digoxin).

Dobutamine, a beta-adrenergic agonist, is the inotropic agent of choice in acute cardiac failure, especially when the etiology is an ischemic injury. Dobutamine acts rapidly, with an inotropic effect similar to that of isoproterenol. However, CO is enhanced without appreciable change in heart rate, blood pressure, arrhythmias, or infarct size if one already has occurred. In addition to increasing contractility, dobutamine decreases preload and afterload. The **starting dose** is 2.5 µg/kg/minute, which can be increased to 10–15 µg/kg/minute.

When low CO is complicated by severe hypotension and oliguria, **dopamine**, another catecholamine, may be preferable to dobutamine. Dopamine not only enhances cardiac contractility but also causes renal and mesenteric vasodilatation at low doses (0.5–2.0 µg/kg/minute). We have found low-dose dopamine especially helpful when urine output is low despite apparent adequate intravascular volume. Higher doses (>10 µg/kg/minute) elevate peripheral resistance and heart rate. If inotropic support appears necessary beyond the immediate postoperative period, **digoxin** should be started, since long-term digitalis therapy appears to improve left ventricular function in heart failure.

c. **Low CO secondary to bradycardia** may require cardiac pacing, since atropine may worsen the risk of arrhythmia.

d. **Arrhythmias** are another cardiac problem encountered in the perioperative period. A few general comments about arrhythmias in vascular patients should provide a basis for their initial management (Table 10-4).

(1) The primary physiologic consequence of an atrial or ventricular arrhythmia is **diminished CO**. Cerebral, mesenteric, and renal blood flows are decreased. The perfusion of these organs may already be chronically reduced by atherosclerotic stenoses. More important, coronary perfusion may fall. Unlike cardiac patients who have undergone coronary artery bypass, peripheral vascular patients often have coronary artery disease that has **not** been corrected. Uncontrolled arrhythmias may result in severe myocardial ischemia and infarction.

(2) Every effort must be made to determine the **etiology** of the arrhythmias. Common causes of

Table 10-4. Emergency treatment of common postoperative arrhythmias

Arrhythmia	Treatment of choice	Dose	Alternatives
Ventricular fibrillation	Cardioversion	200–360 J	Plus cardiopulmonary resuscitation or lidocaine
Ventricular tachycardia	Cardioversion	200–360 J	Lidocaine Procainamide Bretylium 5 mg/kg IV
Premature ventricular contractions	Lidocaine	50–100 mg bolus; repeat in 10 min; 200 mg total	Procainamide 20–30 mg/min; maximum 17 mg/kg
Supraventricular tachycardia	Carotid massage Adenosine	6 mg IV bolus; repeat with 12 mg q1–2 min × 2	Digoxin Propranolol Diltiazem
	If narrow complex: Verapamil If wide complex: Lidocaine Procainamide	5–10 mg IV over 2–3 min 1.0–1.5 mg/kg IV bolus 20–30 mg/min; maximum 17 mg/kg	
Atrial fibrillation	Diltiazem Digoxin	0.25 mg/kg, 5–10 mg/hr 0.5 mg IV 0.125–0.250 mg IV q4–6h to loading dose of 0.5–1.0 mg	Cardioversion Procainamide Anticoagulants
Digitalis-induced tachyarrhythmia	Dilantin Potassium	50 mg IV q5min to 250 mg 10–20 mEq/hr via central line to keep serum potassium at >4.0 mEq/liter	

arrhythmias in the early postoperative setting are hypoxia, hypothermia (<33°C), hypo- or hyperkalemia, acid-base imbalance, and operative cardiac infarction. Each of these etiologies can be explored easily by checking body temperature, arterial blood gases, serum electrolytes, and cardiac isoenzymes, in addition to use of a 12-lead ECG. These tests should be routine on the patient's arrival in the recovery room.

(3) Table 10-4 outlines general principles of emergency arrhythmia treatment.

(a) **Tachycardia**, especially when accompanied by hypertension, requires increased cardiac oxygen consumption, which is poorly tolerated when coronary artery disease is present. Therefore, we strive to keep heart rate below 100 beats/minute.

(b) **Bradycardia** is not as common as tachyarrhythmias in our experience. Heart rates of less than 50 beats/minute also may decrease CO and coronary perfusion. If atropine (0.5–1.0 mg IV) does not speed the rate and if hypotension becomes a problem after adequate volume replacement, cardiac pacing may be necessary.

(c) **Premature ventricular contractions (PVCs)** are a fairly common early postoperative arrhythmia, especially if the patient is cold and acidotic. We treat PVCs when they are multifocal, occur at a rate of more than six per minute, or are associated with runs of ventricular tachycardia or bigeminy. A bolus of lidocaine (50–100 mg IV) will settle many patients. Persistent PVCs may require a continuous lidocaine infusion (1–4 mg/minute) until chronic antiarrhythmics are started.

IV. **Bleeding**. During an operation or in the early recovery period, the most common causes of persistent bleeding are (1) failure of mechanical hemostasis, (2) anticoagulants, (3) dilutional thrombocytopenia, (4) consumptive or disseminated intravascular coagulation, and (5) defects in clotting factors. Table 10-5 lists common laboratory tests to check various steps in the hemostatic scheme. The clinical situation and the results of these tests usually will identify the cause of bleeding. Correction of the bleeding problem may then be accomplished by specific therapy.

A. **Failure of mechanical hemostasis** should be recognized before the wounds are closed. Wound hematomas that appear in the first 6 hours after operation usually are the result of unligated blood vessels. We recommend early evacuation of large wound hematomas and control of the bleeding site by sterile operative technique. Undrained hematomas increase the risk of infection, which can be disastrous if an adjacent graft becomes involved. After intraabdominal vascular surgery, significant internal

Table 10-5. Evaluation of the clotting and fibrinolytic system

Test	Purpose of test	Normal finding	What abnormal test may indicate
Bleeding time (Ivy method)	Measures time to compaction of platelet plug	8 min (2–8 min)	Platelet count <75,000 Abnormally functioning platelets Defective capillaries von Willebrand's disease
Platelet count	Measures number (not function) of platelets	160,000–350,000/mm^3 (50,000 considered adequate for surgical hemostasis if platelet function is normal)	Dilutional thrombocytopenia Consumption of platelets Defective platelet production Heparin-induced thrombocytopenia
Peripheral blood smear	Evaluates number and appearance of platelets	15–20 platelets/HPF of anticoagulated blood 3–4 platelet clumps/HPF of blood smear	Thrombocytopenia (decreased platelets/HPF) Thrombocytopenia (bizarre giant platelets) DIC (fragmented red blood cells)
Prothrombin time	Measures extrinsic pathway of clotting (factors VII, X, V, II) Usual test to monitor warfarin therapy Not affected by platelets	10–12 sec INR 1.0–1.3	Defective extrinsic pathway of clotting DIC Anticoagulation (warfarin)
Partial thromboplastin time	Measures intrinsic pathway of clotting (factors XII, XI, IX, VIII)	44 sec	Defective intrinsic pathway of clotting Congenital abnormalities of clotting (e.g., hemophilia disorders, von Willebrand's disease) Dilutional coagulopathy from blood transfusion DIC Anticoagulation (e.g., heparin)

Thrombin time	Evaluates presence of adequate fibrinogen	12 sec	Thrombolytic drugs Low fibrinogen levels Increased fibrin split products Anticoagulation (heparin) DIC
Fibrinogen assay	Directly measures fibrinogen levels	200–400 mg/100 ml	Thrombolytic drugs DIC
Fibrin split products	Measures fibrin split products (degradation of fibrin)	<1:40	Primary fibrinolysis (platelet count falls with DIC but not with primary fibrinolysis)

HPF = high-powered field; DIC = disseminated intravascular coagulation; INR = international normalized ratio.

hemorrhage should be suspected if more than 2 units of blood have to be given to maintain the hematocrit in the first 6–12 hours after operation.

B. **Anticoagulants** such as heparin or warfarin sodium (Coumadin) may cause oozing from wound edges. Such bleeding usually is not significant when mechanical hemostasis is adequate. Some surgeons prefer to routinely reverse the effect of intraoperative heparin with protamine sulfate given in a dose of 0.5–1.0 mg of protamine per 1 mg (100 units) of heparin. A partial thromboplastin time (PTT) or activated clotting time (ACT) may be checked to ensure reversal of the heparin effect. Fresh-frozen plasma (FFP) also may be used to counteract heparin or Coumadin. The usual dose of FFP is approximately 10 ml/kg of body weight. Rarely, it is necessary to administer intravenous vitamin K (25–50 mg) to help stop frank hemorrhage in a patient on Coumadin.

Oozing from wound edges also may be seen in patients on chronic antiplatelet therapy. The effect of antiplatelet drugs persists for 3–7 days after they are discontinued. Although platelet dysfunction may cause more wound ecchymosis, generally it is not necessary to administer fresh platelets. If intraoperative wound oozing is excessive, a dose of DDAVP (vasopressin or desmopressin acetate, 0.3 µg/kg IV in a single dose) may counteract the antiplatelet effect of aspirin.

C. **Dilutional thrombocytopenia** may present a problem after administration of more than 10 units of stored packed red blood cells. Dilutional thrombocytopenia can be associated with excessive use of autologous blood prepared in a high-speed centrifuge. These rapid autotransfusion machines return packed red blood cells **without** their accompanying platelets. Platelets should be available and administered when packed red blood cell transfusion exceeds 10 units. In general, a platelet count of greater than 50,000 will be adequate for hemostasis during operation. An appropriate starting dose usually is 6 units of platelet concentrate. After operation, spontaneous bleeding usually does not occur until the platelet count is less than 20,000.

D. **Disseminated intravascular coagulation (DIC)** or consumptive coagulopathy occurs in a variety of clinical settings associated with increased formation of tissue thromboplastin. The most common situations are (1) massive blood transfusions, (2) major transfusion reaction, (3) massive soft-tissue trauma or ischemia, and (4) sepsis. Thrombocytopenia and DIC also have been reported as an idiosyncratic reaction that some patients have to systemic heparin. **If heparin-induced thrombocytopenia is suspected (falling platelet count <70,000–80,000 after heparin), all heparin, including small amounts in arterial lines, must be stopped immediately.**

Basically, DIC involves consumption of platelets and coagulation factors (primarily VIII, V, and fibrinogen), increased fibrin split products that act as anticoagulants, and fibrin plugs that damage red blood cells. The **clinical criteria for DIC** include thrombocytopenia, prolonged prothrombin time, low fibrinogen levels, and microangiopathic blood smear. The main feature that differentiates DIC from primary fibrinolysis is the platelet count, which falls with DIC.

Despite past claims that heparin is the drug of choice for DIC, the primary treatment remains correction of the underlying clinical problem. Heparin should be reserved for situations in which efforts to correct the underlying cause or replacement therapy (FFP, platelets) have failed to correct overt hemorrhage.

E. **Defects in clotting factors** may be familial or acquired from liver disease. These coagulation problems usually are evident by history or by abnormal partial thromboplastin or prothrombin times. Specific blood component therapy generally is effective in managing these deficiencies during the perioperative period.

V. **Gastrointestinal stress ulceration and hemorrhage** may complicate major vascular operations. Typically, the most susceptible patients exhibit certain risk factors. The most common associated problems are sepsis, prolonged hypotension, extensive operative tissue trauma, severe respiratory insufficiency, renal failure, or advanced age. The ulcerations generally involve the body of the stomach but may affect the colon. Approximately 10% of patients with mucosal ulcerations have clinically recognized bleeding, usually 6–7 days after the onset of the stress. The bleeding usually is controllable by nonoperative methods and almost always resolves if the risk factor (e.g., sepsis) is eliminated. Surgical mortality for operative intervention to control stress hemorrhage exceeds 50%; clearly, the key to managing gastrointestinal stress bleeding is prevention.

Control of gastric pH is the primary component in stress ulcer prophylaxis. Maintenance of gastric pH above 4 has been associated with less stress bleeding. In severely ill patients, adequate prophylaxis requires hourly measurement of intragastric pH.

Prophylaxis with **antacids** (30–50 ml/hour) is more effective and less costly than with H_2-receptor antagonists such as cimetidine (300 mg IV q6h) or ranitidine (50 mg IV q6–8h). The main possible side effects of antacid therapy are diarrhea and metabolic alkalosis. H_2-receptor antagonists may be helpful in patients with a history of active peptic ulcer disease who must undergo a major vascular operation or for patients whose postoperative care is difficult because antacids are causing severe diarrhea or alkalosis. Sucralfate (Carafate) is another alternative agent for stress ulceration prophylaxis.

VI. **Renal failure** once was one of the main complications following major abdominal vascular surgery, especially following emergency aneurysm repair. Adequate intravascular hydration and mannitol administration before infrarenal aortic clamping have nearly eliminated such renal failure following elective aortic surgery. Postoperative renal failure also is more likely to occur in dehydrated patients with underlying chronic renal insufficiency, diabetes mellitus, or both. Their renal function may deteriorate after arteriography or surgery.

A. **Recognition of renal failure** is relatively simple. The hallmark is falling urine output (<15 ml/hour) and rising serum blood urea nitrogen and creatinine. However, other signs may suggest early renal insufficiency and allow intervention before serious renal deterioration occurs. In general, patients with adequate intravascular volume and CO produce 30–60 ml of urine per hour or 0.5 ml/kg body weight/hour. The normal kidney can concentrate urine as indicated by a urine-plasma osmolarity ratio of more than 1.3 and a urine-plasma creatinine ratio of more than 100. The normal kidney also retains sodium as indicated by a urine sodium of only 20–40 mEq/liter.

Early or imminent renal failure should be suspected when the following occur:

1. Urine output is below 15 ml/hour for longer than 2 hours in a patient with adequate intravascular volume (PCWP ≥12 mm Hg) and adequate CO (2.7–4.3 liters/m^2).

2. Polyuria (>60 ml/hour) occurs in an intravascularly volume-depleted patient (high-output renal failure).

3. Urine-plasma creatinine ratio is less than 10.

4. Rising urinary loss of sodium (urine-plasma sodium ratio approaching 0.9 [e.g., urine sodium 80–110 mEq/liter]).

5. Failure to concentrate urine (specific gravity ≤1.010 or urine-plasma osmolarity ratio <1.3 and usually near 1.0).

This functional assessment of the kidneys (Table 10-6) can be accomplished by a 1-hour urine collection of sodium, creatinine, and total osmolarity and a single serum specimen for the same measurements. When hypoperfusion (prerenal) occurs in an otherwise normal kidney, sodium is retained in an attempt to correct the volume deficit. Thus, urinary sodium is low (<20 mEq/liter). In contrast, the kidney affected by vasomotor nephropathy (acute tubular necrosis [ATN]) cannot effectively conserve sodium, and the urinary sodium concentration is high (>20 mEq/liter). Recently, a more refined measurement of **urinary fractional excretion of sodium** (FE_{Na}) has been used to categorize the probable cause of acute renal insufficiency. Renal hypoperfusion is indicated by a FE_{Na} of less than 1 while values of 2–3 are compatible with acute parenchymal damage (ATN). The FE_{Na} is variable and nondiagnostic when oliguria is caused by urinary tract obstruction. Patients with azotemia in the setting of liver disease (hepatorenal syndrome) will have urinary indices indistinguishable from volume depletion. In clinical situations where acute renal failure is suspected, this fairly quick renal function check may identify impending renal failure and allow prompt treatment that may avoid permanent renal insufficiency.

As soon as renal failure is apparent, the **etiology** must be determined if appropriate therapy is to be

**Table 10-6. Functional
assessment of perioperative renal function**

Type of renal failure	Urine osmolarity (mosm/kg)	Urine Na[a] (mEq/liter)	Urine creatinine/ plasma creatinine	FE_{Na}[b]
Renal hypo- perfusion (prerenal)	>Plasma	<20	≥100	<1
Vasomotor nephropathy (acute tub- ular necrosis)	Isomotic	>20	≤10	>2
Urinary obstruction (postrenal)	Isomotic	Variable		>2

[a]Urine sodium concentration measurement can be misleading if diuretics have been administered shortly before urine collection for analysis.
[b] FE_{Na}=urinary fraction excretion of sodium
$$FE_{Na} = \frac{\text{urinary sodium concentration}}{\text{plasma sodium concentration}} \div \frac{\text{urinary creatinine concentration}}{\text{plasma creatinine concentration}}$$
Source: JD Blachey, WL Henrich. The diagnosis and management of acute renal failure. *Semin Nephrol* 1:11, 1981.

undertaken. Classically, the causes of acute renal failure have been divided into three groups.

6. **Prerenal failure** generally implies inadequate intravascular volume or low CO. This assessment is made by checking blood pressure, PCWP (CVP is less reliable), and CO.

7. **Renal causes** usually include direct toxic injury to the renal parenchyma by prolonged ischemia, angiographic dye, or other medications, especially nephrotoxic antibiotics such as aminoglycosides.

8. **Postrenal failure** is caused by anatomic obstruction of the urinary collective system, usually the ureters. Ureteral obstruction generally results from extrinsic compression of the ureter by an accidental ligature or metal clip, a mass such as an abscess or phlegmon, or a prosthetic material such as the limb of a graft. Imaging tests that may reveal an enlarged or obstructed ureter include an abdominal computed tomography (CT) scan, ultrasound, or renal scan. The precise location and degree of obstruction may require a retrograde cystoureterogram.

B. As soon as a preliminary diagnosis of impending or acute renal failure is made, certain general **principles of therapy** should be followed.

1. **Maintenance of fluid and electrolyte balance** is paramount if fluid overload and hyperkalemia are to be avoided. Daily fluid requirements for oliguric or anuric patients are less than generally appreciated. Insensible water loss from skin and lungs is about 500 ml/day or 10 ml/kg/day. Without supplemental nutri-

tion, the patient should lose approximately 1 lb daily. Other losses, such as from gastrointestinal drainage, should be measured for volume and sodium concentration and then should be replaced.

In addition to fluid overload, hyperkalemia leading to cardiac standstill is the most immediate threat to life in acute renal failure. Increasing amplitude of the T wave and widening of the QRS complex on the ECG are ominous signs that require immediate reduction of the serum potassium level. The most effective means to counteract the cardiac effects of hyperkalemia is slow intravenous administration of a 10% solution of calcium chloride, up to 10 ml over 10 minutes. Calcium must be administered cautiously in patients on digoxin. Another method of acute therapy involves driving serum potassium into cells by intravenous sodium bicarbonate or insulin plus glucose (10 units of regular insulin plus one ampule of 50% dextrose in water). If this therapy is ineffective or if hyperkalemia is recurrent, hemodialysis may be necessary. Control of more chronic hyperkalemia may require oral administration of the exchange resin sodium polystyrene sulfonate (Kayexalate), 20 g tid with 20 ml of 70% sorbitol solution.

2. **Prevention of protein catabolism** by intravenous or oral administration of essential L-amino acids and glucose may shorten the duration of renal dysfunction and improve chances of survival.

3. **Prevention of late complications** involves prophylactic antacid therapy for gastrointestinal ulceration and prompt treatment of any infections. Sepsis remains a leading cause of death in acute renal failure.

4. **Adjustment of dosages** for any medication that is normally excreted by the kidney is essential. Common examples in vascular patients are digoxin and antibiotics such as aminoglycosides. Many of these drugs can be monitored by determination of blood levels.

5. **Hemodialysis** may become necessary if the patient develops (1) hyperkalemia that cannot be controlled by other medical measures, (2) fluid overload with pulmonary edema that is not responding to fluid restriction and diuretics, and (3) uremic symptoms.

VII. **Psychosis.** Postoperative psychosis manifested by agitation, mental confusion, and hallucinations is not uncommon in elderly patients who undergo major vascular surgery. In many patients, this change in mental status is mild and resolves in a few days without any specific treatment.

A. The **etiology** frequently is normal sensory and sleep deprivation in the unfamiliar hospital surroundings. Metabolic changes such as hypoxia, hypoglycemia, hyponatremia, and sepsis may alter mental function. Alcohol withdrawal also must be considered in the differential diagnosis. Narcotics may worsen the problem.

B. **Treatment** depends on the specific etiology and the severity of the psychosis. If no metabolic problem is identified, treatment should focus on reestablishing the normal waking and sleeping pattern. A major tranquilizer such as haloperidol (0.5–2.0 mg PO or IM bid–tid) may help sedate more agitated patients. Sedation must be carefully monitored; otherwise, patients may become obtunded, making them more susceptible to aspiration and atelectasis. The patient's family should be reassured that postoperative psychosis generally clears completely in several days. The patient, who may be bothered by his or her own confusion, hallucinations, or nightmares, also needs reassurance that he or she will soon be better.

Alcohol withdrawal is an important cause of postoperative psychosis. Although some patients will admit to alcoholism, many alcoholics will deny excessive drinking. Agitation and hallucinations caused by alcohol withdrawal may make early postoperative care extremely difficult. Such patients often are difficult to keep in bed. Frequently, they pull out their intravenous lines, gastric tubes, and urinary catheters. Therefore, these support lines should be well secured and the patient should be carefully restrained. A quiet environment with dimmed lights is essential, since noise and light often agitate such patients. In addition, a variety of sedatives may be used. Chlordiazepoxide (Librium) is an effective choice in our experience. Initially, large doses of Librium (25–100 mg PO or IV q6h) may be necessary. Intramuscular absorption may vary, so intramuscular administration is not recommended. Since the Librium doses are cumulative and alcohol withdrawal is self-limited, doses should be rapidly tapered (e.g., to 300 mg, 150 mg, and finally 75 mg over 3–5 successive days). Other important therapeutic measures include adequate hydration and administration of thiamine (100 mg IM qd) and multivitamins. Hypomagnesemia and hypoglycemia are common electrolyte problems in alcoholics. True delirium tremens with autonomic overactivity and cardiovascular instability is uncommon in our experience, but if it occurs, the previously outlined supportive care must be undertaken promptly and must be carefully monitored in an intensive care setting.

VIII. **Sepsis.** Perioperative sepsis is an uncommon problem after most vascular reconstructions. Patients at increased risk of infectious complications are those with preoperative chronic lung disease, liver cirrhosis, malnutrition, graft infections, and ruptured aneurysms. After operation, prolonged use of intravascular and urinary catheters, extended endotracheal intubation, ischemic colitis, and wound hematomas or tissue necrosis often precede local or systemic sepsis. Early recognition and treatment remain the keys to success when sepsis occurs. Specific types of infection tend to present at certain times after operation, and knowledge of these patterns is important in deciding which examinations or tests are most likely to identify the septic source.

  A. **Pulmonary atelectasis** is the most common cause of fever in the first 24–48 hours after operation. Generally the chest examination and x-ray will document the problem, and deep breathing exercises and endotracheal suction will resolve it. In the presence of fever, rales, and an infiltrate that persist beyond 24 hours, we culture the sputum and continue broad-spectrum antibiotics until the results are available for a more specific antibiotic regimen.

B. The second most common source of sepsis in the first few days after surgery is **central venous catheters**—in particular, triple-lumen catheters, since they have multiple ports through which bacteria may gain entry during infusion or blood sampling. The typical presentation of catheter sepsis is a sudden fever spike, chills, and a drop in blood pressure and systemic vascular resistance. The catheter must be removed, and the catheter tip and blood should be cultured. Since bacteremia may seed a new synthetic graft, we generally use broad-spectrum antibiotics that are effective against gram-positive, gram-negative, and anaerobic organisms. Enterococcus is one organism that requires specific treatment (e.g., ampicillin). Usually fever resolves quickly after catheter removal, and culture-specific antibiotics are continued for 5–7 days and until repeat blood cultures are negative.

C. Following aortic surgery, any signs of sepsis associated with diarrhea must raise one's suspicion of **ischemic colitis**. Proctosigmoidoscopy should be done to inspect the left colon. Evidence of extensive mucosal ischemia, localized tenderness, and systemic sepsis mandate resection of the involved bowel. Mild mucosal ischemia with no signs of sepsis is usually managed with bowel rest, maintenance of normal CO, and antibiotics.

D. Peripheral intravenous site thrombophlebitis is another common source of fever, usually occurring in 3–5 postoperative days. Removal of the intravenous catheter and application of local heat will be sufficient therapy for most cases. A tender, erythematous venous cord with pus at the intravenous site requires operative excision of the septic vein.

E. A urinary tract infection (UTI) should be suspected when patients develop a fever after a Foley catheter has been in place or after its removal when urinary retention occurs. The clinical presentation of a UTI is often delayed until postoperative days 7–10, when the patient may be out of the hospital.

F. Wound infections generally do not become apparent until 5–7 postoperative days. Because lower-extremity infections may involve underlying grafts, these infections may require drainage and debridement in the operating room.

G. Intraabdominal sepsis also may not become apparent until 10–14 days after laparotomy. Patients with fever at this time and no other explanation should undergo an abdominal CT scan to search for an abscess. If acute acalculous cholecystitis is suspected by upper abdominal tenderness, hepatobiliary scintigraphy (technetium-iminodiacetic acid scan) or ultrasound may help confirm the diagnosis before operation.

H. Finally, unexplained fever after 5–14 postoperative days may be related to a superficial or deep **venous thrombophlebitis** of the lower limb. Usually a careful examination of the leg will reveal some tenderness, swelling, or venous cord. A duplex ultrasound can be used to establish the diagnosis. Diagnosis and treatment are presented in more detail in Chaps. 4, 5, and 21.

I. Some patients succumb to so-called **multiorgan failure** and **sepsis**. They generally manifest simultaneous and progressive failure of the heart, lungs, kidneys, and sometimes liver. Generally, the common denominator in multiorgan failure is a period of shock or a low CO state. Recent studies document that cardiogenic shock results in severe splanchnic vasoconstriction that is mediated by the renin-angiotensin system. Manifestations of the selective splanchnic vasoconstrictive response to shock may include stress ulceration of the stomach, centrilobular liver necrosis, nonocclusive small bowel ischemia, ischemic colitis, and perhaps ischemic pancreatitis and acalculos cholecystitis. Obviously, prevention of **multiple splanchnic organ failure** depends on maintaining adequate CO throughout the perioperative period. In addition, any septic focus, such as an abdominal abscess, must be eliminated to reverse the downhill clinical course.

Selected Reading

Barie PS, Shires GT. *Surgical Intensive Care*. Boston: Little, Brown, 1993.

Beal AL, Cerra FB. Multiple organ failure syndrome in the 1990s. *JAMA* 271:226, 1994.

Gilman AG, Rall TW, Nies AS, Taylor P. *The Pharmacological Basis of Therapeutics* (8th ed). New York: Pergamon, 1990.

Myers BD, Moran, SM. Hemodynamically mediated acute renal failure. *N Engl J Med* 314:97, 1986.

Marino PL (ed). *The ICU Book*. Philadelphia: Lea & Febiger, 1991.

National Conference on Standards and Guidelines for Cardiopulmonary Resuscitation and Emergency Cardiac Care. Adult advanced cardiac life support. *JAMA* 268:2172, 1992.

Niemann JT. Cardiopulmonary resuscitation. *N Engl J Med* 327:1075, 1992.

Tobin MJ. Mechanical ventilation. *N Engl J Med* 330:1056, 1994.

Woodley M, Whelan A (eds). *Manual of Medical Therapeutics* (27th ed). Boston: Little, Brown, 1992.

Specific Arterial Problems

Cerebrovascular Disease

A surgeon with vascular expertise is a key member of the health care team that treats patients with cerebrovascular disease. This involvement in the care of such patients has been the direct result of the success of carotid, aortic arch branch, and vertebral artery reconstructions for the relief of symptomatic stenotic or ulcerated arterial lesions, aneurysms, and vascular tumors located in the neck. The surgeon may also be consulted to evaluate patients with asymptomatic but high-grade (>70% stenosis) carotid disease.

In this chapter, we discuss the management of common clinical presentations that suggest extracranial carotid or vertebral artery disease. We have also selected certain principles of operative care that facilitate a smooth, safe operation for the patient. Finally, the management of the most common early and late postoperative complications of carotid operations is summarized.

Common Clinical Presentations

I. **Transient ischemic attacks.** Approximately 75% of patients who suffer a stroke have experienced some type of preceding transient neurologic symptom. For strokes that occur in the carotid artery distribution, these transient ischemic attacks (TIAs) are usually hemiparesis, hemiparesthesias, transient monocular blindness, or difficulties with speech. TIAs of the vertebrobasilar artery distribution generally are characterized by dizziness, bilateral eye symptoms, ataxia, facial numbness, or some bilateral extremity weakness and numbness. Classically, a TIA is defined as acute neurologic symptoms that last less than 24 hours and completely resolve. However, the duration usually is measured in minutes, not hours. The term **reversible ischemic neurologic deficit (RIND)** has been used to describe neurologic symptoms that last longer than 24 hours but then rapidly resolve completely.

   A. The **outcome of TIAs** depends on the underlying etiology. TIAs are not specific for carotid artery stenosis or ulcerated plaques. Only about 50% of patients with TIAs will have a tight carotid stenosis (<2 mm), occlusion, or ulcerated plaques. If untreated, TIAs associated with significant carotid disease will result in a stroke for 1 of 3 patients in 5 years. **Most of these associated strokes, however, occur within days to weeks, especially when the TIAs are frequent.** The remaining 50% of patients with TIAs have thromboembolism from the heart, aortic arch, intracranial vascular disease, or no evident etiology. TIAs from thromboembolism or hypercoagulability also commonly lead to a stroke. However, patients with no evident etiology for their TIAs and normal carotid arteriograms may follow a more benign course; they seldom suffer a stroke.

Visual symptoms occur in approximately 25% of patients presenting with symptomatic carotid bifurcation atheroma. Transient monocular blindness (amaurosis fugax) is the most common ocular symptom. Rarely, the deterioration in visual acuity is due to ischemic neurovascular glaucoma. Unfortunately, permanent visual loss without warning affects 1 of 4 patients with ocular manifestations. This tragic outcome emphasizes the importance of identifying severe carotid stenosis or ulceration and correcting it before retinal artery occlusion or ischemic optic neuropathy has caused permanent visual loss.

B. The **natural history of TIAs** can be altered by **anticoagulation** or surgical therapy in selected patients. Antiplatelet drugs (aspirin, dipyridamole, sulfinpyrazone) retard platelet aggregation and thus may prevent the microemboli that cause TIAs. Aspirin therapy reduces the risk of continuing TIAs, stroke, and death by 19% compared to controls. Of special interest was the finding by the Canadian Cooperative Study Group that aspirin benefits men with TIAs but not women. This finding may be explained by sex differences in platelet sensitivity to aggregating stimuli. Heparin or warfarin sodium (Coumadin) can control TIAs in at least 90% of patients with recent onset. Coumadin also has proved effective in reducing serious cerebral infarct from 45% in untreated patients to 24% in treated individuals over 5 years. Of course, the main disadvantage of long-term Coumadin therapy is compliance and bleeding complications in about 15% of patients.

Surgical therapy also provides excellent long-term relief of TIAs that are the result of carotid stenosis of greater than 70% in diameter reduction. In general, the symptoms of 90% of patients with classic carotid symptoms of contralateral motor or sensory loss, ipsilateral eye symptoms, or dysphasia are relieved by carotid endarterectomy. In contrast, relief of nonspecific symptoms such as dizziness, syncope, and mental confusion is achieved in less than 50% of such patients. However, the chance of relief of such nonhemispheric symptoms is greater in patients whose carotid stenosis is hemodynamically significant by ocular pneumoplethysmography (Gee-OPG) than in those individuals with OPG-negative lesions (72% versus 32%, respectively). The total incidence of perioperative and late stroke is about 5–10% in operated patients compared to 25–35% in nonoperated patients.

C. Because untreated TIAs may lead to stroke, we recommend some type of anticoagulation or surgery for patients with TIAs. The **choice of therapy** is influenced by answers to the following questions:

1. **Are the symptoms actually transient ischemic episodes or some other neurologic or psychosomatic complaint?** This question is not always easy to answer. TIAs in the carotid distribution classically present with unilateral hemiparesis, hemiparesthesias,

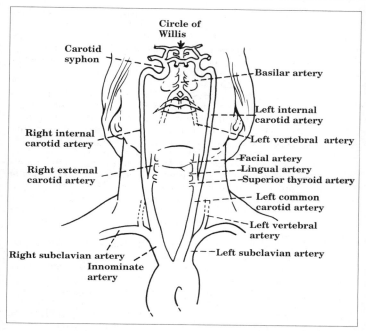

Fig. 11-1. Anatomy of the aortic arch and extracranial cervical arteries. The internal carotid artery has no branches in the neck.

speech disturbance, or amaurosis fugax. Amaurosis fugax is described as a graying out of vision, sometimes compared to pulling a shade down over the visual field. The symptoms that present confusion in determining whether a true TIA is being experienced are atypical complaints, especially dizziness and unsteady gait. These vertebrobasilar symptoms are rather common in elderly patients who may experience postural hypotension when arising quickly from a lying, sitting, or stooping position. If a psychosomatic problem is suspected, a careful inquiry about family or work situations may disclose emotional stress that initiates the symptoms. If the patient is unsure of the symptoms, a family member who may have observed an attack should be asked. Noninvasive carotid tests may assist in the selection of patients with atypical neurologic symptoms for arteriography. If these tests indicate a hemodynamically significant carotid lesion, we may suggest arteriography. Correction of a carotid stenosis in the presence of vertebral occlusion may alleviate vertebrobasilar symptoms by improving collateral flow to the posterior brain via the circle of Willis (Fig. 11-1).

2. **Are the transient neurologic attacks chronic and stable or repetitive and progressive?** If the

TIAs are chronic and not progressive, elective evaluation is appropriate. Noninvasive tests generally detect hemodynamically significant carotid lesions. Duplex ultrasonography allows visualization of plaques and measurement of the degree of stenosis. In selected patients, carotid duplex scanning may provide sufficient anatomic and functional information to proceed with carotid bifurcation endarterectomy without arteriography, but this approach is controversial. Currently, we still recommend good-quality arteriograms showing the aortic arch, cervical, and intracranial cerebrovasculature in most symptomatic patients.

Complete elective evaluation for TIAs also may require electrocardiographic monitoring (Holter monitor) to detect arrhythmias or echocardiography to rule out a diseased valve or mural thrombus. Transesophageal echocardiography may also reveal ulcerative atherosclerosis of the aortic arch, which is now recognized as a source of thromboembolic stroke in some patients.

We also have found consultation with a neurologist or neuroophthalmologist to be helpful in evaluating our patients, particularly if atypical neurologic or eye symptoms are present. In such cases, computed tomography (CT) or magnetic resonance imaging (MRI) of the brain is used to diagnose intracranial mass lesions and cortical atrophy. Electroencephalography (EEG) is appropriate if a seizure disorder is suspected.

If the TIAs are ongoing or have progressed in the past 24–72 hours, we hospitalize the patient immediately. These patients generally are systemically anticoagulated with heparin (loading dose of 5,000–10,000 units, with a continuous hourly infusion of 750–1,000 units). If the patient's overall medical condition is stable, an urgent arteriogram usually is done within 24 hours after admission. Heparin is withheld for 2–4 hours before the study. Operative candidates with severe (>70%) carotid stenosis or shaggy, irregular ulcerative plaques undergo carotid endarterectomy. The exact timing of arteriography and surgery must be individualized; it depends on the patient's medical condition and the availability of an experienced anesthesiologist and operating team.

Management becomes more difficult if the neurologic symptoms are progressing without complete resolution. These patients should be considered to have a stroke in evolution. Anticoagulation and emergent carotid surgery for severe carotid lesions may reduce the stroke rate and mortality in this group. However, the differentiation between a **stroke in evolution** or a **completed stroke** is not always clear. Surgery for a completed stroke seldom reverses any established neurologic deficit and may lead to worsening of the stroke and death. A CT scan may help determine whether cerebral infarction has occurred, but CT findings of a stroke may not be positive until 12–24 hours after the incident. MRI may be superior to CT scan in the early detection of brain infarction, but CT may be better for identification of hemorrhage.

Although carotid endarterectomy for acute stroke has been discouraged, there has been renewed interest in a more aggressive approach to selected patients with acute stroke. In one series from the Mayo Clinic, carotid revascularization for acute carotid occlusion and profound stroke resulted in a normal neurologic exam (27%) or minimal deficit (12%) in nearly 40% of patients. The surgical mortality of 20% was comparable to the natural history of untreated stroke. Others have also demonstrated good results from early carotid endarterectomy in patients with small, fixed neurologic deficits, even when CT scan has been positive. These more aggressive approaches have been balanced by other studies suggesting that carotid endarterectomy for stroke should be delayed for at least 5 weeks and until the deficit is stable or reaches a plateau in its improvement. Currently, we favor this more delayed approach to carotid surgery for stroke. Long-term follow-up supports the value of carotid endarterectomy in reducing the morbidity and mortality of recurrent stroke. Surgical patients have a recurrent stroke rate of 3–5% and a 5-year survival of about 80%, compared to unoperated patients who have a recurrent stroke rate of 25–60%.

3. **What is the patient's operative risk?** Combined mortality and stroke morbidity for elective carotid endarterectomy should be 2–4%. If the patient with chronic TIAs is a poor surgical risk, antiplatelet and/or Coumadin therapy is the initial treatment of choice. Arteriography and surgery should be reconsidered if anticoagulant therapy fails to control the TIAs. For good surgical candidates with classic carotid TIAs, we recommend elective cerebrovascular arteriography and elective surgical correction of an ulcerative or stenotic plaque (>70% diameter reduction) that correlates with the exhibited symptoms. **There have now been three randomized clinical trials documenting the superiority of carotid endarterectomy over anticoagulation in preventing neurologic events in symptomatic patients with high-grade (>70%) carotid stenosis** (North American Symptomatic Carotid Endarterectomy Trial [NASCET], European Carotid Surgery Trial, and Veterans Affairs Symptomatic Carotid Endarterectomy Trial). The benefit amounted to a cumulative 2-year stroke rate of 9% for endarterectomy patients compared to 22% for the medically treated patients in the NASCET trial.

II. **Asymptomatic cervical bruits.** Controversy continues over the natural history and management of asymptomatic cervical bruits.

A. The **natural history** of a cervical bruit depends on what underlying cardiovascular lesion is causing the noise. A neck bruit may originate from the carotid arteries or be transmitted from the aortic arch or heart (see Fig. 11-1). Precise location of the source of the bruit generally requires an ultrasonic duplex scan (see Chap. 5). An echocardiogram (transthoracic or transesophageal) also helps differentiate carotid bruits from transmitted cardiac murmurs.

The degree of narrowing of a carotid stenosis determines whether cerebral blood flow on that side is reduced. Unfortunately, the loudness of a bruit does not correlate with the degree of stenosis. In fact, a tight carotid stenosis with severely diminished flow may have a minimal or inaudible bruit. At present, an accurate noninvasive method to determine the **hemodynamic significance of a carotid bruit** is ocular pneumoplethysmography (OPG) or carotid duplex scanning. OPG pressures correlate with internal carotid pressure. Duplex scanning provides a B-mode ultrasound image plus a pulsed Doppler analysis of the flow velocity pattern across a lesion. The degree of stenosis can be categorized, and a high-grade (80–90%) lesion or occlusion can be identified. These tests are discussed in detail in Chap. 5.

B. Our **clinical management** of patients with asymptomatic neck bruits is determined by answers to the following questions:

1. **Is the patient a good operative risk?** If so, we recommend noninvasive carotid testing to help determine the location and hemodynamic significance of the bruit. If the patient is not, we generally do not pursue further evaluation. The risk of carotid endarterectomy in high-risk patients, especially those with symptomatic cardiac disease, generally exceeds the risk of stroke from an asymptomatic carotid stenosis. Such patients generally should be followed until they become symptomatic with TIAs.

2. **Do noninvasive carotid tests suggest a hemodynamically significant carotid stenosis?** If the answer is yes and the patient is a good surgical candidate, we recommend arteriography and subsequent carotid endarterectomy for carotid stenosis (>50% diameter or 75% cross-sectional area). The combination of an asymptomatic pansystolic carotid bruit and an abnormal OPG on the same side has been correlated with an 3–5% incidence of stroke per year. In our experience, the risk of stroke in such cases is considerably higher than the risk of postoperative stroke for elective carotid endarterectomy (1–2%). Patients with a normal OPG have a better prognosis, with only a 1% per year incidence of stroke. Patients with asymptomatic carotid bruits in whom noninvasive carotid tests do not suggest a hemodynamically significant stenosis usually are followed. They undergo arteriography if symptoms develop subsequently or if noninvasive tests demonstrate that the stenosis is progressing into the 80–99% stenotic category. The appropriate frequency of such follow-up visits is debatable, but a visit every 6–12 months is reasonable.

Although some physicians are hesitant to recommend carotid endarterectomy for patients with asymptomatic carotid bruits, the natural history of this group does not appear to support this nonoperative approach in otherwise healthy adults with a reasonable life expectancy. The rationale for prophylactic carotid endarterectomy for high-grade asymptomatic carotid stenosis began with the classic clinical observations of Dr. Jesse Thompson of Dallas. In his nonoperated group, 26.8% eventually had TIAs, 15.2% experienced a nonfatal stroke, and 2.2% had a fatal stroke. On the other hand, 90% of operated patients remained asymptomatic. Only 4.5% of the operated patients developed TIAs and 2.3% experienced a nonfatal stroke.

More recently, Strandness and colleagues at the University of Washington used duplex scanning prospectively to study the natural history of carotid arterial disease in asymptomatic patients with cervical bruits. The presence of or progression to a greater than 80% internal carotid stenosis was highly correlated with development of TIA, stroke, and asymptomatic internal carotid occlusion in 46% of patients compared to those lesions of 0–79% stenosis (1.5%). The majority of adverse events occur within 6 months of the findings of an 80–99% stenosis.

Three randomized clinical trials have addressed the benefit of prophylactic carotid endarterectomy for asymptomatic high-grade carotid stenosis (Carotid Artery Surgery Asymptomatic Narrowing Operation Versus Aspirin [CASANOVA], Veterans Affairs Asymptomatic Carotid Endarterectomy Trial, and Asymptomatic Carotid Atherosclerosis Study [ACAS]). The CASANOVA trial excluded patients with stenosis greater than 90% and those with bilateral high-grade stenoses, two groups most likely to benefit from endarterectomy. A substantial portion (57%) of the medical group crossed over into the surgical arm, but neurologic endpoints leading to this switch were not considered in the final analysis. Thus, the CASANOVA trial did not resolve the dilemma of the critical asymptomatic carotid stenosis. **The Veterans trial found a significant reduction in combined TIAs and stroke in the surgical group (8%) versus the medical group (20.6%).** However, there was not a statistically significant difference when stroke alone was analyzed (surgical versus medical, 4.7% versus 9.4%). The relatively small sample size was one limitation of this study. Finally, the ACAS trial is the largest of the three studies and has analyzed the outcomes of 1,500 patients with no cerebral symptoms and a greater than 60% diameter reduction of the carotid artery. Results of the ACAS trial favor carotid endaterectomy over medical therapy.

The decision to recommend elective carotid endaterectomy for asymptomatic carotid stenosis also must be influenced by the experience of the available anesthesiologists and the surgical team. Mortality generally does not exceed 2–3% if surgery is performed by an experienced team, and permanent neurologic deficits at the time of operation also should remain in this low range.

3. **Is the patient scheduled for other major surgery?** Controversy also continues over whether patients with asymptomatic carotid bruits are at increased risk for perioperative stroke at the time of other major surgery, especially any operation in which prolonged hypotension may occur. The major surgery of most concern has been cardiac and aortic operations. Only 0.5–1.0% of patients who undergo major cardiovascular surgery suffer a perioperative stroke. Several studies have shown that cervical bruits are not a good predictor of perioperative stroke. In fact, perioperative strokes often occur in patients who were not suspected of having carotid disease. These strokes also are more commonly diffuse than focal. The conclusion of these studies is that major cardiovascular surgery can be performed on patients with asymptomatic carotid bruits who have not had carotid endarterectomy.

However, we follow a selective approach to such patients. Noninvasive carotid testing is performed to determine the hemodynamic significance of the carotid stenosis. Poorly compensated lesions generally are corrected before elective aortic surgery is attempted. Combined carotid endarterectomy and heart operations, such as coronary artery bypass or valve replacement, are reserved for patients with unstable cardiac disease and severely stenotic or symptomatic carotid disease. Most surgeons agree that patients with symptomatic carotid disease should have carotid endarterectomy before other elective surgery is performed.

III. **Asymptomatic contralateral carotid artery stenosis.** Another controversial area in carotid surgery is the management of patients with the asymptomatic contralateral carotid artery stenosis following a carotid endarterectomy. These patients may be at increased risk of TIAs and stroke. The outcome of such lesions again may depend on the hemodynamic significance of the asymptomatic lesion. Conservative management of nonoperated vessels opposite an endarterectomy appears appropriate until symptoms develop or a lesion greater than 80% is detected. We generally repair a hemodynamically significant contralateral carotid stenosis as a staged procedure. The endarterectomies are performed at least 5–7 days apart, although some patients require a longer recovery period between operations. If the contralateral stenosis is not hemodynamically significant, or if the patient is not a good surgical risk, or if the first endarterectomy was complicated by cranial nerve injury, we follow the patient until symptoms occur or noninvasive studies document progression of the stenosis.

IV. **Asymptomatic ulcerated lesions.** The natural history of asymptomatic ulcerated carotid lesions is not easy to define. First, ultrasound cannot accurately detect plaque ulceration.

It can define plaque morphology (homogeneous versus heterogeneous), but these characteristics do not always correlate with surface ulceration. Arteriography also is not particularly accurate in defining ulceration. The ulceration may vary from a slight nonstenotic irregularity to a complicated ulcerated stenosis.

V. Asymptomatic Hollenhorst plaque. Occasionally a patient is referred for evaluation of an asymptomatic Hollenhorst plaque (cholesterol embolus in a retinal arteriole) noted incidentally on routine retinoscopy, often by an ophthalmologist. Such asymptomatic findings do not appear predictive of future transient or fixed retinal or cerebral symptoms. We generally screen such patients with a carotid duplex scan and do not proceed with further evaluation or treatment unless a high-grade carotid stenosis is detected. Surgically remediable lesions are found in only about 15% of such patients.

VI. Subclavian steal syndrome. Left subclavian stenosis or occlusion is a common atherosclerotic lesion. Generally, it is asymptomatic and is discovered because the left brachial blood pressure is lower than the right. Left arm claudication seldom is a significant problem, since the collateral flow to the left arm usually is well developed. However, for a few patients proximal left subclavian occlusion may cause subclavian steal syndrome. Its clinical features are dizziness, syncope, visual blurring, or ataxia, classically associated with vigorous left-arm exercise. The mechanism of the syndrome appears to be retrograde flow from the left posterior cerebral circulation down the left vertebral artery to the distal subclavian artery and arm. Theoretically, this "stealing" of blood from the brain to the left arm causes intermittent posterior cerebral ischemia.

In our experience, classic subclavian steal syndrome is uncommon. Although many patients with subclavian occlusive disease have retrograde left vertebral flow on arteriography, few have cerebral symptoms with arm claudication. If they do have cerebral ischemic symptoms, we perform noninvasive evaluation of the carotid system. Subclavian steal syndrome sometimes is relieved simply by correcting a severe left carotid stenosis, which improves collateral flow via the circle of Willis to the posterior brain. Significant arm claudication may be relieved by carotid-subclavian bypass, subclavian-subclavian bypass, subclavian-to-carotid transposition, or transluminal angioplasty.

VII. Totally occluded internal carotid artery. It is uncertain whether thromboendarterectomy of an occluded internal carotid artery is advisable. Certainly, surgical repair of a thrombosed internal carotid artery in the setting of a completed stroke may be associated with intracranial hemorrhage and a high mortality risk. The natural history of untreated carotid occlusion is still debated. Approximately 25% of patients have subsequent TIAs, and 10–15% have a stroke. Many patients, however, remain asymptomatic.

  A. A few reports indicate that **thromboendarterectomy** of a totally occluded internal carotid artery can be achieved with a low morbidity and mortality rate and a 65–70%

overall patency in severely symptomatic patients. Retrograde filling of the ipsilateral intracranial internal carotid artery to its petrous or cavernous segment appears to be a good sign of operability. Timing of such surgery seems critical. Operation within 2 hours of acute symptoms or after a wait of 1–3 weeks has been recommended.

B. Another approach to management of the symptomatic patient with a totally occluded internal carotid artery is **external carotid artery endarterectomy** or bypass revascularization when an external carotid stenosis is present. External carotid revascularization may relieve symptoms of internal carotid artery occlusion by increasing both the total and regional cerebral blood flow.

C. Finally, symptomatic patients with total internal carotid occlusion also may be relieved by **extracranial-to-intracranial (EC-IC) anastomosis** of the temporal artery to the middle cerebral artery. EC-IC bypasses generally are performed by a neurosurgeon experienced in microsurgical technique. We continue to see gratifying results in selected patients. However, the international randomized EC-IC bypass study failed to confirm that EC-IC anastomosis is effective in preventing ischemic stroke in patients with atherosclerotic disease in the carotid and middle cerebral arteries. Consequently, EC-IC bypass is rarely performed anymore.

VIII. Vertebrobasilar insufficiency. Vertebrobasilar insufficiency or nonhemispheric TIAs are characterized by instability of the patient in the upright position, visual changes, and bilateral paresthesias with occasional paresis. They are the result of hypoperfusion of the basilar artery and its branches. Left subclavian stenosis proximal to the left vertebral artery or stenosis of the origin of either vertebral artery may decrease vertebrobasilar flow. Vertebrobasilar insufficiency is especially likely to occur when carotid occlusive disease also is present and collateral flow via the circle of Willis is inadequate. In such cases, we generally repair the carotid lesions in the hope that increased collateral flow will alleviate the vertebrobasilar symptoms. If carotid occlusive disease is not present or the circle of Willis is not intact, direct vertebral artery reconstruction should be considered. Proximal subclavian stenosis is usually corrected by carotid-subclavian bypass, subclavian-subclavian bypass, or subclavian-to-carotid reimplantation. Stenosis at the origin of either vertebral artery may be managed by endarterectomy or reimplantation of the vertebral artery into the side of the common carotid artery. Extracranial-to-intracranial anastomosis also may improve the posterior cerebral circulation. Finally, percutaneous balloon angioplasty of focal subclavian stenosis can be successful, but vertebral artery embolization is one potential risk.

IX. Pulsatile masses. Pulsatile masses near the carotid artery usually are true aneurysms, carotid body tumors, adjacent lymphadenopathy, or a tortuous carotid artery. Sonography, CT scanning, or MRI can generally differentiate between these etiologies. Carotid aneurysms are rare but dangerous since they may lead to rupture, cerebral embolization, thrombosis, and local pressure symptoms. The best surgical approach is resection and arterial restoration by direct end-to-end anastomosis or an interposition graft. Carotid body tumors generally are slow-growing, but they are relentless neoplasms. Periadventitial excision or carotid artery replacement is recommended for all carotid body tumors. Radiation therapy appears to be of little value in their management. Observation is appropriate only for asymptomatic elderly patients who are poor surgical risks.

X. Carotid fibromuscular dysplasia (FMD) is a relatively benign, often incidental finding that rarely causes ischemic infarction during prolonged observation. Although carotid FMD may be associated with TIAs, the incidence of subsequent stroke is less than that seen with atherosclerotic carotid occlusive disease. Patients with FMD are more prone to internal carotid dissection. When neurologic or visual symptoms can be attributed to carotid FMD, they generally resolve without operation and recurrence is uncommon. High-grade symptomatic FMD stenoses can be treated by intraoperative internal carotid dilation, and large or symptomatic aneurysms can be resected with vein graft reconstruction.

Operative Management

Because carotid endarterectomy is the most common operation for extracranial cerebrovascular disease, we focus on principles of operative care for carotid reconstructions. These same principles also apply to other types of vertebral and subclavian revascularization.

I. Preoperative preparation. For elective cases, anticoagulants and antiplatelet medications are usually discontinued at least 48 hours before surgery. The main exception is a patient with multiple recent TIAs or a severe carotid stenosis (<2 mm), who usually remains on heparin or aspirin until operation.

Although neck infection is rare, several preventive measures are taken. The chin, neck, and anterior chest are shaved on the side of endarterectomy. This area is washed with a surgical scrub solution within 6–12 hours of operation. Preoperative parenteral antibiotics are started when the patient goes to the operating room; the antibiotic of choice usually is a cephalosporin or semisynthetic penicillin.

The patient is made NPO after midnight. Stable or asymptomatic patients are admitted on the morning of operation. Some symptomatic patients will already be hospitalized for heparin anticoagulation. An intravenous infusion of balanced salt solution (e.g., 5% dextrose in Ringer's solution at 100–125 ml/hour) is begun to maintain hydration. General narcotic premedications that may cause hypotension are avoided.

On the day of surgery, a responsible member of the operating team is present in the operating room from the time the patient enters the room until the patient is transported to the recovery area. An arterial line is generally inserted in the operating room. Selected patients with severe cardiac disease (see Chap. 8) may also receive a Swan-Ganz catheter. A Foley bladder catheter is optional but may assist with blood pressure control since bladder distention may exacerbate hypertension in a labile patient.

II. Operative principles

A. General endotracheal anesthesia is our preference, since it both provides the best control of the airway and best facilitates management of cardiorespiratory function. Other experienced surgeons prefer regional cervical block and local anesthesia.

B. Carotid exposure (see Fig. 11-1) must be gentle and meticulous to avoid venous or nerve injury and dislodgement of atheromatous material from a plaque. Figure 11-2 demonstrates the relative positions of the major nerves of the neck that surround the carotid artery.

1. Branches of the **ansa cervicalis** (hypoglossis) may be divided for better exposure, without a resulting neurologic deficit.

2. The **hypoglossal nerve** usually crosses the carotid artery at or near the carotid bifurcation. Most hypoglossal injuries are caused by retraction of the nerve. Clamp injuries may occur if the hypoglossal nerve is not dissected free from the common facial vein before it is divided. Hypoglossal injury results in weakness of the tongue on the operated side, with tongue deviation toward the side of the injury. This deficit may cause biting of the tongue while chewing, and the patient may have some difficulty swallowing or speaking. Bilateral hypoglossal nerve injury may be life-threatening, since the tongue may prolapse posteriorly and obstruct the airway when the patient is supine.

3. The **vagus nerve** usually runs in the posterior carotid sheath behind the carotid artery. Occasionally, it swings anteriorly along the anterolateral surface of the carotid artery. The vagus nerve must be dissected free from the carotid artery, especially at the proximal and distal extent of carotid dissection, where clamps may accidentally injure it.

   a. Vagal injury is most commonly manifested by hoarseness, since the **recurrent laryngeal nerve** normally originates from the vagus in the chest and runs back to the vocal cord in the tracheoesophageal groove. The recurrent laryngeal nerve loops around the subclavian artery on the right side and the ligamentum arteriosum on the left. Occasionally, the laryngeal nerve is nonrecurrent and originates from the vagus nerve in the neck and passes posteriorly to the carotid artery.

   b. The **superior laryngeal nerve** travels behind the carotid bifurcation to the true vocal cord. This nerve innervates the cricothyroid muscle, which maintains the tone of the vocal cord. Injury may be avoided by careful dissection around the external carotid and superior thyroid arteries. Injury results

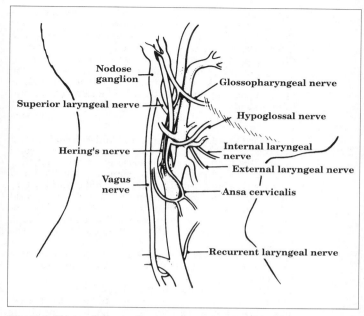

Fig. 11-2. Nerves that may be encountered or injured during carotid endarterectomy. Specific nerve function is discussed in the text.

in voice tone fatigue, especially after prolonged speaking or singing.

4. The **greater auricular nerve** is a sensory nerve to the skin overlying the mastoid process, the concha of auricle, and the earlobe. It lies on the anterior surface of the sternocleidomastoid muscle and may be injured when the neck incision is carried toward the mastoid process. Injury results in skin numbness around the lower ear and earlobe.

5. The **mandibular branch** of the facial nerve runs forward from the angle of the mandible and parallel to the mandible. Injury results in weakness of the perioral musculature on the injured side. The patient may drool from the corner of the mouth.

C. **Prevention of thromboemboli** obviously is essential if neurologic deficits are to be avoided. We take several measures to avoid thrombus accumulation and embolism.

1. During gentle carotid dissection, **suction** is used rather than blotting with sponges to keep the operative field dry. Vigorous manipulation of the carotid bifurcation may dislodge loose atheromatous material from an ulcerated plaque.

2. Before carotid clamping, **heparin** is administered intravenously and allowed to circulate for at least 5 minutes. Our usual dose is 5,000 units.

3. The inside of the carotid artery is **irrigated** with heparinized saline to wash out any loose atheroma or clot both before a shunt is inserted and before the internal carotid artery is reopened.

4. Since the endarterectomy surface may be thrombogenic, low molecular weight dextran is begun in the recovery room as an antiplatelet and anticoagulant drug. A loading dose of 100 ml is administered, and administration is continued at 20 ml/hour until aspirin can be reinstituted orally on the first postoperative day.

5. Backward bleeding of the internal and external carotid arteries and forward bleeding of the common carotid artery flush out any clot or loose atheroma that may accumulate behind vascular clamps. Carotid blood flow also is reinstituted up the external carotid artery for a few seconds before opening the internal carotid artery. This sequence of reopening the carotid branches should allow any thromboemboli to go out through the external carotid artery and not directly to the brain.

D. **Cerebral protection** from clamp ischemia probably is best achieved by two methods: careful blood pressure control and shunting.

1. In Chap. 8, we emphasized that cerebral perfusion is directly related to **systemic blood pressure.** Therefore, during carotid clamping, we remind the anesthesiologist to maintain the blood pressure in a normotensive to mildly hypertensive range. If continuous EEG monitoring is used, a diffuse slowing pattern often can be eliminated by simply raising the patient's systemic blood pressure.

2. **Shunting** during carotid endarterectomy remains controversial. Experienced surgeons have demonstrated that with or without shunting, carotid endarterectomy can be performed with a low incidence of permanent postoperative neurologic deficit (1–3%). The key question is how to identify the few patients who will not tolerate carotid clamping long enough for the surgeon to complete endarterectomy without a shunt. The two most common methods to assess adequate cerebral perfusion during carotid clamping are carotid stump pressures and EEG monitoring (see Chap. 9). Our experience suggests that carotid stump pressures may not correlate with adequate cerebral perfusion as indicated by EEG monitoring. Consequently, we insert a shunt after carotid clamping if focal EEG changes occur and are not corrected by manipulation of anesthetic agents or blood pressure. If EEG monitoring is not available, a carotid stump pressure below 50 mm Hg may indicate inadequate cerebral collateral flow during carotid clamping. Even without EEG changes, we often insert a shunt to allow for an unhurried endarterectomy and to provide an intraluminal stent which, in our experience, facilitates a better closure of the internal carotid artery. In a teaching situation, we

prefer routine shunting. We also believe that routine shunting is advisable when the contralateral internal carotid artery is occluded. Finally, in patients in whom the internal carotid plaque extends high into the carotid artery, an intraluminal shunt may make endarterectomy excessively difficult. In such cases, the endarterectomy of the distal plaque probably should be performed without a shunt in place. A shunt may subsequently be inserted to complete the operation.

E. The **endarterectomy technique** should achieve the two main goals of carotid artery reconstruction. The first goal is adequate removal of the stenotic or ulcerated plaques. Since atherosclerotic lesions involve the intima and media, we generally remove the plaques down to the external elastic membrane. In our experience, such a deep endarterectomy plane has resulted in the removal of retained media fibers, which may cause recurrent myointimal restenosis, but it has not been associated with late aneurysm formation. The second goal is closure of the arteriotomy so that stenosis or thrombosis does not occur. A primary closure of the arteriotomy usually is possible. Patches are used when primary closure would cause stenosis or when the endarterectomy is being repeated. Patch angioplasty may protect against early thrombosis. Recent clinical trials indicate that patching is beneficial in the following situations: (1) small internal carotid artery (<3.5 mm), (2) long internal carotid arteriotomy (>3 cm), (3) women who tend to have small arteries, and (4) reoperative endarterectomies. In our opinion, low-power magnifying glasses (2–4×) help us perform a more meticulous endarterectomy and arterial closure. Flow through the internal and external carotid arteries is assessed by a sterile continuous-wave Doppler probe. Absence of flow or an obstructed, monophasic signal indicates thrombosis or stenosis, which requires immediate thrombectomy and a patch. Other methods of intraoperative assessment include arteriography or B-mode ultrasound (see Chap. 9).

F. **Recognition of postoperative neurologic deficit** ideally is made in the operating room if the anesthesiologist can awaken and extubate the patient early. Otherwise, the patient is moved to the recovery area and a neurologic examination of general motor function is made as soon as the patient is responsive. In our experience, the earliest signs of a neurologic deficit may be severe hypertension, difficulty in being awakened from anesthesia, or clumsiness of fine hand movement.

The proper management of an immediate postoperative neurologic deficit must be individualized.

1. First, the patient's general **cardiorespiratory status** must be stabilized expeditiously. This includes stabilization of heart rate, blood pressure, pulmonary ventilation, and blood oxygenation.

2. Treatment then depends on the **location** of the neurologic deficit.

a. If the deficit is a **contralateral hemiparesis**, a technical problem at the endarterectomy site may exist. We generally have returned these patients immediately to the operating room to examine the endarterectomy site. Two tests may help determine whether the arteriotomy should be reopened. First, duplex ultrasound is a sensitive method to ascertain carotid thrombosis or a major filling defect due to thrombus or a technical problem (e.g., residual plaque). Second, an intraoperative carotid arteriogram may also be done if ultrasound is not available or equivocal. If these tests are not satisfactory, reexploration of the artery remains the only way to rule out a technical error.

    b. If the neurologic deficit is diffuse, the patient may have suffered an **internal capsule stroke**, usually caused by a hypotensive episode. Patency of the carotid arteries should be assessed by either an OPG or ultrasound. If the operated side appears occluded, then reoperation is appropriate. If both carotid arteries appear widely patent, the patient should receive supportive care. A CT brain scan should be performed in approximately 12–24 hours to localize the cerebral infarct area and assess the amount of cerebral edema or hemorrhage.

III. Postoperative care

  A. Day of surgery. All patients spend the first 12–24 hours after cerebrovascular surgery in an intensive recovery area, where vital signs and neurologic status can be continuously monitored. The head of the bed is elevated 30–45 degrees to diminish cerebral edema and facilitate deep breathing. The patient is kept NPO until the first postoperative morning since reexploration is occasionally necessary. While the patient is NPO, a maintenance intravenous infusion of 5% dextrose in water and one-half normal saline is run at 1 ml/kg/hour. Hyponatremia and water intoxication must be avoided in those patients who occasionally develop cerebral edema because of inappropriate secretion of antidiuretic hormone. Patients who have undergone staged bilateral carotid endarterectomies may be insensitive to hypoxia as a result of carotid baroreceptor trauma. Therefore, they must be observed closely for bradycardia, hypotension, and respiratory distress.

  B. Postoperative day 1. If a wound drain has been used, it is removed on the first postoperative day. Patients who are doing satisfactorily are transferred to the appropriate ward, where diet and ambulation are resumed. Supplemental oxygen is continued if arterial blood gases indicate hypoxia (PO_2 less than 60 mm Hg). The infusion of low molecular weight dextran is discontinued. The efficacy of long-term antiplatelet therapy after carotid endarterectomy is not known. However, we tend to prescribe a low dose of aspirin (80–325 mg daily), especially if the patient has known coronary artery disease, a Dacron patch angioplasty, or contralateral uncorrected carotid disease.

  C. Postoperative days 2–3. The patient's general well-being recovers quickly (by the second to third postoperative day) if no serious complications have occurred. During the final few days of hospitalization, the dosages of antihypertensive medication, if needed, should be adjusted as the patient becomes more active. Skin sutures or metal clips usually can be removed by the fifth postoperative day on an outpatient basis. A postoperative OPG may be obtained for future follow-up.

D. Discharge instructions. By the second or third postoperative day, the patient is ready for discharge. Because the patient's full physical strength may not recover for 2–4 weeks, we generally advise patients to convalesce for that period of time before resuming normal working activities. All patients are rechecked as outpatients in 3–6 weeks after surgery. They return to their local referring physician for long-term management of any medical problems.

Complications

I. Early postoperative problems usually are apparent on the day of surgery and require prompt recognition and treatment.

A. Immediate postoperative neurologic deficits are discussed in the section on Operative Management. Occasionally, a patient will do well in the immediate recovery period but develop TIAs between the first postoperative day and the day of discharge. These patients should undergo a head CT scan; if it is negative for intracerebral hemorrhage, they should be anticoagulated with heparin. They should undergo urgent cerebral angiography for detection of any surgically correctable problems. If no anatomic problem is seen, heparin should be continued until symptoms resolve and antiplatelet therapy is established.

B. Hypertension is a common postoperative problem occurring in approximately 20% of patients who have carotid endarterectomy. Patients who were hypertensive before operation, especially if poorly controlled, are more likely to have severe postoperative hypertension. The incidence of neurologic deficit and death is significantly higher in these hypertensive patients. Therefore, we strive to maintain postoperative systolic blood pressure in a range from the minimal normal preoperative recording to a maximum of 180 mm Hg. Chapter 10 discusses the specific use of nitroprusside and other antihypertensives in detail.

C. Neck hematomas may compromise breathing and swallowing. Patients with large neck hematomas should be returned to the operating room for evacuation. If a patient's respiratory status and hematoma are stable, no attempt at intubation should be made until the surgical team is ready to operate. In cases where respiration is desperately compromised or bleeding is profuse, nasotracheal intubation and control of bleeding in the recovery room may be necessary to save the patient. Smaller neck hematomas may be left alone and usually resolve in 7–14 days. They seldom are complicated by infection. If a pulsatile mass persists after the major portion of the hematoma resolves, a pseudoaneurysm should be suspected and confirmed by ultrasonography.

D. **Local nerve injuries** following carotid operations probably are more common than generally is recognized or reported. Some degree of cranial nerve dysfunction affects 5–20% of patients. The mechanism of injury usually is nerve retraction or clamping and not transection. Most injuries involve the hypoglossal or recurrent laryngeal nerves. The injuries often are mild or asymptomatic and will not be detected unless one specifically examines for them. For example, one-third of recurrent laryngeal nerve injuries will go unrecognized unless direct laryngoscopy is performed. **Therefore, all patients who undergo staged carotid endarterectomy should be tested by direct laryngoscopy before their second operation.** Fortunately, most cranial nerve injuries resulting from retraction trauma will resolve in 2–6 months. Time and reassurance are all the treatment most patients require.

II. **Late complications** of carotid artery reconstructions are uncommon or at least seldom cause symptoms.

A. **Recurrent carotid stenosis** that is symptomatic is rare, affecting only 1–3% of patients after carotid endarterectomy. Asymptomatic restenosis is detectable in 10–20% of patients followed by noninvasive carotid testing, and is more common in women. The risk of a future stroke in this asymptomatic group appears to be low. Recurrent lesions have a striking predilection for the internal carotid artery near its origin and within the confines of the original endarterectomy site. Early recurrent lesions (<36 months) are predominantly a combination of neointimal fibromuscular hyperplasia and surface thrombus. Features of atherosclerosis (abundant collagen, calcium deposits, and foam cells) are more pronounced in late recurrences. An important feature that differentiates primary and recurrent carotid lesions is the presence of surface and intraplaque thrombus in 90% of recurrent stenoses. Recurrent symptoms after carotid endarterectomy generally require repeat angiography. Recurrent stenosis is repaired by repeat endarterectomy and patch angioplasty, by patch angioplasty if an endarterectomy plane is not available, or by segmental carotid resection and an interposition vein graft.

The need for long-term ultrasound surveillance of carotid endarterectomy sites is debatable. Since early restenosis is often a relatively benign fibroplastic lesion, asymptomatic restenosis does not mandate reoperation. However, contralateral atherosclerotic asymptomatic 50–79% stenoses have a significant risk of becoming symptomatic, especially if they progress. Consequently, we recheck such lesions every 6–12 months and caution patients to report any ipsilateral neurologic or ocular symptoms.

B. **Carotid pseudoaneurysm** may occur after primary arterial closure or patch angioplasty. In general, such pseudoaneurysms should be repaired since a mural thrombus may accumulate and cause cerebral thromboembolism. Large pseudoaneurysms also may cause local pressure symptoms.

Selected Reading

Barnett HJM, Eliasziw M, Meldrum HE. Drugs and surgery in the prevention of ischemic stroke. *N Engl J Med* 332:238, 1995.

Bower TC et al. Advanced carotid disease in patients requiring aortic reconstruction. *Am J Surg* 166:146, 1993.

Brewster DC et al. Innominate artery lesions: Problems encountered and lessons learned. *J Vasc Surg* 2:99, 1985.

The CASSANOVA Study Group. Carotid surgery vs. medical therapy in asymptomatic carotid stenosis. *Stroke* 22:1229, 1991.

Chervu A, Moore WS. Carotid endarterectomy without arteriography (general review). *Ann Vasc Surg* 8:296, 1994.

Clagett GP et al. Morphogenesis and clinicopathologic characteristics of recurrent carotid disease. *J Vasc Surg* 3:10, 1986.

EC/IC Bypass Study Group. Failure of extracranial-intracranial arterial bypass to reduce the risk of ischemic stroke: Results of an international randomized trial. *N Engl J Med* 313:1191, 1985.

Eliasziw M et al. for the North American Symptomatic Carotid Endarterectomy Trial. Significance of plaque ulceration in symptomatic patients with high-grade carotid stenosis. *Stroke* 25:304, 1994.

European Carotid Surgery Trialists' Collaborative Group. MRC European Carotid Surgery Trial: Interim results for symptomatic patients with severe (70–99%) or with mild (0–29%) carotid stenosis. *Lancet* 337:1235, 1991.

Evans BA, Sicks JD, Whisnant JP. Factors affecting survival and occurrence of stroke in patients with transient ischemic attacks. *Mayo Clin Proc* 69:416, 1994.

Gertler JP et al. Carotid endarterectomy for unstable and compelling neurologic conditions: Do results justify an aggressive approach? *J Vasc Surg* 19:32, 1994.

Hobson RW et al. Efficacy of carotid endarterectomy for asymptomatic carotid stenosis. *N Engl J Med* 328:221, 1993.

Hobson RW II, Krupski WC, Weiss DG and the VA Cooperative Study Group on Asymptomatic Carotid Stenosis. Influence of aspirin in the management of asymptomatic carotid artery stenosis. *J Vasc Surg* 17:257, 1993.

Mayberg MR, Wilson SE, Yatsu F. for the Veterans Affairs Cooperative Studies Program 309 Trialist Group. Carotid endarterectomy and prevention of cerebral ischemia in symptomatic carotid stenosis. *JAMA* 266:3289, 1991.

McCrory DC et al. Predicting complications of carotid endarterectomy. *Stroke* 24:1285, 1993.

Meyer FB, Sundt TM Jr. (eds). *Occlusive Cerebrovascular Disease*. Philadelphia: Saunders, 1994.

Moore WS et al. Carotid endarterectomy: Practice guidelines—report of the Ad-Hoc Committee of the Joint Council of the Society for Vascular Surgery and the North American Chapter of the International Society for Cardiovascular Surgery. *J Vasc Surg* 15:469, 1992.

Myers SI et al. Saphenous vein patch versus primary closure for carotid endarterectomy: Long-term assessment of a randomized prospective study. *J Vasc Surg* 19:15, 1994.

North American Symptomatic Carotid Endarterectomy Trial Collaborators. Beneficial effect of carotid endarterectomy in symptomatic patients with high-grade carotid stenosis. *N Engl J Med* 325:445, 1991.

Roederer GO et al. The natural history of carotid arterial disease in asymptomatic patients with cervical bruits. *Stroke* 15:605, 1984.

Wilson SE, Mayberg MR, Yatsu F, Weiss DG and the Veteran Affairs Trialists. Crescendo transient ischemic attacks: A surgical imperative. *J Vasc Surg* 17:249, 1993.

Lower-Extremity Claudication

Intermittent claudication of the lower limbs is the most common manifestation of peripheral arterial occlusive disease. The term **claudication** actually means "a limp." The patient may limp or claudicate for several reasons. The patient's calf muscles may develop cramping pain with walking. The hip and thigh muscles may cramp or tire. Walking also may be limited because of a feeling of diffuse lower-extremity weakness and numbness.

Although claudication usually is associated with vascular disease, degenerative hip disease or neurospinal conditions also may cause a patient to claudicate. Therefore, in the evaluation of lower-extremity claudication, the physician must first question the underlying etiology. Is the claudication caused by arterial occlusive disease or some other problem? The history and physical examination often can answer this question (see Chap. 3). Treadmill walking with measurement of resting and postexercise ankle systolic blood pressures provides objective data to support or refute the clinical impression (see Chap. 5).

If the initial evaluation defines arterial occlusive disease as the cause of claudication, the next question is how should the claudication be managed. Should therapy be medical, or should an invasive procedure such as percutaneous balloon angioplasty or an operation be recommended? Finally, if an operation is recommended, what operation should be performed?

I. **Patterns of disease.** Vascular claudication of the lower limb generally is caused by an arterial stenosis or occlusion in one of two main anatomic sites (Fig. 12-1). A common location of stenosis or occlusion is the superficial femoral artery, frequently at the exit of the adductor canal. Some patients have occlusive disease localized primarily to the distal abdominal aorta and iliac arteries with open distal arteries.

Patient history, physical examination, and noninvasive segmental leg pressures and pulse volume recordings usually can identify the primary location of disease (see Chaps. 3 and 5). Since therapeutic decisions are influenced by the location of occlusive lesions, we attempt to categorize patients into three basic patterns of peripheral arterial disease (Fig. 12-2).

A. **Aortoiliac disease (type 1).** Type 1, the least common pattern (10–15%), is limited to the distal abdominal aorta and common iliac arteries. Patients with focal aortoiliac disease are characteristically age 35–55, with a low incidence of hypertension and diabetes but a high frequency of heavy cigarette smoking and hyperlipidemias. There has been an alarming increase in premature atherosclerotic aortoiliac disease in younger women (age 35–50) who have smoked since adolescence. These patients generally complain of proximal lower-extremity claudication involving the hip and thigh muscles with progression to the calf

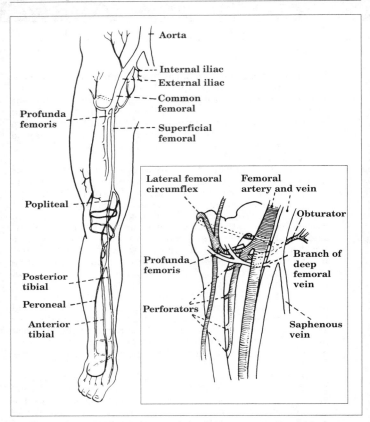

Fig. 12-1. Arterial anatomy of the lower extremity. The most common locations of atherosclerotic occlusive disease are the aortoiliac region and the superficial femoral artery. Enlarged drawing of the femoral region demonstrates the major collateral channels of the profunda femoris artery. Branches of the deep femoral vein cross the anterior surface of the profunda femoris artery and must be carefully divided before extensive profundaplasty is attempted.

muscles. In about 15% of such patients, however, the claudication affects only the calves. Diminished femoral pulses and femoral bruits are characteristic physical findings. Weak pedal pulses often are palpable, since the femoropopliteal system is open. Some men have the triad of bilateral leg claudication, impotence, and absent femoral pulses, which is commonly called **Leriche's syndrome**. Patients with type 2 disease (20%) have aortoiliac atherosclerotic lesions that also involve the external iliac arteries extending to the groins. Final definition of whether the patient has type 1 or 2 aortoiliac disease must be made by arteriography.

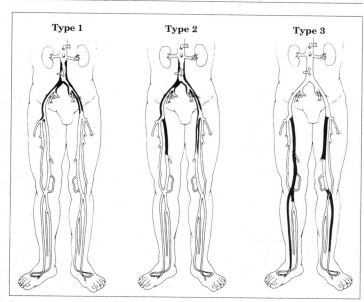

Fig. 12-2. Patterns of aortoiliac and femoropopliteal arterial occlusive disease. Type 1 is limited to the distal abdominal aorta and common iliac arteries. Type 2 is a combination of aortoiliac and femoropopliteal disease. Type 3 involves primarily the superficial femoral, popliteal, and tibial arteries.

B. **Combined aortoiliac and femoropopliteal disease (type 2).** The majority of patients with lower-extremity claudication (66%) have combined aortoiliac and femoropopliteal disease (type 2). This type usually occurs in patients with multiple cardiovascular risk factors: smoking, hypertension, hyperlipidemia, and sometimes adult-onset diabetes mellitus. They usually have more incapacitating leg claudication than is seen in aortoiliac or femoropopliteal disease alone and often progress to more severe ischemia problems, such as rest pain, foot ulcers, or toe gangrene.

C. **Isolated femoropopliteal disease (type 3).** Patients with isolated femoropopliteal disease generally present with calf claudication that starts after the patient walks a certain distance and is relieved by simply stopping for a few minutes. These patients often are older (age 50–70) and have a higher prevalence of hypertension, adult-onset diabetes mellitus, and associated vascular disease of the coronary and carotid vessels than do those with aortoiliac disease. Like patients with aortoiliac disease, they frequently are cigarette smokers. They generally have good femoral pulses but no palpable popliteal or pedal pulses. Their claudication usually is improved by a walking program and remains stable for long periods of time if significant proximal aortoiliac disease is not present. In fact, the following observations support initial nonoperative management: Patients over 60 years of age with superficial femoral artery occlusive disease (1) have a low likelihood of limb loss (2–12% in a 10-year follow-up) if followed closely on conservative treatment, (2) can expect improvement in symptoms (80%) if the initial ankle-to-brachial systolic pressure index (ABI) is greater than 0.6, and (3) should undergo evaluation for angioplasty or reconstructive surgery if the ABI falls below 0.5. Five-year survival is 70–80%, and only 20% will require surgical revascularization.

II. **Initial management.** The following principles are crucial in determining the best treatment for a patient with intermittent vascular claudication. For most patients, initial treatment is nonoperative. Only 5–10% of patients with claudication will require amputation of an extremity due to progression of the disease in 5 years. Most patients who progress to amputation are those who continue to smoke or who have diabetes mellitus. Surgical indications are discussed in sec. **III.**

A. **Determination** of initial treatment is based on the duration, disability, and progression of the claudication. Initial management also is influenced by the patient's general medical condition.

1. **Duration**. If the leg claudication is of recent onset and is not incapacitating, a trial period of nonoperative therapy is indicated. This approach is recommended particularly for patients who are suspected of having a recent superficial femoral artery occlusion. Although they may experience sudden severe calf claudication when the superficial femoral artery occludes, their claudication generally improves in 6–8 weeks if profunda femoris arterial collaterals are well developed. In general, we prefer to follow patients with recent onset of claudication for at least 3–6 months to determine whether the claudication will stabilize, improve, or worsen.

2. **Disability**. We generally ask two important questions of the patient about the disability imposed by the leg claudication: Does the leg claudication prevent normal activity, especially the performance of essential daily activities or a job? Does the claudication limit leisure activities that the patient enjoys? In our experience, the answers to these two questions are more helpful in determining patient management than is the distance the patient can walk before he or she is stopped by claudication.

3. **Progression**. It is extremely important to determine whether the claudication is stable or progressing. Patients who have noted rapid progression of claudication over the past 6 months to 1 year are more likely to need elective arterial reconstruction than are stable claudicators. Patients with progressive claudication also are more likely to appreciate any relief an operation may provide.

4. **Assessment of the patient's general medical condition** is essential for determining the proper initial management of claudication. Elective operations for intermittent claudication should be reserved for patients who appear to have a low risk of mortality (2–3%) and morbidity. This assessment is discussed in detail in Chap. 7. Patients with multiple medical problems and stable leg claudication should be followed until symptoms become incapacitating or the limb is threatened by rest pain, nonhealing ulcers, or gangrene.

B. **Nonoperative management** includes a walking program and control or elimination of cardiovascular risk factors.

1. **Regular lower-extremity exercise** increases metabolic adaptation to ischemia caused by walking and may enhance collateral blood flow. The result is stabilization or improvement of claudication. A variety of exercise programs can alleviate claudication. A relatively simple program that has helped 80% of our patients emphasizes the following concepts:

   a. Patients are asked to set aside a definite period and frequency of exercise **in addition** to normal daily activities (e.g., 30 minutes, 3–5 days per week). Exercise every day may be too much activity for many older patients; consequently, an every-other-day exercise program is ideal.

   b. Patients are instructed to walk at a comfortable (not too fast) pace and stop for a brief rest whenever claudication becomes severe.

   c. This walk-rest routine should be continued for 30 minutes. As the leg muscles adapt to anaerobic metabolism, the frequency and length of rest stops will decrease. After 6–8 weeks, most claudicators can double or triple their comfortable walking distance. In bad weather, the patient may use an indoor treadmill, walk inside a shopping mall, or use a stationary exercise bicycle.

2. **Elimination of cigarette smoking** improves blood flow to the legs and increases skin temperature. The main vasoconstrictive agent in tobacco is nicotine. Convincing chronic smokers to quit is not easy; many patients enjoy their tobacco addiction too much to be convinced to stop. Although many techniques are available to help patients discontinue smoking, none of them will succeed unless the patient really **wants** to stop. Patients who are convinced that smoking is related to vascular disease and who have good motivation generally will completely stop smoking and not resume tobacco use. Unfortunately, such patients are in the minority. Only 40% of men and 30% of women who stop smoking remain off tobacco use after 1 year. Nicotine skin patches may enhance these discouraging abstinence rates by 10–15%.

3. **Control of hyperlipidemias** may retard the progression of peripheral atherosclerosis, although the

data are controversial. Certainly, young adults (age 20–45) with severe hyperlipidemias need treatment, since control of hyperlipidemia may retard coronary and peripheral vascular disease. Normal plasma cholesterol is arbitrarily defined as less than 200 mg/100 ml. However, the risk from serum cholesterol is continuous and increases as the cholesterol level rises. Normally, triglycerides should be below 150 mg/100 ml. In general, serum measurements of cholesterol and triglycerides should be determined after a 12-hour fast. Simple inspection of a standing serum specimen refrigerated for 12–24 hours allows phenotypic determination of the lipoprotein type. Lipoprotein electrophoresis usually is unnecessary. A low-fat (35% of calories), low-cholesterol (<300 mg daily) diet remains the cornerstone of treatment. Alcohol may exacerbate hypertriglyceridemia in susceptible persons. The current recommendation is at least a 3-month trial of diet management before drugs are added.

The details of drug therapy can be reviewed in other medical or pharmacologic reference sources. Briefly, cholesterol may be lowered 15–20% by bile acid sequestering resins (cholestyramine, colestipol), lovastatin, probucol, niacin, and clofibrate. Fibrates (e.g., clofibrate [Atromid-S] and gemfibrozil [Lopid]) are effective in lowering triglyceride levels. Partial ileal bypass also can interrupt cholesterol absorption but should be reserved for patients in whom medical treatment has failed.

4. **Control of diabetes mellitus** may not retard peripheral atherosclerosis. However, strict control may help the diabetic to more quickly resolve infections and heal minor sores of the lower extremities.

5. **Control of hypertension** also is important, since stress on the arterial wall is directly related to blood pressure (see Chap. 1). Controlled hypertension also reduces a patient's risk of stroke, congestive heart failure, and renal small-vessel damage.

6. **Pentoxifylline** (Trental) is the first Food and Drug Administration–approved drug for the treatment of intermittent claudication. This rheologic agent is a methylxanthine that reduces blood viscosity by improving red blood cell membrane flexibility and inhibits platelet aggregation. In a multicenter trial, pentoxifylline significantly increased the distance patients could walk before the onset of claudication. Its effect on the progression of atherosclerosis remains unclear.

In our practice, pentoxifylline, 400 mg PO bid or tid with meals, has been combined with a walking program and smoking reduction for selected patients with mild to moderate claudication. If walking is improved after 6–8 weeks, the pentoxifylline is often stopped to ascertain whether exercise and abstinence from tobacco will maintain improvement. If claudication worsens, pentoxifylline may be restarted. Common side effects of pentoxifylline are gastrointestinal upset and dizziness. Some patients can tolerate only 400 mg bid. However, our experience has been that pentoxifylline cannot prevent the need for surgical revascularization or balloon angioplasty in patients with severe progressive claudication or resting ischemia.

III. **Indications for invasive therapy.** Patients must be selected carefully for angioplasty or surgery for lower-extremity claudication. Impairment of occupational performance and significant limitation on a low-risk patient's life-style are reasonable indications, but only if a favorable anatomic situation for percutaneous angioplasty or surgical reconstruction exists. The best results are obtained when the occlusive disease is localized to the aorta and iliac arteries with open distal vessels. A focal superficial femoral artery stenosis is also a favorable anatomic lesion for angioplasty.

Occasionally, an active individual with an incapacitating above-the-knee superficial femoral artery occlusion may require an elective femoropopliteal bypass. However, in such cases it must be ascertained that significant proximal aortoiliac disease does not coexist, since inadequate inflow may jeopardize the long-term success of a femoropopliteal graft. A femoral artery pressure study may help detect significant iliac occlusive disease (see Chap. 6).

We generally discourage elective arterial reconstruction for **stable** claudication if the primary disease is (1) combined diffuse aortoiliac and femoropopliteal arterial disease or (2) severe below-the-knee popliteal and tibial artery disease. An aortofemoral bypass without addition of a femoropopliteal bypass generally will not completely relieve claudication when multilevel occlusive disease (type 3) exists. An aortofemoral bypass for claudication in patients with combined aortoiliac and femoropopliteal disease should be recommended only when claudication is rapidly progressive and the aortoiliac disease has advanced to critical stenoses or occlusions. Likewise, below-the-knee femoropopliteal or femorotibial bypasses should be primarily limb salvage procedures, and only occasionally should they be used to treat claudication alone.

IV. **Preoperative evaluation**
   A. The principles of assessing **operative risk** and stabilizing chronic medical problems are discussed in Chap. 7. Mortality for percutaneous angioplasty should be negligible. Operative mortality for elective aortoiliac reconstruction or femoropopliteal bypass for claudication should not exceed 2–3%. The primary risk to life during vascular reconstructions is coronary artery disease. Significant coronary artery disease exists in at least 40% of patients with peripheral vascular disease. In general, we recommend that the necessary surgical procedures for significant coronary artery disease be performed before elective aortic surgery is attempted.
   B. The importance of **weight reduction** before elective aortic surgery cannot be overemphasized (see Chap. 7). Truly elective operations (e.g., aortofemoral bypass for life-style–limiting claudication) should be delayed until

excess weight is reduced. Weight reduction alone frequently alleviates some claudication.

C. Before elective surgery, patients should be asked to make a commitment to **stop smoking** before operation and not to resume tobacco use after recovery. They should be informed that the chance of graft failure approaches 30% in patients who continue to smoke regularly.

D. **Angiography is performed only after a decision has been made to undertake arterial reconstruction.** Arterial reconstruction includes both operative procedures and percutaneous transluminal angioplasties. Nonoperative management generally can be selected and followed by patient history, physical examination, and noninvasive testing, without performance of an arteriogram.

V. **Selection of proper procedure.** The proper choice of operation or transluminal angioplasty for claudication depends on the general condition of the patient, the extent of the atherosclerotic process, and the experience of the surgeon. The preoperative arteriogram and papaverine femoral artery pressure measurements are the single best determinants of which procedure should be undertaken in a given patient (Table 12-1). A well-trained vascular surgeon should understand the indications and limitations for the following procedures: aortoiliac endarterectomy, aortoiliac or aortofemoral bypass graft, femoropopliteal bypass, lumbar sympathectomy, transluminal angioplasty, and extraanatomic reconstruction such as axillofemoral and femorofemoral bypasses.

A. **Aortoiliac endarterectomy.** In patients with occlusive disease limited to the distal aorta and common iliac arteries, **aortoiliac endarterectomy** gives excellent long-term results, provided the patient eliminates or controls his or her vascular risk factors. Endarterectomy will be suitable in approximately 10% of the patients with aortoiliac disease and is preferred because of the advantages of autogenous tissue and the absence of a prosthesis. Disease should terminate at or just beyond the common iliac bifurcation, allowing a satisfactory endpoint without extending more than 1–2 cm into the external iliac segment. Endarterectomy is contraindicated in the presence of any of three complications: (1) aortic or iliac aneurysmal disease, (2) aortic occlusion to the level of the renal vessels, or (3) any occlusive disease in the external iliac or femoral arteries. The 5- and 10-year patency rates are 95% and 85%, respectively.

B. **Percutaneous transluminal angioplasty** (e.g., balloon dilatation plus stenting) is currently the initial treatment of choice for focal arterial stenoses that cause claudication (see Chap. 6). A focal common iliac stenosis of less than 3 cm in length has been a lesion well suited to treatment by percutaneous transluminal angioplasty. Recanalization of total iliac occlusions and dilatation of distal aortic stenoses also have been reported. Angioplasty results can be enhanced by the addition of stents where plaque resists balloon dilatation or where stenosis is recurrent. In addition, excellent results have been achieved with superficial femoral artery stenoses. The appropriate role

Table 12-1. Aortofemoral graft for multilevel occlusive disease: Predictors of success and need for distal bypass

Emphasis of evaluation	Predictors of good result with AF bypass alone	Predictors of need for distal bypass
Proximal disease	Absent or severely reduced femoral pulse	"Normal" femoral pulse
	Severe stenosis/occlusion (arteriogram) (positive femoral artery pressure study)[a]	Mild-moderate inflow disease (arteriogram) (Negative femoral artery pressure study)
Distal disease	Good outflow tract (arteriogram)	Poor outflow tract (arteriogram)
	Index runoff resistance <0.2	Index runoff resistence ≥0.2[b]
Intraoperative	Improved pulse volume recorder amplitude	Unimproved/worse pulse volume recorder amplitude
Clinical	Nonadvanced ischemic symptoms (i.e., claudication, rest pain)	Advanced ischemia (necrosis/sepsis)

[a]Femoral artery pressure study (see Chap. 6). An iliac stenosis is significant when the resting pressure gradient across the iliac segment is greater than 5 mm Hg or falls more than 15% after reactive hyperemia or papaverine injection.
[b]Index runoff resistance = $\dfrac{\text{thigh-ankle pressure difference}}{\text{brachial pressure}}$
Source: Modified from DC Brewster, BA Perler, JG Robinson, RC Darling. Aortofemoral graft for multilevel occlusive disease: Predictors of success and need for distal bypass. *Arch Surg* 117:1593, 1982.

of transluminal angioplasty in the treatment of lower-extremity claudication is still debated. Current results indicate that it may allow repeated treatment of focal occlusive lesions with postponement of a definitive operation until more diffuse or severe disease is present.

C. The majority of patients with incapacitating claudication will require a **bypass graft of the aortoiliac segments** for durable relief (>5 years). Aortofemoral bypass grafts are preferred to aortoiliac bypass grafts, because, not uncommonly, the external iliac segment eventually is obliterated by progressive arteriosclerosis. Subsequent downstream repair becomes necessary in approximately 25–30% of patients who are initially treated by aortoiliac bypass, compared to 10–15% of patients who undergo aortofemoral bypass initially. In selected patients with unilateral iliac occlusive disease, ilioiliac and iliofemoral bypass grafts or endarterectomy may be performed through a retroperitoneal approach. Five-year patency rates of 70–80% are encouraging and indicate that iliac-origin arterial grafts are useful in situations where one wants to avoid transabdominal aortofemoral grafting or extraanatomic femorofemoral or axillofemoral bypasses.

D. Femoropopliteal bypass for stable claudication is being performed less frequently now than it was in the early

1980s. Long-term follow-up of patients with leg claudication from a solitary superficial femoral artery occlusion indicates that nonoperative treatment often stabilizes the problem. In addition, progression of proximal aortoiliac disease may lead to poor inflow to a femoropopliteal bypass and eventual hemodynamic graft failure, often within 5 years. Therefore, patients who undergo femoropopliteal bypass for claudication alone should have a good anatomic situation, which includes normal aortoiliac inflow, a patent popliteal artery above the knee with a two- or three-vessel runoff, and a high likelihood of an available saphenous vein. Autogenous saphenous vein remains superior to all other graft materials for durability of a femoropopliteal bypass.

E. **Lumbar sympathectomy** alone is not considered adequate treatment of lower-extremity claudication. However, sympathectomy may be beneficial occasionally for ischemic rest pain, microembolic phenomenon, or foot sores when poor runoff and inadequate vein for a bypass are present and the ABI is greater than 0.35.

F. **Extraanatomic axillofemoral or femorofemoral bypasses**, in our practice, are useful only in a limited group of patients with claudication. The most suitable candidates are those with the following:

1. Iliac occlusion and a normal iliac artery and normal hemodynamics of the contralateral (donor) leg.
2. Previous postirradiation intestinal obstructions or fistulas that discourage intraabdominal aortofemoral reconstruction.
3. Known extensive postsurgical abdominal adhesions.

Direct aortoiliac arterial reconstruction for claudication is preferable to extraanatomic bypasses. When done by experienced hands, aortoiliac reconstruction is safe and provides a durable result in 85–90% of patients at 5 years. In contrast, 5-year patency for femorofemoral bypass and axillofemoral bypass for claudication approaches 50–75% in the best reports.

G. **Elective aortoiliac reconstruction** for occlusive disease is generally **not combined** with other nonvascular operations. For example, we favor leaving asymptomatic gallstones alone despite the recommendations of others to do a cholecystectomy if there are no mitigating circumstances. Although the morbidity of adding cholecystectomy may be low, additional procedures do increase the risks of complications. Also, postoperative cholecystitis secondary to cholelithiasis is a rare entity in our experience. Most postoperative cholecystitis is acalculous and occurs in patients who have been in shock and have the so-called splanchnic shock syndrome. Occasionally, however, we discover incidentally a gallbladder with cholelithiasis **and** chronic smouldering cholecystitis during operative exploration. If the aortic reconstruction goes well, we may perform cholecystectomy **after** the retroperitoneum and femoral wounds have been closed to cover the prosthetic graft.

VI. **Preoperative preparation.** In our clinical practice, patients who are scheduled for elective arterial operations for claudications will need the following preparation.

A. Prior to hospital admission. A complete history, physical examination, and routine diagnostic studies are performed before hospital admission. Baseline studies include a complete blood count, urinalysis, chest x-ray, 12-lead electrocardiogram (ECG), serum electrolytes, creatinine, blood sugar, liver function tests (bilirubin, serum glutamic-oxaloacetic transaminase, alkaline phosphatase, total protein, albumin), platelet count, prothrombin time (PT), partial thromboplastin time (PTT), uric acid, fasting serum cholesterol and triglycerides, calcium, phosphorus, and pulmonary function tests in patients with chronic lung disease. Any preoperative consultations with other specialists are arranged, preferably before admission.

B. Preoperative angiography. Preoperative angiography (see Chap. 6) is accomplished at least 24–48 hours before elective operation. Arteriography can often be done on an outpatient basis with a short period of postprocedural observation and intravenous hydration. Ideally, a day's delay before operation is necessary after angiography, to be certain that renal function does not deteriorate after the angiographic contrast load.

C. Day before operation. Final preparations on the day before operation include the following:

1. The patient is typed and cross-matched for 2–4 units of packed red blood cells for aortic operations and typed and held for femoropopliteal reconstructions. If autotransfusion is planned, arrangements are made for its availability.

2. For bowel preparation the patient receives clear liquids and a laxative (e.g., magnesium citrate, 120 ml PO) the evening before surgery.

3. Since elective arterial patients may have chronic intravascular volume depletion from diuretics and acute dehydration from the angiogram and the bowel preparation, an intravenous infusion of Ringer's lactated solution at 100–125 ml/hour is started before surgery. Depending on individual patient requirements, such hydration may take 6–12 hours prior to operation. Thus, many patients will require hospital admission on the evening prior to aortic surgery.

4. Skin preparation includes shaving hair in the operative field as close to the time of operation as possible to minimize colonization of shaved areas by hospital-acquired bacteria. A shower with hexachlorophene, chlorhexidine gluconate, or povidone-iodine soap also is done as close to the time of operation as possible, usually just before the intravenous infusion is started.

5. Patients are instructed in deep breathing and coughing, as well as in the use of an incentive spirometer. We also teach the patient leg exercises that are used as prophylaxis against deep venous thrombosis, for stimulation of lower-extremity blood flow, and for maintenance of leg muscle tone prior to ambulation.

6. Preoperative prophylactic antibiotics are administered intravenously when the patient is called to the operating room. A semisynthetic penicillin or a cephalosporin is used. For patients with a history of penicillin allergy, the cephalosporins are avoided and the patient receives another antibiotic (e.g., vancomycin, 500–1,000 mg) with good coverage for hospital-acquired organisms.

VII. **Operative principles.** The details of operative technique are beyond the scope of this handbook. Other operative atlases describe techniques for arterial reconstruction. Certain principles of intraoperative care, however, do warrant emphasis in a book on patient care.

A. **Patient positioning.** The patient is kept in the supine position with the electrocautery ground beneath the buttocks. The arms generally are adducted to the sides. Ischemic heels are elevated or wrapped with a soft dressing to prevent pressure sores.

B. **Skin preparation.** The operating room should be heated to a warm (70–75°F) temperature during the skin preparation, to reduce heat loss from the patient. The skin preparation extends from the nipples to the knees for aortofemoral reconstructions and to the toes for patients who may require an associated femoropopliteal bypass. Care must be taken to avoid pooling of the preparatory solution beneath the patient, especially in contact with the electrocautery ground. Full-thickness chemical skin burns can result from pooling and prolonged contact with the solution. After application of the antiseptic preparatory solution, the skin is covered with a plastic Steri-Drape. Although Steri-Drapes may not reduce the incidence of wound infection, we recommend their use to prevent contact of graft materials with the skin, which may contaminate the graft.

C. **Intraoperative monitoring.** All lower-extremity arterial reconstructions are monitored with the pulse volume recorder (PVR) or a Doppler flow detector (see Chap. 9). As a general rule, PVR cuffs are placed one limb segment below the anticipated reconstruction site (i.e., at the calf for aortofemoral bypass and at the ankle for femoropopliteal bypass). A baseline recording is made. Additional recordings are made immediately following the arterial reconstructions and before the patient leaves the operating room. Sterile cuffs should be used in the operative field.

D. **Systemic anticoagulation.** Heparin is used for systemic anticoagulation while the aorta and distal arteries are clamped. Our experience has indicated that an adequate heparin dose is 3,000–5,000 units given intravenously at least 5 minutes before aortic clamping. Although monitoring of heparin effect may not be necessary, we prefer to check an activated clotting time (ACT) before and after heparinization. An ACT of 200–300 seconds is adequate for most cases. Smaller additional doses of heparin (500–1,000 units) often are given during regional irrigation of the iliac and major femoral artery branches. Reversal of heparin is optional at the termination of the procedure. In general, heparinization with the above doses does not require reversal, since the heparin effect diminishes in about 90 minutes. However, if one

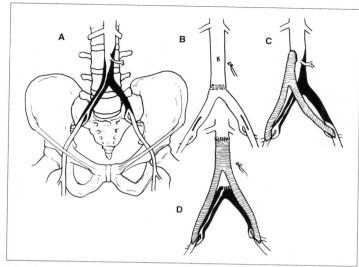

Fig. 12-3. Types of aortoiliac reconstruction. Aortoiliac endarterectomy (B) is our preferred operation for occlusive disease localized to the distal abdominal aorta and common iliac arteries (A). For aortofemoral grafting, we recommend the proximal end-to-end anastomosis (D) rather than the end-to-side technique (C) (see text). (Modified from RC Darling et al. Aorto-iliac reconstruction. *Surg Clin North Am* 59:565, 1979.)

chooses to reverse heparinization, ACTs are the primary method used to monitor reversal with protamine sulfate (0.5–1.0 mg/1 mg heparin).

E. Intraoperative diuretics. A good urinary diuresis (0.5–1.0 mg/kg body weight) must be established prior to aortic clamping. Infrarenal aortic clamping diminishes renal cortical blood flow (see Chap. 8). This reflex cortical ischemia can be prevented by adequate intravascular volume expansion and administration of the osmotic diuretic mannitol. We administer 12.5–25.0 g mannitol just before clamping the aorta. When needed, small (10–20 mg) doses of furosemide are added. In addition, dopamine (2–3 µg/minute IV) causes renal vasodilatation.

F. Proximal aortic anastomosis. Controversy continues over whether the proximal aortic graft anastomosis should be end-to-end or end-to-side (Fig. 12-3). Our experience strongly favors end-to-end aortic anastomosis. Its primary advantages are as follows:

1. The origin of the graft is from a higher and less diseased part of the infrarenal abdominal aorta.

2. There is a better hemodynamic situation, since the main infrarenal aortic blood flow is directed through the graft without competitive flow with the distal abdominal aorta.

3. There is better retroperitoneal coverage of the graft. Because a small segment of infrarenal aorta is resect-

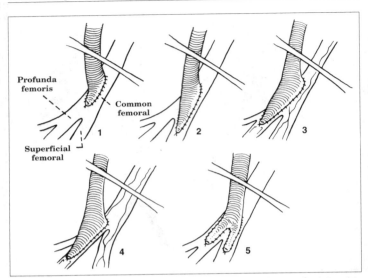

Fig. 12-4. Types of femoral anastomosis for aortofemoral bypass grafts. 1. Type 1 anastomosis to the common femoral artery. 2. Type 2 anastomosis, in which the graft is carried onto the proximal superficial femoral artery. 3. Type 3 anastomosis, in which the graft is carried onto the profunda femoris artery. 4. Type 4 anastomosis, involving only the profunda femoris artery. 5. Type 5 anastomosis, involving a patch angioplasty of both the superficial and deep femoral arterial orifices. (Modified from RC Darling et al. Aorto-iliac reconstruction. *Surg Clin North Am* 59:565, 1979.)

ed before graft insertion, the graft lies in a better anatomic position for coverage with retroperitoneal tissue. The onlay or end-to-side aortic anastomosis leaves the graft protruding more anteriorly. For this reason, the end-to-side graft seems more likely than the end-to-end graft to adhere to the adjacent duodenum and cause aortoenteric fistula.

G. **Distal anastomosis** for aortofemoral bypass also has a significant influence on graft patency. Basically, there are five methods of distal anastomosis (Fig. 12-4).

1. **Type 1, anastomosis to the common femoral artery**, is preferred for patients with widely patent profunda femoris and superficial femoral arteries.

2. **Type 2 anastomosis carries the graft onto the proximal superficial femoral artery** and is recommended when the orifice of the superficial femoral artery is stenotic but the distal arteries and profunda femoris artery are otherwise normal.

3. **Type 3 anastomosis (also known as profundaplasty) carries the graft onto the profunda femoris artery.** It is recommended for all patients with extensive superficial femoral artery occlusion. For most patients, the profunda femoris artery is of ade-

quate diameter (3–4 mm) and length (15–20 cm) to maintain aortofemoral graft flow and adequately perfuse the lower leg via collaterals.

4. **Type 4 anastomosis is done only to the profunda femoris artery.** It is necessary when the common femoral and superficial femoral arteries are extensively obliterated.

5. **Type 5 anastomosis splits the hood of the graft** to patch open proximal stenoses of both the proximal superficial femoral artery and the profunda femoris artery.

H. **Gastrointestinal decompression** with a nasogastric tube is often necessary for 24–72 hours.

1. Gastrointestinal ileus may be prolonged after aortic reconstruction, especially if extensive lysis of adhesions or dissection of the duodenum is necessary. In our experience, patients generally have sluggish intestinal peristalsis for at least 2–3 days after operation. Although nasogastric decompression was once used routinely for this entire period, the vast majority (90%) of patients can tolerate the removal of the nasogastric tube on the first postoperative morning. After removing the tube, we generally wait 24–48 hours to be certain that peristalsis is adequate before commencing an oral liquid diet. This is progressed to solid food in the subsequent 24–48 hours.

2. Appetite after major aortic reconstruction usually is poor. Consequently, patients generally do not resume normal caloric intake for at least 5–7 days. A weight loss of 5–10 lb is not uncommon in the first month following surgery. Patients who have marginal nutrition prior to operation or a complicated postoperative course may not tolerate further weight loss, so their caloric intake may require parenteral supplementation.

VIII. **Postoperative care.** Despite multiple medical problems and sometimes long, extensive operations, most patients who undergo major aortic or peripheral arterial reconstruction can expect an uncomplicated postoperative recovery if certain principles of care are followed.

A. **Initial stabilization** of the patient should be done in an intensive care recovery room where vital signs, urine output, ECG rhythm, and respiratory status should be monitored continuously for at least 12–24 hours.

On arrival in the intensive care unit, the patient should be checked immediately for systemic blood pressure, heart rate and rhythm, and arterial blood gases. If the patient is intubated, the ventilator settings should be adjusted after review of the initial blood gases. The criteria for extubation are discussed in Chap. 10.

After these vital functions have been stabilized, additional baseline tests may be obtained, including a portable chest x-ray to check endotracheal tube position and to ensure adequate lung expansion. In addition, a 12-lead ECG should be compared with the preoperative ECG for any changes indicative of intraoperative myocardial ischemia or infarction. Cardiac isoenzymes should be sent for laboratory study if any intraoperative myocardial ischemia was detected. A blood specimen also should be sent for measurement of hematocrit, serum electrolytes, blood sugar, PT, PTT, and platelet count.

Management of common early postoperative problems is outlined in Chap. 10.

B. Fluid management must be meticulous, since many vascular patients have coronary artery disease and do not tolerate fluid overload. Several simple observations about fluid and electrolyte balance after major aortic or peripheral arterial surgery and a few guidelines for fluid administration should make fluid management easy.

1. Patients undergoing major peripheral arterial reconstructions, especially aortic procedures, often leave the operating room after large amounts of fluid resuscitation. A great deal of this fluid is sequestered in the interstitial spaces and will remain there until it is gradually mobilized and excreted in 48–72 hours. In addition, inappropriate secretion of antidiuretic hormone results in sodium and water retention. Therefore, maintenance intravenous fluids should be limited to approximately 80 ml/hour or 1 ml/kg body weight per hour of 5% dextrose in half normal saline with 20–30 mEq potassium chloride per liter. When needed, intravenous fluid can always be increased.

2. Some patients are cold and vasoconstricted when they first arrive in the recovery area. As they rewarm and vasodilate, additional fluid may be necessary, indicated by falling urine output, lower blood pressure, tachycardia, and low filling pressures. If hemoglobin is less than 8 g/dl or hematocrit is less than 25%, packed red blood cells should be infused. Otherwise, volume replacement may be made with a bolus (5–10 ml/kg of a balanced salt solution [e.g., Ringer's lactated solution]).

3. When patients begin to mobilize excess fluid on the second or third postoperative day, maintenance intravenous rates may need to be reduced to an amount just sufficient to keep veins open (KVO). If the patient is edematous and urine output has not increased, a small dose (10–20 mg) of furosemide may initiate a good diuresis.

C. Pulmonary care after extubation is discussed in Chap. 10.

D. Wound care requires special attention, since local infection may rapidly extend to a prosthetic graft or cause a bacteremia that could seed the graft surface. Initial dressings should be removed on the first postoperative day. If the wound is sealed, no further dressing is needed. If serosanguineous fluid is still leaking from the wound, a sterile gauze dressing should be applied until the drainage stops. Lymph leaks from groin incisions may be treacherous, since infection of the deeper inguinal lymphatics may also infect an adjacent graft. Most minor lymph leaks will resolve in 3–5 days. If a groin lymph leak is copious and not decreased or closed in 3–5 days, wound exploration and reclosure should be done. Prolonged lymph leakage increases the risk of bacterial invasion of the perigraft lymphatics and may result in an early prosthetic graft infection.

E. The proper time to **ambulate** a patient after aortic or other peripheral arterial reconstruction is another controversial area. Proper timing must be individualized. The following factors must be considered.

1. Many patients are not hemodynamically stable for 24–48 hours. Tachycardia and wide swings in blood pressure are not well tolerated, since many of these patients have heart disease. Immediately after operation, incisional pain may cause tachycardia and hypertension. Within 48–72 hours, mobilization of excess fluids may expand intravascular volume, placing additional stress on the heart. If hemodynamically labile patients attempt to ambulate before tachycardia is controlled and excess fluids are mobilized, they may experience myocardial ischemia or infarction. Myocardial infarction occurs most commonly on the third day after major surgery.

2. If the patient has an inguinal lymph leak, it is most likely to stop if lower-extremity activity is curtailed by bed rest. Since ambulation may be delayed for 24–72 hours, we insist that patients do leg exercises (flexion and extension of calf and thigh muscles) for at least 5 minutes every hour. (Figure 12-5 shows several important features of the patient's bed position and equipment.) These exercises improve venous emptying from calf muscles and thus are prophylaxis for deep venous thrombosis. The leg exercise also increases blood flow to the legs and consequently through any graft. Finally, these exercises help maintain leg muscle tone prior to ambulation. In our experience, delayed ambulation in some patients has not increased either pulmonary complications or venous thromboembolism, provided coughing, deep breathing, and footboard exercises are done routinely.

F. **Convalescence** following major aortic or peripheral arterial surgery generally takes 6–8 weeks. However, patients often expect a quicker recovery. Therefore, we inform them that normal appetite may not return for 3–4 weeks, that their weight may not stabilize for 1 month or so, and that their general strength and well-being may not fully recover for 2–3 months. We generally recheck these patients in the outpatient office 4–6 weeks after discharge from the hospital. The main exception is the need to check wounds and remove skin clips or sutures after early hospital discharge.

G. **Long-term success** of lower-extremity arterial reconstruction and patient survival depends on many factors. For simplicity, we emphasize to the patient three things that we expect him or her to do to ensure long-term success:

1. All tobacco use must be eliminated. Although most patients will stop at the time of operation, at least 50% eventually return to some tobacco use. Those who smoke again are definitely at increased risk of graft

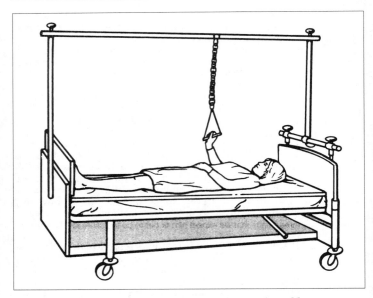

Fig. 12-5. Postoperative bed position following aortic and lower-extremity arterial reconstructions. Important features include a foam mattress to alleviate pressure sores, an overhead trapeze to assist with movement in bed, and a footboard for lower-leg exercises.

   failure and other cardiovascular events, especially myocardial infarction and stroke.

 2. Weight must be controlled with a low-fat, low-cholesterol diet. It often is helpful for a dietitian to discuss such a diet with the patient and family.

 3. Physical and mental activities must be engaged in regularly. Regular exercise, such as walking, maintains cardiorespiratory conditioning and enhances lower-extremity blood flow. Keeping the mind occupied gives the patient a better sense of well-being and productivity. Many patients experience postoperative depression and need reassurance that with time their general strength and well-being will improve. When indications for lower-extremity revascularization are analyzed, 60–70% of previously employed patients with claudication and 50% of patients presenting for limb salvage return to work. The remaining patients are often retired but resume normal daily activities in 6–8 weeks.

 H. Postoperative outpatient checkups are the primary means to determine long-term graft patency and to detect new manifestations of cardiovascular disease at other locations. Reevaluation generally is done at 4–6 weeks after surgery and subsequently at 6 months postoperatively, and then yearly.

IX. Postoperative complications. Early graft-related complications following arterial operations for lower-extremity claudication affect about 3% of patients. Late complications such as anastomotic aneurysm, graft thrombosis, or graft infection are more common, involving approximately 10% of patients. We focus here on the recognition of such complications and the principles of management.

A. Early graft-related complications

1. **Hemorrhage** from an arterial graft anastomosis generally is manifested by a groin or leg hematoma for femoral or popliteal anastomosis and signs of shock for intraabdominal aortic or iliac anastomosis. Treatment is early reoperation, evacuation of the hematoma, and suture control of the bleeding site. Failure to follow this approach may result in infection of the hematoma, eventual pseudoaneurysm formation, or death from hemorrhagic shock.

2. **Thrombosis** may be the result of a technical error at the anastomosis, a thromboembolus, or inadequate runoff to maintain graft flow. Routine perioperative vascular monitoring (see Chap. 9) should recognize thrombosis before severe ischemia occurs. Proper management includes operative reexploration and thromboembolectomy. It often also includes operative arteriography if the adequacy of runoff is questioned.

3. **Infection** of an aortofemoral or femoropopliteal graft often originates in the groin area. In many cases, superficial wound infection may be managed by local drainage and antibiotics if there is no underlying graft infection. If the graft becomes visible in the wound, the graft also must be considered infected. Extensive exposure of the suture line, especially when associated with intermittent hemorrhage, makes removal of the infected graft and either local reconstruction with autogenous grafts or extra-anatomic bypass mandatory.

4. **Colon ischemia** may affect at least 1–5% of patients who undergo aortic reconstruction for occlusive disease. The etiology is inadequate left colon perfusion following inferior mesenteric artery ligation, sometimes exacerbated by low cardiac output states and/or inadequate collateral blood flow from the superior mesenteric or internal iliac arteries. Superficial mucosal or muscularis ischemia usually causes transient diarrhea and resolves spontaneously without mortality. Late colon stricture may occur. Transmural colon ischemia will progress to bowel perforation, sepsis, and death in at least 70% of cases.

   Clinical manifestations vary with the severity of ischemia. Bloody diarrhea, lower abdominal pain, and signs of unexplained sepsis suggest the diagnosis of colon ischemia. Flexible lower-gastrointestinal endoscopy may reveal mild changes of patchy hemorrhage and edema or the more severe signs of ulceration and pseudomembranes. Milder cases need bowel rest, antibiotics, and hydration until the diarrhea resolves. Resection of the necrotic colon is necessary in the presence of severe ischemia manifested by peritonitis or sepsis.

B. Late graft-related complications

1. **Gastrointestinal hemorrhage,** especially hema-teme-sis, in a patient who has received a prosthetic aortic graft must raise a high suspicion of an aortoenteric fistula. Although the initial hemorrhage may stop and not recur for days or weeks, untreated aortoenteric fistulas eventually lead to exsanguination and death. Therefore, such patients should be resuscitated and undergo emergency endoscopy. Aortography in cases of aortoenteric fistula is more often normal than abnormal and thus is not the most helpful diagnostic test. If the source of hemorrhage is located in the stomach or duodenal bulb, appropriate therapy is instituted. However, if no gastric or duodenal lesions are evident and blood is coming from the distal duodenum, the patient should undergo emergency abdominal exploration for diagnosis and repair of a suspected aortoduodenal fistula. Repair generally requires closure of the intestine and removal of the adjacent graft with extraanatomic bypass. If graft-enteric erosion is not associated with local abscess, however, in situ graft replacement, bowel repair, and an omental coverage of the new graft will succeed in 85% of patients according to the experience of Walker, Cooley, and their colleagues in Houston.

   If gastrointestinal hemorrhage is minor, a more elective evaluation may be accomplished. An indium white blood cell scan and computed tomography (CT) scan are sensitive tests for localization of an abnormality at the fistula site. Although arteriography seldom shows the aortoenteric fistula, the arteriogram may demonstrate a local pseudoaneurysm and does provide anatomic information that is useful in reconstruction. Angiography also may delineate other causes of hemorrhage, such as angiodysplasias of the intestine.

2. **Chronic aortic or lower-limb graft infection** may present as an aortoenteric fistula, femoral pseudoaneurysm, groin abscess, or chronically draining sinus tract. Most infections of aortic prostheses originate in the groin and are most commonly caused by *Staphylococcus* species. Although the infection may originate at one anastomosis, it rarely remains localized, spreading its way along the perigraft plane to eventually involve the entire graft.

   Sometimes infection is not obvious and diagnosis is difficult. Infections may be indolent, with negative fluid and blood cultures, no fever, and no leukocytosis. An arteriogram should be done to define the involved anatomy. An indium white blood cell scan may be positive at the infected site. A CT scan or high-resolution ultrasound may define intraabdominal perigraft collections.

   Although removal of a focally infected segment of a graft may succeed in eliminating infection, resolution of many graft infections will require extraction of the entire prosthesis and an extraanatomic bypass. Putting off or limiting operations often allows a local infection to spread, and eventually life-threatening graft hemorrhage or sepsis may occur.

Patients with infected abdominal aortic grafts have discouraging 30-day and 1-year survival rates of 70–80% and 40–50%, respectively. Staged revascularization (i.e., axillofemoral bypass) followed by infected abdominal graft removal in 24–48 hours accounts in part for improved perioperative survival seen in recent series. A recent literature review concluded that mortality is lower when a new remote revascularization precedes removal of an infected abdominal aortic graft or treatment of an aortoenteric erosion or fistula. Such a staged approach substantially reduces major amputation from 40% when graft removal precedes revascularization to 5–10% when the extraanatomic bypass is done first. When extraanatomic revascularization precedes removal of an infected graft, subsequent infection of the new bypass has been rare.

3. **Graft thrombosis** that occurs within a few weeks to months of operation often is the result of some technical problem of graft placement or anastomosis. Graft occlusion after this time generally is caused by disease progression at or beyond the distal anastomosis. Impending graft failure may be recognized by recurrent progressive claudication or falling Doppler ankle pressures, especially after exercise. Duplex ultrasound surveillance is currently an excellent method to detect hemodynamically significant anastomotic or graft stenoses. These warning signs are an indication for arteriography to define correctable lesions before total thrombosis occurs. Reoperations to maintain patency of failing or thrombosed aortofemoral grafts succeed in nearly 80% of patients and result in long-term limb preservation in 60–70%. Operative mortality for revision of femoral anastomotic problems is only 1.5% in our experience.

4. **Anastomotic pseudoaneurysm** occurs most frequently at the common femoral artery. The causative factors are complex and include atherosclerotic deterioration of the artery and anastomotic disruption due to tension, inadequate suture bites, local infection, graft dilation, or suture deterioration. Clinically asymptomatic anastomotic aneurysms of less than 2.5 cm may be safely followed by observation only. However, large false aneurysms or symptomatic aneurysms should be electively repaired before they are complicated by thrombosis, distal emboli, or rupture.

5. **Sexual dysfunction** in men following aortoiliac operations may be manifested by impaired or absent penile erection and lack of ejaculation after otherwise normal coitus. Previously normal sexual function may be altered by the interruption of preaortic sympathetic fibers, the parasympathetic pelvic splanchnic nerves, or the internal iliac artery flow. It is obvious that the surgeon must know whether any sexual dysfunction existed before surgery. If impotence is a significant problem to the patient, he may be referred to a urologist for evaluation and treatment.

6. **Spinal cord ischemia** following operations on the abdominal aorta has been rare and is considered unpredictable. However, a recent review emphasized that the problem appears to occur in patients in whom internal iliac artery perfusion was impaired, when atheromatous embolism is evident, and when early postoperative hypotension or low cardiac output may further compromise marginal spinal cord perfusion.

Selected Reading

Brewster DC, Darling RC. Optimal methods of aorto-iliac reconstruction. *Surgery* 84:739, 1978.

Brewster DC. Clinical and anatomic considerations for surgery in aortoiliac disease and results of surgical treatment. *Circulation* 83(Suppl I): I–42, 1991.

Cambria RP et al. Transperitoneal versus retroperitoneal approach for aortic reconstruction: A randomized prospective study. *J Vasc Surg* 11:314, 1990.

Carter SA et al. Walking ability and ankle systolic pressures: Observations in patients with intermittent claudication in a short-term walking exercise program. *J Vasc Surg* 10:642, 1989.

Couch NP. On the arterial consequences of smoking. *J Vasc Surg* 5:807, 1986.

Crawford ES et al. Aorto-iliac occlusive disease: Factors influencing survival and function following reconstructive operation over a 25-year period. *Surgery* 90:1055, 1981.

Darling RC et al. Is the iliac artery a suitable inflow conduit for iliofemoral occlusive disease: An analysis of 514 aortoiliac reconstructions. *J Vasc Surg* 17:15, 1993.

Dormandy JA, Murray GD. The fate of the claudicant—A prospective study of 1969 claudicants. *Eur J Surg* 5:131, 1991.

Hallett JW Jr, Greenwood LH, Robison JG. Lower extremity arterial disease in young adults: A systematic approach to early diagnosis. *Ann Surg* 202:647, 1985.

O'Hara PJ et al. Surgical management of infected abdominal aortic grafts: Review of a 25-year experience. *J Vasc Surg* 3:725, 1986.

Nevelsteen A, Wouters L, Suy R. Aortofemoral Dacron reconstruction for aorto-iliac occlusive disease: A 25-year survey. *Eur J Vasc Surg* 5:179, 1991.

Reilly LM et al. Improved management of aortic graft infection: The influence of operation sequence and staging. *J Vasc Surg* 5:421, 1987.

Ricco JB. Unilateral iliac artery occlusive disease: A randomized multi-center trial examining direct revascularization versus crossover bypass. *Ann Vasc Surg* 6:209, 1992.

Szilagyi DE et al. A thirty-year survey of the reconstructive surgical treatment of aorto-iliac occlusive disease. *J Vasc Surg* 3:421, 1986.

Threatened Limb Loss

Threatened limb loss is a general term that implies an acute or chronic vascular problem that, if left untreated, may result in an amputation. The term does not specify any particular etiology, and the underlying problem may be diabetic neuropathy, arterial thromboembolism, atherosclerotic arterial occlusive disease, or a peripheral aneurysm thrombosis.

Early recognition of the signs of acute or chronic threatened limb loss and prompt initiation of therapy are necessary if the lower extremity is to be saved. The initial patient evaluation, therefore, must determine whether the patient needs emergency treatment or a more routine diagnostic work-up before therapy begins. This determination is based primarily on the patient history and physical examination (see Chap. 3) supplemented by the results of noninvasive vascular tests (see Chap. 5) and radiologic studies (see Chap. 6).

In Chap. 12, we discussed the management of claudication of the lower extremities. Special attention was given to principles of aortoiliac revascularization (angioplasty or surgery). In this chapter, we concentrate on femoropopliteal and tibial reconstructions, which are more frequently needed for limb salvage. However, since many aortoiliac bypasses also are performed as limb salvage procedures, Chap. 12 should be reviewed in conjunction with this one for a complete overview of lower-extremity arterial revascularization.

I. **Common clinical presentations.** Patients with threatened limb loss generally present with one or more of the following problems:

A. **Chronic rest pain** in the lower extremity may be the first symptom of severe lower leg ischemia (Table 13-1). There are a variety of causes of chronic leg and foot pain; the differential diagnosis includes diabetic neuropathy, osteoarthritis, chronic venous insufficiency, and causalgia-type syndromes. The arterial circulation to the leg may be normal in these conditions.

Certain features suggest the rest pain is ischemic in origin. First, chronic ischemic rest pain is localized primarily to the forefoot and not above the ankle. Second, the forefoot generally has rubor on dependency and pallor on elevation. Third, pedal pulses are absent. **Chronic ischemic rest pain usually does not occur unless the patient has at least two hemodynamically significant arterial occlusive lesions.** Most individuals with rest pain will have one of two distinct anatomic patterns of occlusive disease (Fig. 13-1). The physician or surgeon must identify which anatomic pattern exists in order to select the proper therapy.

1. Combined aortoiliac and superficial femoral arterial occlusive disease, or

2. A femoropopliteal arterial occlusion with distal tibial occlusive disease.

B. **Nonhealing skin ulcers** of the foot or lower leg also may be the result of arterial insufficiency. However, in the presence

Table 13-1. Clinical categories of chronic limb ischemia

Grade	Category	Clinical description	Objective criteria
0	0	Asymptomatic—no hemodynamically significant occlusive disease	Normal treadmill/stress test
I	1	Mild claudication	Completes treadmill exercise*; AP after exercise <50 mm Hg
	2	Moderate claudication	Between categories 1 and 3
	3	Severe claudication	Cannot complete treadmill exercise and AP after exercise <50 mm Hg
II	4	Ischemic rest pain	Resting AP <40 mm Hg, flat or barely pulsatile ankle or metatarsal PVR; TP <30 mm Hg
III	5	Minor tissue loss—nonhealing ulcer, focal gangrene with diffuse pedal ischemia	Resting AP <60 mm Hg, ankle or metatarsal PVR flat or barely pulsatile; TP <40 mm Hg
	6	Major tissue loss—extending above TM level, functional foot no longer salvageable	Same as category 5

AP = ankle pressure; BP = brachial pressure; PVR = pulse volume recording; TP = toe pressure; TM = transmetatarsal.
*Five minutes at 2 mph on a 12% incline.
Source: Modified from RB Rutherford et al. Suggested standards for reports dealing with lower extremity ischemia. *J Vasc Surg* 4:80, 1986.

of adequate arterial perfusion, healing may be retarded by local cellulitis, underlying osteomyelitis, traumatic pressure from improper footwear, or improper medical treatment. A good history and physical examination should provide adequate information for sorting out the various reasons for poor healing. Because of peripheral sensory neuropathy, diabetics are especially susceptible to foot ulcers. Unfortunately, they often do not feel the initial sore and consequently may not present until the ulcer is deep and infected.

   C. **Gangrene** is the classic sign of inadequate blood supply to the skin and subcutaneous tissue. Dry gangrene is characterized by a noninfected black eschar. Wet gangrene is associated with tissue maceration and purulence.
   D. **Microemboli** cause distinctive bluish, mottled spots that often are randomly scattered over the toes. They are usu-

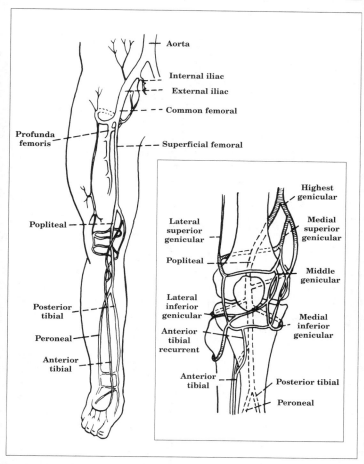

Fig. 13-1. Arterial anatomy of the leg and popliteal region.

ally painful. They also may be mistaken for local traumatic bruises, so their true significance may be overlooked. Microemboli may originate from any point in the proximal arterial system. Most commonly they arise from the heart, aneurysms, or ulcerated plaques.

E. Acute arterial ischemia (Table 13-2) is characterized by the sudden onset of extremity pain, pallor, paresthesia, pulselessness, and sometimes paralysis. If the patient has a history of claudication or a previous lower-extremity arterial graft, the acute symptoms may be caused by thrombosis of a stenotic artery or the arterial graft. **If the patient previously had no symptoms of peripheral vascular disease, the acute ischemia is more probably caused by a thromboembolus to the leg.**

Table 13-2. Clinical categories of acute limb ischemia

Category	Description	Capillary return	Muscle weakness	Sensory loss	Doppler signals	
					Arterial	Venous
Viable	Not immediately threatened	Intact	None	None	Audible (AP >30 mm Hg)	Audible
Threatened	Salvageable if promptly treated	Intact, slow	Mild, partial	Mild, incomplete	Inaudible	Audible
Irreversible	Major tissue loss, amputation regardless of treatment	Absent (marbling)	Profound, paralysis (rigor)	Profound, anesthetic	Inaudible	Inaudible

AP = ankle pressure.
Source: Modified from RB Rutherford et al. Suggested standards for reports dealing with lower extremity ischemia. *J Vasc Surg* 4:80, 1986.

II. Diagnostic evaluation. A number of diagnostic tests may help determine the optimum treatment for the threatened limb. Tests should be carefully selected to provide the maximum amount of information with the minimum amount of discomfort and delay for the patient, who often is experiencing considerable chronic or acute pain.

   A. Noninvasive vascular testing. The Doppler system and a pulse volume recording (PVR) are simple yet accurate methods to determine the criteria for ischemic rest pain and the likelihood of healing (see Chap. 5). Ischemic rest pain generally is associated with a Doppler ankle pressure below 35 mm Hg in nondiabetics and below 55 mm Hg in diabetics. Ischemic rest pain is unlikely when ankle pressures exceed 55 mm Hg in the nondiabetic and 80 mm Hg in the diabetic. Foot ulcers that are not infected and not associated with osteomyelitis have a favorable chance of healing if the ankle pressure is above 65 mm Hg in the nondiabetic and above 90 mm Hg in the diabetic. Ankle and forefoot PVRs that are less than 5 mm or flat are predictive of ischemic rest pain and poor tissue healing. Resting supine transcutaneous oxygen (TcO_2) measurements of less than 20–30 mm Hg are indicative of severe ischemia, especially if forefoot TcO_2 levels fall to less than 10 mm Hg with leg elevation. Postoperative measurements can be used to assess the adequacy of revascularization.

   B. Plain x-ray of the bone underlying a skin ulcer may show signs of osteomyelitis. These signs include bone rarefaction, periosteal elevation, and new bone formation. A bone scan is indicated when osteomyelitis seems likely but a plain x-ray is negative. Bone changes may not be apparent until osteomyelitis has been active for 2–3 weeks.

   C. Cultures and **Gram's stains** should be made of all ulcers to identify the predominant organism. Histologic stain also may reveal fungi.

   D. An **electrocardiogram** (ECG) is essential when arterial embolism is suspected, since atrial fibrillation with a mural thrombus is a common underlying condition. For cases in which intermittent arrhythmia is suspected, a 24-hour continuous ECG monitor (Holter) may be used.

   E. An **echocardiogram** should be done as part of the diagnostic work-up for arterial embolism that may originate from the heart. The echocardiogram may reveal a diseased heart valve or a mural thrombus.

   F. Ultrasound of the abdominal aorta also should be performed in the evaluation of thromboemboli, since emboli may be shed from a thrombus in an abdominal aortic aneurysm. If a femoral or popliteal aneurysm is suspected as a result of physical examination, ultrasound is an accurate method to confirm peripheral aneurysms that also may shed emboli or acutely thrombose, placing the leg in jeopardy.

   G. Arteriography remains the definitive method to delineate the exact level of arterial occlusion and to define vascular anatomy that must be known before selecting a proper intervention (i.e., thrombolytic therapy, balloon angioplasty, or surgical revascularization). If the femoral pulses are weak or absent, an aortogram with runoff is needed. If femoral pulses are normal and the arterial occlusive disease appears localized to the leg alone, a transfemoral arteriogram of the affected leg may suffice. A femoral artery pressure study may be done to assess the adequacy of the proximal aortoiliac inflow (see Chap. 6). Routine angiography may not clearly visualize distal tibial or plantar arch vessels and thus will discourage any attempt at revascularization. However, we have found that simple preoperative transcutaneous Doppler examination will usually reveal which tibial arteries are patent at the ankle and which one has the best flow signals. Although the presence of a patent pedal arch on arteriography was once considered predictive of success for femorodistal bypass, more recent studies report reasonable patency rates and limb salvage in patients in whom the pedal arch appears absent or diseased.

H. Coagulation and **platelet function** should be analyzed in all patients who present with atypical arterial thrombosis. This group includes young adults (age 20–40) with severe arterial occlusive disease and other individuals with recurrent arterial thromboembolism that cannot be explained by common etiologies. Antithrombin deficiency has been documented as one cause of unexplained thrombosis and graft failure. In some cases of recurrent arterial thrombosis, a familial enhanced platelet aggregability has been identified. Plasminogen abnormalities should also be considered. Other coagulation defects that must be checked include protein C and protein S deficiencies, anticardiolipin antibody, lupus-like anticoagulant, and antiphospholipid antibody.

III. Management may begin after it has been determined by the initial patient evaluation whether the patient has acute or chronic threatened limb loss. In our experience, the following principles of treatment provide the best assurance of limb salvage.

A. Acutely threatened limb loss usually is caused by a thromboembolus, popliteal aneurysm thrombosis, or a sudden graft occlusion. Thrombosis of a chronic arterial stenosis may cause temporary pain, pallor, and paresthesia, but usually it does not progress to paralysis. In fact, these acute symptoms often rapidly resolve in minutes to a few hours because of previously developing collateral vessels.

1. Immediate treatment should include systemic heparinization (5,000–10,000 units IV, then 1,000 units/hour) to prevent further propagation of thrombi. If leg pain is severe, a narcotic may be administered while further tests are being arranged.

2. Initial diagnostic tests should include routine blood counts, electrolytes, glucose, and baseline coagulation studies (prothrombin time, partial thromboplastin time, and platelet count). An ECG should be done to check for atrial fibrillation and any sign of acute myocardial infarction.

A Doppler flow detector may be used to localize the level of obstruction and record ankle pressures. The absence of ankle Doppler signals almost always means that urgent surgical intervention will be necessary. If the ankle has monophasic Doppler signals and the foot has sensation and movement, 2–3 hours of observation is acceptable. If the leg does not continue to improve during this time, surgical intervention will be necessary.

3. An **emergency arteriogram** usually is performed to determine the location of the arterial occlusion as well as the inflow and outflow on either side. However, arterial exploration in the operating room should be undertaken immediately if the acute occlusion is clearly an embolus. Intraoperative arteriograms can be performed if necessary. Time is an important factor in acute arterial occlusion, since irreversible nerve and muscle damage may occur within 6 hours.

4. The **choice of operation** for an acute arterial occlusion will depend on the underlying etiology. **Thromboembolectomy** with Fogarty balloon catheters is the operation of choice for thromboemboli. Adequate thrombectomy of the femoral or iliac arteries can be accomplished through a femoral arteriotomy. A popliteal embolus should generally be extracted through a popliteal arteriotomy, so that each individual tibial artery may be checked for clot. Passing a catheter from the groin will not necessarily clean out all the tibial arteries. Extracted thromboemboli should be sent for pathologic examination, since occasionally arterial tumor embolism will be the first manifestation of an atrial myxoma. After embolectomy, the patient should be continued on heparin, followed by long-term warfarin sodium (Coumadin) therapy.

If the acute arterial ischemia is caused by a graft occlusion, **graft thrombectomy** may be possible. Generally graft occlusions are the result of an intrinsic graft or juxta-anastomotic stenosis. Consequently the thrombectomy will not succeed unless the stenosis is corrected simultaneously.

Bypass grafting of an arteriosclerotic occlusion of the iliac or superficial femoral artery may be necessary to salvage the acutely ischemic leg. A few seriously ill cardiac patients who are dependent on a transfemoral intraaortic balloon assist device will develop limb-threatening ischemia. An emergency femorofemoral bypass may be necessary if the balloon must remain in place for cardiac support.

Finally, an acute arterial thrombosis or graft occlusion may be opened by **thrombolysis** with streptokinase, tissue plasminogen activator, or urokinase (see Chap. 6). This method of treatment must be used on carefully selected patients by physicians familiar with the administration of these agents and their bleeding complications. After thrombolysis, balloon angioplasty may be used to correct a causative focal arterial steno-

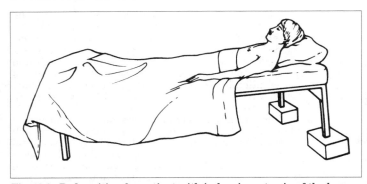

Fig. 13-2. Bed position for patient with ischemic rest pain of the lower extremity. The head of the bed is elevated 6 inches to improve arterial perfusion of the pedal circulation by gravity. Sheets are draped over a footboard to alleviate pressure on the feet.

sis. Although we were initially enthusiastic about thrombolytic therapy for occluded grafts and still use it initially in some patients, bleeding and thromboembolic complications have caused us to favor surgical thrombectomy plus graft revision or replacement in most cases. Surgical correction of the causative arterial lesion is usually necessary to ensure long-term graft patency even after thrombolysis. Occasionally we use intraoperative urokinase (250,000–500,000 units) infused intraarterially into a thrombosed tibial outflow tract where Fogarty balloon thromboembolectomy has been incomplete.

B. Chronic threatened limb loss generally is associated with arteriosclerotic occlusive disease of the aortoiliac region, femoropopliteal segment, or distal tibial arteries.

   1. Foot protection from further injury is the first order of care. The heel should be protected from pressure sores by a soft gauze pad (ABD pad) secured with a gauze roll, **not** tape. Commercially made vascular "boots" (e.g., Rooke boot) are also available. Lamb's wool or gauze pads should be placed between the toes to prevent "kissing" ulcers caused by toes and toenails rubbing against one another. A lanolin-base lotion should be applied daily to the foot to keep the skin soft and prevent cracking, especially over the heel. If pressure bothers the foot, bed sheets may be draped over a footboard (Fig. 13-2). Elevating the head of the bed 6 inches may relieve ischemic rest pain by the simple effect of gravity on arterial perfusion. We do not recommend so-called metal bed cradles or tents, as a patient may inadvertently abrade the lower leg or foot against the metal frame, causing skin ulceration.

   2. Preventive foot care must be taught to the patient (see Chap. 14).

   3. Local infection should be controlled before insertion of synthetic bypass grafts. Local debridement of infected toes and parenteral antibiotics should precede graft procedures by several days. Otherwise, graft infection may occur in the groin, where lymphatics may be laden with bacteria.

4. **Arteriography** is discussed in sec. **II.G** and in Chap. 6.

5. The **choice of operation or percutaneous transluminal angioplasty** depends on the location of the occlusive disease and the condition of the patient.

   a. **Combined severe aortoiliac and femoropopliteal occlusive disease** should be treated by bypass grafts of the aortoiliac disease. When the superficial femoral artery is diseased, the femoral anastomosis should be carried down onto the profunda femoris artery. Long-term limb salvage will be accomplished in the majority of patients by aortofemoral bypass alone. Approximately 20% of patients, however, will need an additional distal bypass. Determining which patients will need simultaneous aortofemoral and femoropopliteal bypasses is not always easy. Preoperative factors that suggest a combined procedure is indicated are extensive below-the-knee femoropopliteal-tibial occlusions combined with open foot lesions and an ankle pressure below 30 mm Hg. In high-risk patients, extraanatomic axillofemoral or femorofemoral bypass may be used to correct severe iliac occlusive disease.

   b. **Occlusive disease of the common femoral artery, profunda orifice, and superficial femoral artery** may be managed by local endarterectomy and profundaplasty. Profundaplasty is most likely to succeed when (1) aortoiliac inflow is normal, (2) the distal profunda femoris artery is normal and has well-developed collateral pathways to the popliteal artery, and (3) the popliteal artery is patent with at least two- to three-vessel runoff. This anatomic situation is not common, so we seldom use profundaplasty as the primary operation for limb salvage.

   c. **Femoropopliteal artery occlusion** can be managed by bypass grafting, endarterectomy, or percutaneous transluminal angioplasty. Our method of choice is saphenous vein bypass grafting, since this operation has proved superior to endarterectomy and synthetic bypasses. Current synthetic choices for femoropopliteal bypass include Dacron, human umbilical vein, and polytetrafluoroethylene (PTFE). These grafts provide excellent long-term patency when the distal anastomosis is above the knee, but significantly poorer patency is found in below-the-knee anastomosis. In a prospective multicenter randomized comparison of autologous saphenous vein and expanded PTFE grafts, primary patency of vein was clearly superior to PTFE for infrapopliteal bypass (49% versus 12% at 4 years). However, there was no significant difference in limb salvage (vein versus PTFE, 57% versus 61%). Although 2-year patency was similar for both grafts to the popliteal artery (64–70%), vein was superior at 5 years (vein, 68%; PTFE, 38%). Umbilical vein grafts have had a patency rate similar to PTFE, but umbilical grafts may manifest aneurysmal degeneration in long-term follow-up. Percutaneous transluminal angioplasty can recanalize total superficial femoral artery occlusions of less than 10 cm long and may be the first procedure to attempt in seriously ill patients who need limb salvage (see Chap. 6).

d. Some poor-risk patients will have **both an iliac stenosis and a superficial femoral artery occlusion.** A combined aortofemoral and femoropopliteal procedure carries a high rate of morbidity and mortality for them. A good alternative is transluminal dilatation of the iliac stenosis, followed by femoropopliteal bypass under regional (e.g., epidural) anesthesia.

e. The most challenging group of patients who require operation for limb salvage have **severe distal tibial and peroneal occlusive disease.** It appears that acceptable long-term patency (50–60% at 5 years) and excellent limb salvage rates (50–73% at 5 years) may be achieved by femorotibial, femoroperoneal, and pedal vein bypass grafts. Multisegment femorodistal occlusive disease also has been successfully treated by sequential anastomoses of a vein graft to several patent segments. **Patency of femoroinfrapopliteal vein bypasses is comparable for each tibial artery and is similar in diabetics and nondiabetics.** Whether in situ or reversed saphenous vein is better remains controversial.

Several factors have rejuvenated enthusiasm for **in situ saphenous vein bypass grafting** after its original description in 1962 (Fig. 13-3). Its proponents claim a higher use of smaller veins, a lesser degree of endothelial damage, better size match at the anastomoses, improved hemodynamics, and superior early and late patency. Recently, these advantages have been challenged. Current series show similar early and late patency rates for in situ versus reversed infrapopliteal bypasses (1-year, 87–90%; 3-year, 82–85%; and 5-year, 77–85%). Preparation of vein grafts and the technique of anastomoses are probably more important than whether the vein is in situ or reversed. In our practice, the most appealing advantages of the in situ technique have been higher use of small veins (3–4 mm) and the technical ease of leaving the vein in situ and using the smaller end for the distal anastomosis.

Because a vein remains the best conduit for early and late patency, extra effort to obtain a suitable vein seems justified. These options include the con-

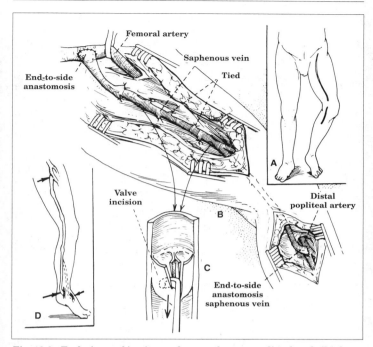

Fig. 13-3. Technique of in situ saphenous femoropopliteal and tibial bypass grafting. A. Greater saphenous vein is exposed through one or two long incisions along the medial aspect of the thigh and calf. B. Saphenous vein is left in its natural bed. Its valves are cut with special instruments. C. Its branches are tied to prevent arteriovenous fistulas. Proximal anastomosis is made to the common femoral or superficial femoral artery, and distal anastomosis is constructed to the distal popliteal artery or to the tibial or peroneal branches. D. Long bypasses to the level of the ankle are possible by this technique.

tralateral leg vein, arm veins, composite synthetic and vein grafts, and shorter bypasses using less vein (e.g., popliteal-tibial or tibiotibial bypasses). In our experience, vein grafts to isolated popliteal segments have been a good alternative to femorodistal bypass in certain patients. These grafts have a 5-year patency rate similar to femorotibial bypasses (65% versus 66%, respectively). Provided that tissue necrosis of the foot is not extensive, such grafts are adequate to relieve severe ischemia, especially when a limited length of vein is available and the tibial arteries appear marginal for a suitable distal anastomosis.

f. With the increasing age of the general population, more elderly patients are presenting **with ischemic rest pain and gangrene of the foot.** Attempts to salvage such a limb usually require a long hospitalization and considerable expense. However, limb salvage is possible in 70% at 1 year and 60% at 3 years, but generally about 30% at 5 years after surgery. Successful revascularization results in lower costs than primary amputation. In patients over 80 years of age, limb salvage is comparable to younger groups, with a 3-year survival of about 50% and a limb preservation rate of 70%. Consequently, present data support an attempt at arterial reconstruction in most elderly patients with severe ischemia. Primary amputation is appropriate when gangrene extensively involves the forefoot and heel. Whether a failed below-knee femoropopliteal bypass changes the level of amputation depends on numerous factors, but generally an unsuccessful reconstruction does not alter final amputation level.

  g. Sympathectomy alone generally is not sufficient to salvage many limbs at risk. Good relief of rest pain has been achieved when the preoperative ankle-brachial artery pressure index is relatively high (i.e., >0.35). Results are less favorable when tissue necrosis is present.

  h. Creation of a **distal arteriovenous fistula** as an adjunct to maintaining arterial and synthetic bypass graft patency remains controversial. The physiologic advantage of this technique is questionable; consequently, we have not embraced it.

6. Angioscopy has been evaluated as an adjunct to in situ vein grafting, arterial embolectomy, femoropopliteal bypass surgery, and laser recanalization. Clinical trials by Miller and colleagues at Harvard have supported its effectiveness, but the technology has had a limited impact so far in most practices.

IV. Perioperative care

A. Preoperative preparation. The routine laboratory tests for limb salvage cases are the same studies outlined for aortic cases in Chap. 12. The patient should be typed and cross-matched preoperatively for 2 units of packed red blood cells. All patients should take nothing by mouth after midnight and should be hydrated with an intravenous infusion (5% dextrose in Ringer's lactated solution, 100–125 ml/hour) before operation. Skin preparation should include the abdomen and both legs, since an opposite leg vein sometimes is harvested. We recommend a cephalosporin or semisynthetic penicillin as a prophylactic antibiotic to be administered as the patient goes to the operating room.

B. Intraoperative care. Certain points of intraoperative patient care and surgical management deserve mention.

  1. Patient positioning. Most lower-extremity arterial revascularizations are performed with the patient supine. The heels must be protected from pressure sores by elevating the calves on soft towels or placing soft pads on the heels. If the pulse volume recorder is being used for intraoperative monitoring of lower-extremity perfusion, the PVR cuffs should be placed at the ankles and baseline tracings should be recorded (see Chap. 9).

2. **Surgical exposure.** Certain features of surgical exposure facilitate anastomotic construction and prevent postoperative wound complications.

   a. The incisions for exposure of the **great saphenous vein** must be made directly over the vein. There is a tendency to bevel the incision and bring it too far anterior to the course of the vein. The result is medial skin flap necrosis.

   b. The **above-knee popliteal artery** can be exposed through a medial distal thigh incision going over the top (lateral) edge of the sartorius muscle and then beneath the adductor magnus tendon. **Three noteworthy anatomic features occur at the adductor magnus tendon: the superficial femoral artery becomes the popliteal artery, the supreme geniculate artery (an important collateral) originates from the proximal popliteal artery, and the saphenous nerve becomes superficial.** Injury to the nerve can result in a bothersome chronic medial leg neuralgia.

   c. The **below-knee popliteal artery** can be exposed via a medial proximal leg incision just below the knee joint. The medial head of the gastrocnemius muscle must be retracted inferiorly. The popliteal vein and tibial nerve are also medial and posterior to the artery. More extensive exposure of the popliteal artery may require detachment of the semimembranosus and semitendinosus muscle tendons.

   d. Occasionally the **entire popliteal artery** requires exposure for repair of a large popliteal aneurysm (Fig. 13-4). This generous exposure allows easier and safer performance of aneurysm evacuation and obliteration of feeding collaterals into the aneurysm sac.

   The tendons can be anatomically reattached at the conclusion of the operation. Such an extensive exposure appears to increase postoperative leg edema but does not result in knee instability in most patients.

   e. The **tibioperoneal trunk and proximal posterior tibial artery** can be exposed through the medial knee approach by detaching some of the soleus muscle from the tibia. Exposure of the proximal anterior tibial artery generally requires a separate anterior lateral leg incision, which is made approximately one finger-breadth lateral to the edge of the tibia and carried 8–10 cm distally. The artery is located in the groove between the anterior tibial and extensor digitorum longus muscles.

   f. Bypasses can also be taken to the pedal arteries (Fig.13-5) in selected patients. The most common pedal arterial target for distal anastomosis is the dorsalis pedis artery followed by the common plantar and lateral plantar arteries.

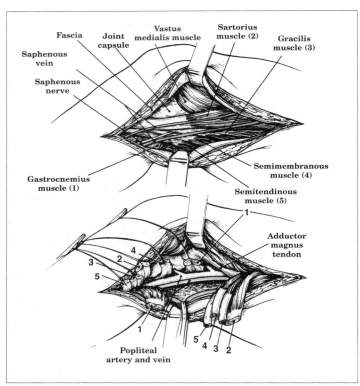

Fig. 13-4. Medial approach to the popliteal artery. The saphenous nerve should be gently retracted to minimize postoperative saphenous neuralgia. Division of the medial knee tendons and medial head of the gastrocnemius muscle provides clear popliteal artery exposure with minimal morbidity. Most patients have a single great saphenous vein, although an accessory saphenous vein may be present as this illustration indicates.

3. **Preparation of the saphenous vein.** Endothelial damage during preparation of saphenous vein grafts is an important factor in early and late graft failure. Optimum preparation includes gentle dissection of the vein, careful ligation of side branches away from the vein wall, minimal warm ischemia time if the vein is removed from the leg, and limited distention. Gentle dilation of the vein can be achieved with a papaverine solution (1 ml [30 mg] of papaverine in 9 ml of saline). Immersion of the vein in cold Ringer's lactate or blood also minimizes endothelial damage.

4. **Distal arterial control** can be accomplished with minimal damage to the arteries by using a **pneumatic thigh tourniquet** inflated to 300 mm Hg after the

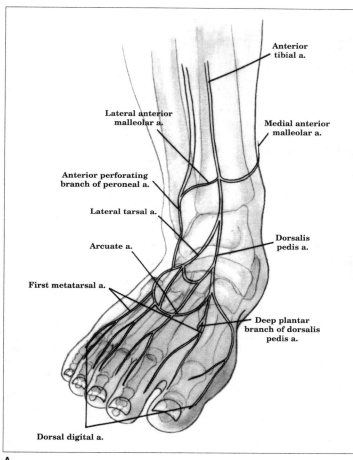

A

Fig. 13-5. Anatomy of the pedal arteries. A. Dorsum of foot. B. Plantar surface of foot. (Adapted from P Gloviczki et al. Prospective evaluation of 100 consecutive microscope-aided pedal bypasses revealed an effective and low risk operation to salvage the ischemic foot. *Am J Surg* 168:76, 1994.)

lower limb is wrapped tightly with an elastic Esmarch's bandage.
5. **Anastomotic technique** should emphasize a long gentle anastomotic angle to minimize turbulence. Distal popliteal and tibial arterial anastomoses are constructed more accurately under low-power magnification.
6. **Vascular monitoring.** See Chap. 9.
7. **Postoperative dressings** should be applied so that they are not constricting at the knee. A tight dressing

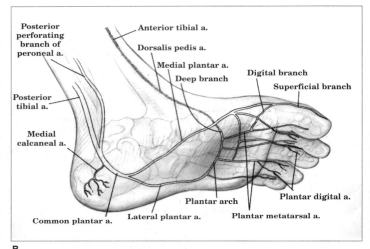

B
Fig. 13-5 *(cont.)*

can compress a graft enough to diminish or occlude blood flow.

C. **Postoperative care.** Patients generally should remain under intensive observation for at least 6–12 hours after lower-extremity revascularization. It is during this immediate postoperative period that most early graft occlusions occur, so hourly checks of pedal pulses, PVRs, or Doppler ankle pressures should be made. To enhance early perioperative patency, we generally use low-molecular weight dextran 40 for 24 hours. Our regimen has been a 100-ml IV in the recovery room and 20 ml/hour for one 500-ml bottle. Subsequently, patients receive aspirin, 80–325 mg qid, and low-dose heparin, 5,000 units subcutaneously, until discharge. Long-term anticoagulation with warfarin and children's aspirin (80 mg) is often used for below-knee synthetic grafts and redo grafts to the tibial arteries.

Guidelines for postoperative laboratory tests, fluid administration, and antibiotic use are outlined in Chap. 12.

1. **Postoperative day 1.** The initial dressings should be removed, and new dressings are applied only if serosanguineous or lymph drainage continues. Strict bed rest is continued for any patient with a popliteal or tibial bypass. Lower-extremity footboard exercises are done every hour to increase lower-extremity arterial and venous flow. Those patients with severe popliteal artery trifurcation and distal disease must be monitored closely for perioperative myocardial and cerebral ischemia. The incidence of myocardial infarction and cerebrovascular events appears higher in this anatom-

ic subgroup than in patients with only superficial femoral arterial occlusive disease.

2. **Postoperative days 2–5.** Bed rest for 1–2 days allows the early popliteal space and calf swelling to resolve. The initial incisional pain usually is improved enough by the second or third postoperative day to allow comfortable ambulation. Some patients with more distal tibial bypasses to the ankle or foot may require 3–5 days of bed rest before pedal and ankle edema has resolved sufficiently to allow ambulation. If such patients are ambulated too early, swelling may compromise or disrupt tenuous incisions. Continuous epidural anesthesia followed by epidural analgesia for 24–48 hours has been an excellent method in our experience to keep these patients comfortable. Initially, we encourage the patient to use crutches or a walker to help with weight-bearing. We discourage prolonged sitting, since this position worsens early postoperative leg swelling. Most patients will have lower-leg edema for 6 weeks to several months after lower-extremity revascularization. Below-the-knee support hose may alleviate this swelling.

3. **Associated amputations.** Some patients will require an amputation after lower-extremity arterial reconstruction to remove necrotic tissue that was present before surgery. Whether associated amputations should be done simultaneously with arterial reconstruction is debatable. Certainly, infected lesions or abscesses need debridement and drainage prior to grafting. Superficial dry gangrene may autoamputate after foot circulation is improved. Thus, we normally wait 5–7 days after arterial reconstruction to perform necessary digital or foot amputations. This time seems to allow better demarcation of the proper amputation level. Although this approach has been our general philosophy, we have combined femoropopliteal revascularization with toe or forefoot amputations in selected patients.

V. **Postoperative complications**

A. **Early problems.** As with aortoiliac reconstructions, the most common early postoperative graft-related complications in limb salvage cases are hemorrhage, thrombosis, and infection.

1. **Hemorrhage** usually follows one of two patterns. In the first pattern, bleeding frequently occurs within 24 hours from the vein graft or an anastomosis. Early repair and hematoma evacuation usually do not lead to graft failure or infection. The second pattern of postoperative hemorrhage occurs from 3–28 days after operation and in most cases is caused by graft infection. Hemorrhage usually occurs at the proximal or distal anastomosis. These patients are at greater risk of eventual limb loss.

2. **Thrombosis** in the first 24 hours after operation is most often the result of a technical problem, most commonly a poorly constructed anastomosis. Other possi-

ble technical problems include graft kinking, extrinsic muscle or tendon compression, elevation of an intimal flap, or clamp injury to a proximal or distal artery. Some frequent causes of early thrombosis other than technical problems are inadequate outflow and inadequate vein graft size (<4 mm). Occasionally early graft thrombosis is due to a previously unknown hypercoaguability. In our experience, the long-term prognosis of early graft failure has been poor, even if the graft is successfully opened.

3. **Infection** usually occurs in the groin. The most common underlying factors are obesity and fat necrosis or hematoma after operation. If the infection is superficial and the graft is not exposed, the graft usually can be salvaged by local wound care and antibiotics. Deeper infection, especially involving a synthetic graft, may lead to serious hemorrhage. Therefore, graft removal and extraanatomic bypass when possible are the preferred methods of management.

4. **Compartment syndrome** is caused by prolonged ischemia (>8–12 hours) that is present before lower-extremity revascularization and that may cause serious swelling of the calf muscles. Since these muscles are enveloped in fixed fascial compartments, swelling may lead to myonecrosis and permanent nerve damage. The anterior compartment is most susceptible to this ischemic syndrome. The earliest clinical signs are lower-leg pain with decreased skin sensation on the dorsum of the foot between the first and second toes (deep peroneal nerve) and weakness of toe dorsiflexion. Optimum treatment is fasciotomy. Prophylactic fasciotomy should be considered for all cases of acute arterial ischemia in which revascularization is delayed beyond 6–8 hours.

5. **Femoral nerve injury** may occur after groin operations, especially in repeat procedures or extensive dissections of the profunda femoris artery. The injury may not be apparent until the patient tries to ambulate and discovers that the knee joint cannot be extended because of quadriceps weakness. Treatment requires a flexible knee brace. Many femoral nerve apraxias will resolve in 3–6 months.

B. **Late problems.** Late postoperative graft-related complications occur in about 30% of patients who undergo arterial procedures below the inguinal ligament. The most common problem is graft thrombosis. Two main factors seem to contribute to late graft failure. One factor is progression of atherosclerotic disease in proximal and distal arteries. However, increasing evidence documents that alterations in the vein graft may also eventually lead to graft thrombosis. Mills and colleagues have emphasized that 10–15% of reversed saphenous vein grafts develop a hemodynamically significant inflow, intrinsic graft or outflow stenosis at a mean follow-up of 2 years. The peak incidence of early hemodynamic graft failure occurs within 12 months of graft implantation. Intrinsic graft stenosis causes the majority of failures (60%). These lesions are predominantly focal intimal hyperplasia distributed equally at the proximal and distal juxta-anastomotic areas. The remaining causes are inflow failure (13%), outflow failure (9%), muscle entrapment (4%), and hypercoagulable state (4%).

If these vein graft alterations are detected before graft thrombosis, successful repair and long-term patency can be accomplished in 75–85% of cases over 5 years. **Current emphasis is on detecting failing grafts before they occlude.** Periodic reevaluation (3–6 months) should focus on any recurrent symptoms and objective signs of a failing graft. These signs include a 0.15 fall in the ankle-brachial pressure index. Important duplex ultrasound predictors of graft failure include a decrease in peak systolic flow velocity to less than 45 cm/second in the graft plus an increased peak systolic velocity across a stenotic area (2–3 × normal graft velocity).

When infrainguinal bypasses fail, reoperative surgery can achieve extended limb salvage in about 50% of patients. Late cumulative graft patency is better for revised, pseudo-occluded grafts than revised, thrombosed grafts (65–75% versus 5–15% at 5 years). There is a significant improvement in early patency rates when a new bypass graft is inserted as compared to thrombectomy and patch angioplasty of the original graft.

Selected Reading

Abbott WM et al. Arterial embolism: A 44-year perspective. *Am J Surg* 143:460, 1982.

Andros G et al. Arm veins for arterial revascularization of the leg: Arteriographic and clinical observations. *J Vasc Surg* 4:416, 1986.

Bandyk DF et al. Monitoring functional patency of *in situ* saphenous vein bypasses: The impact of a surveillance protocol and elective revision. *J Vasc Surg* 9:296, 1989.

Brewster DC et al. Factors affecting patency of femoropopliteal bypass grafts. *Surg Gynecol Obstet* 157:437, 1983.

Brewster DC, LaSalle AJ, Robison JG, Darling RC. Femoropopliteal graft failures: Clinical consequences and success of secondary reconstructions. *Arch Surg* 118:1043, 1983.

Gloviczki P et al. Prospective evaluation of 100 consecutive microscope-aided pedal bypasses revealed an effective and low risk operation to salvage the ischemic foot. *Am J Surg* 168:76, 1994.

Green RM et al. Revision of failed infrainguinal bypass graft: Principles of management. *Surgery* 100:646, 1986.

Mills JL, Fugitani MD, Taylor SM. The characteristics and anatomic distribution of lesions that cause reversed vein graft failure: A five-year prospective study. *J Vasc Surg* 17:195, 1993.

Moody AP, Edwards PR, Harris PL. *In situ* versus reversed femoropopliteal vein grafts: Long-term follow-up of a prospective, randomized, trial. *Br J Surg* 79:750, 1992.

Harris PL et al. Prospective randomized comparison of in-situ and reversed infrapopliteal vein grafts. *Br J Surg* 80:173, 1993.

Leather RP, Shah DM, Chang BB, Kaufman JL. Ressurection of the *in situ* saphenous vein bypass: 1000 cases later. *Ann Surg* 208:435, 1992.

Ouriel K et al. A comparison of thrombolytic therapy with operative revascularization in the initial treatment of acute peripheral arterial ischemia. *J Vasc Surg* 19:1021, 1994.

Pevec WC, Darling RC, L'Italien GJ, Abbott WM. Femoropopliteal reconstruction with knitted, nonvelour Dacron versus expanded polytetrafluoroethylene. *J Vasc Surg* 16:60, 1992.

Taylor RS et al. Improved technique for polytetrafluoroethylene bypass grafting: Long-term results using anastomotic vein patches. *Br J Surg* 79:348, 1992.

Veith FJ et al. Six-year prospective multicenter randomized comparison of autologous saphenous vein and expanded polytetrafluoroethylene grafts in infrainguinal arterial reconstructions. *J Vasc Surg* 3:104, 1986.

Veterans Administration Cooperative Study Group. Johnson WC. Comparative evaluation of PTFE, HUV, and saphenous vein in fempop AK vascular reconstruction. *J Vasc Surg* 15:1070, 1992.

Foot Care

Foot sores can become major problems in patients with diabetes mellitus or atherosclerotic peripheral vascular disease. Serious infection and extensive tissue necrosis may complicate apparently minor foot lesions. Too frequently, the eventual outcome is amputation. Proper foot care can prevent many foot problems that threaten the lower extremity. Unfortunately, numerous patients never learn the basic principles of foot care because many physicians have received minimal formal instruction in this area. The purpose of this chapter, then, is to summarize general principles of foot care.

I. **Magnitude of the problem.** Foot problems due to diabetic neuropathy or arterial ischemia not only consume a great deal of the patient's time but also devastate financial resources if prolonged hospital care is required. Foot lesions are the primary problem of one of every five diabetics who are hospitalized. About 50% of diabetics who have one leg amputated eventually will lose the other extremity. For at least 50–75% of our patients with atherosclerotic peripheral vascular disease, foot lesions or rest pain are the primary indication for a vascular operation. Despite hospital care and operation in some patients, limb salvage is not achieved in 10–20% of cases. Amputation often is necessary in such situations. Rehabilitation after lower-extremity amputation usually takes 1–3 months and costs thousands of dollars. The benefits of preventing foot problems in these patients should be obvious. Fortunately, the time and cost of preventive foot care are relatively minor compared to the great expenditures incurred once a foot lesion occurs.

II. **The susceptible foot.** Certain patients with diabetes and atherosclerosis are especially susceptible to developing nonhealing foot lesions. The diabetic with **peripheral sensory neuropathy** probably is the most susceptible. Because of diminished sensation, minor foot lesions such as blisters, skin cracks, and ingrown toenails may not be noticed by the patient. Even foreign bodies that penetrate the foot may not be felt. The classic example is the diabetic who is not aware of a nail or piece of glass in the foot. Many such diabetics also have retinopathy and may not be able to see such minor lesions.

   Anatomic foot deformities also predispose a person to development of foot problems, especially corns, calluses, and pressure sores. Improperly fitted shoes may cause too much pressure over certain anatomic points (Fig. 14-1). **Dry, hyperkeratotic skin**, especially over the heels, tends to crack. At the base of these cracks, subcutaneous infections often originate and undermine the skin. The result is subcutaneous soft tissue necrosis, cellulitis, or abscess, and larger nonhealing ulcers. Finally, **arterial ischemia** impedes wound healing. Minor foot ulcerations often fail to heal in

---

*Special credit for this chapter must be given to the Joslin Diabetic Clinic, Boston, where so many of these principles of foot care originated.

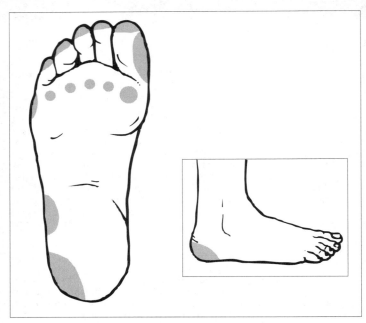

Fig. 14-1. Common locations for pressure-related ulcerations of the foot. Properly fitted footwear is an important factor in preventing pressure sores.

patients with absent pedal pulses and dependent forefoot rubor. As indicated in earlier chapters, healing of superficial foot lesions is unlikely if ankle pressures are less than 80 mm Hg in diabetics and 55 mm Hg in nondiabetics. Toe pressures less than 30 mm Hg and forefoot transcutaneous oxygen (TcO_2) tensions less than 10–20 torr are also predictive of slow or no healing.

III. **Prevention.** Each physician who cares for patients with diabetes and vascular disease is responsible for educating these patients in proper foot care. The principles of proper foot care are easily learned by most people. We have found a printed booklet of general directions for foot care to be especially helpful for outpatients. The physician or office nurse should explain specific instructions and demonstrate proper care of foot lesions to both the patient and the patient's family. A family member often is the best physician's assistant in detecting and treating minor foot problems at home. Additional professional home care may be provided by a visiting nurse.

Prevention of serious foot problems may be discussed conveniently under the following general categories: daily foot care, footwear, exercise, and first aid treatment.

A. **Daily foot care**
  1. **Washing.** The feet should be washed daily with warm **(never hot)** water and a mild soap. Feet should not be

soaked. Soaking tends to macerate skin and may cause burns if the patient has a sensory neuropathy and the water is too hot. After washing, the foot should be thoroughly dried, especially between the toes, where moisture promotes fungal infections.

2. **Inspection.** The foot should be examined for cuts, blisters, ingrown toenails, discolored skin, and cracks. In particular, the heel and spaces between the toes should be checked, since lesions are commonly overlooked in these locations. If the patient has poor vision, a family member or friend should inspect the foot. A physician should be notified of any problems.

3. **Moisturizing the skin.** Dryness leads to cracking of the skin. Therefore, daily application of a lanolin-base moisturizing lotion to the foot, especially the heel, is essential to good foot care. A few examples are lanolin, Eucerin, Nivea, Alpha Keri, Vanicream, and Vaseline Intensive Care lotion. These lotions should not be applied between the toes, since they may cause excess moisture and thus promote fungal infection.

4. **Foot powder.** An antifungal powder such as Desenex should be applied between the toes if foot perspiration is excessive or "athlete's foot" is suspected. Common signs of fungal infection are itching, small blister formation, and skin scaling between the toes or on the sole of the foot.

5. **Toenails.** Toenails should be cut or filed straight across, never shorter than the end of the toe. If nails are cut shorter than the lateral nail groove, they tend to become ingrown. The best time to trim nails is after a foot bath when the foot is clean and the nail usually is softer. A podiatrist should cut thick nails or ones that split easily.

6. **Corns and calluses.** Corns and calluses are the result of friction and pressure from footwear. They usually occur over bony prominences. A podiatrist or physician should care for them. An improperly treated corn or callus often results in an ulcer and infection that involves underlying bone (osteomyelitis). Patients should be cautioned not to trim them and not to apply plasters or chemicals to remove them.

7. **Toe care.** If one toe is causing pressure on another, a small piece of lamb's wool or absorbent gauze between the toes may prevent a pressure ulcer.

8. **Avoidance of trauma.** Foot protection should be worn at all times. Excessive heat from heating pads, hot packs or soaks, and heating lamps must be avoided, particularly if peripheral neuropathy is present. Adhesive tape is not recommended, since it may denude superficial skin. If tape is necessary, paper tape is preferred.

B. **Footwear**
  1. Patients with peripheral neuropathy and arterial ischemia **should never go barefoot!**
  2. Feet should be kept warm and dry with **socks or stockings.** Woolen socks are best in cold weather and

cotton socks when it is warm. Nylon socks or hose that cause excess perspiration should be avoided. Clean socks should be worn each day.

3. Shoes should fit comfortably and allow plenty of room for the toes. Many diabetics prefer specially made footwear. Soft, spacious canvas or tennis shoes often are adequate. Women should avoid pointed shoes that cramp the toes. New shoes should be broken in gradually to avoid blisters.

C. Exercise. Exercise promotes the development of collateral circulation and maintains normal venous and lymphatic flow by the musculovenous and lymphatic pumping mechanism.

1. Walking is the safest exercise for the feet, provided shoes fit properly.

2. Patients should be encouraged to walk daily. If they have intermittent claudication, they should be instructed to walk slowly, rest when claudication occurs, and then resume walking. They should be encouraged to gradually increase their walking distance each week.

3. Ambulation and dependency of the extremity should be curtailed when foot sores are present. Dependency leads to swelling that impedes healing and the resolution of infection.

D. First aid treatment. When the patient first notices a foot sore, he or she should begin certain types of first aid. Even if the lesions seem minor, the patient should be encouraged to promptly notify his or her physician, who generally should inspect the problem and prescribe definitive therapy. Procrastination on the part of the patient often results in inappropriate self-treatment of a foot problem and a consequent complication.

1. Foot lesions or injuries should be washed with warm water and mild soap. **Injuries should not be soaked for prolonged periods, especially in hot solutions that may macerate or burn tissue.** The foot should be carefully dried.

2. In general, strong topical antiseptic solutions such as iodine should **not** be used. An ointment such as bacitracin may be applied to the lesion.

3. The best dressing is simply a clean gauze bandage secured with a roll of gauze or paper tape.

4. The next step of treatment should be examination by a physician.

IV. Definitive treatment. Definitive treatment of foot problems may require the efforts of the primary physician, podiatrist, or surgeon. When the patient with a foot problem is first seen, several basic questions must be considered. First, what is the likelihood that the foot problem is curable and will not lead to limb loss? Second, what is appropriate therapy? Finally, can this therapy be accomplished on an outpatient basis or is hospitalization necessary?

A. Likelihood of healing. We generally rely on several sources of information to predict the likelihood of healing: physical examination, noninvasive vascular tests (Doppler ankle or toe pressures, forefoot TcO_2 tensions, and/or pulse volume recordings [PVRs]), and bone studies (x-ray or bone scan).

1. Small (<2 cm in diameter) superficial skin ulcers, corns, calluses, and ingrown toenails detectable by **physical examination** alone usually heal or are manageable without amputation. Exposed bone at the base of any lesion generally indicates osteomyelitis, even if the x-ray appears normal. Such lesions are unlikely to heal without some type of amputation. Lesions in an area of dependent rubor or ischemic rest pain also seldom heal. A continuing problem is predicting which foot ulcers will heal when pedal pulses are not palpable. An absent femoral pulse and dependent forefoot rubor generally indicate that an open foot lesion is unlikely to heal without surgical intervention.

2. **Noninvasive vascular tests** provide some predictive value in the healing of foot lesions. Noninfected foot ulcers may heal in patients with good femoral pulses but absent distal pulses when ankle pressures are greater than 65 mm Hg in the nondiabetic and 90 mm Hg in the diabetic. PVRs at the ankle of greater than 15 mm are favorable for healing. In our experience, flat or severely diminished (<5 mm) forefoot PVRs generally have correlated with nonhealing. Favorable Doppler pressures or PVRs do not ensure healing, but they at least suggest that initial treatment may be conservative. TcO_2 measurements are also helpful in determining whether ulcers are primarily neuropathic or ischemic. TcO_2 forefoot levels less than 40 mm Hg suggest ischemia. When TcO_2 is 20–30 mm Hg at rest and drops to less than 10 mm Hg with foot elevation, a foot lesion is unlikely to heal unless a revascularization procedure is performed.

3. The use of **radiologic studies** to detect bony change of osteomyelitis should be considered for patients with ulcers over bones. Plain x-ray may not show signs of osteomyelitis for at least 2–3 weeks. These signs include bony rarefaction, local periosteal elevation, and new bone formation. A bone scan may be a more sensitive indicator in equivocal cases.

B. **Principles of treatment**

1. **Corns and calluses** are pressure-induced lesions. Corns represent a traumatic keratosis or overgrowth of the epidermis. They generally occur over a bony prominence (e.g., at the dorsal aspect of the fifth toe). They are conical in shape, the base being superficial and the apex deep, and press against deeper structures. Calluses are flat keratoses that generally occur on the bottom of the foot over bony prominences. Poorly fitted footwear often is the cause of corns and calluses. The danger of these lesions is infection, which may occur beneath them where a bursa or space may form between the superficial keratosis and underlying bone.

Optimum treatment for corns begins with removing the **superficial** corn surface with a scalpel or similar cutting instrument. Care must be taken not to cut into the deep vascular layer of the corn, which may not heal. After removing the cornified layer, a U-shaped felt pad may be applied behind the corn to alleviate local pressure that originally caused the corn. These pads disperse local pressure. Footwear should be changed to ensure no pressure on the corn. Calluses also should be managed primarily by redistributing pressure with inlay pads.

2. **Ingrown toenails** (onychocryptosis) may be complicated by infection. Three basic types of lateral nail problems occur and threaten the diabetic and vascular patient with serious infection and gangrene.

   a. The **incurved** or simple inverted nail curves into the lateral nail groove, causing tenderness and pain with ambulation. To force the lateral nail edge forward and prevent it from digging into the toe pulp, any debris must be cleared from beneath the leading edge of the nail and then cotton must be gently packed beneath the nail edge. If cotton is simply packed along the lateral nail groove, the incurved nail will worsen as the packing pushes the nail down.

   b. An **ingrown nail** is the result of not trimming the nail straight across and leaving a sharp, jagged lateral edge on the nail. This pointed spicule of nail is called a **shard**. Shards tend to penetrate the lateral nail groove and cause infection, so they should be removed. Infection at a shard location may be treated with warm boric acid soaks for 20–30 minutes every 4 hours. A broad-spectrum oral antibiotic (e.g., cephalexin [Keflex]) may be needed if local infection is present.

   c. **Hypertrophic ungualabium** represents an overgrowth of chronic granulation tissue over the lateral nail plate. Hypertrophic ungualabium may follow any incurved nail or ingrown nail or partial excision of the nail. The hypertrophic tissue tends to grow over the lateral nail edge, making local infection more difficult to clear. Proper treatment may require partial or complete removal of the nail and antibiotics for cellulitis.

3. **Minor foot ulcers** (superficial, <2 cm in diameter, and with no exposed bone) should receive the same daily hygiene described in sec. **III.A.** For established clean lesions, bacitracin ointment and a small dry gauze dressing applied twice daily may be used. For ulcers with necrotic debris or crusting, wet-to-dry saline dressings changed four times a day are most useful and clean up and debride the lesion. Sharp debridement should be done by a physician and be limited to necrotic tissue. If the ulcer has a dry eschar, callus around the ulcer edge should be trimmed to allow adequate drainage of moisture or pus from beneath the eschar. Otherwise, pus may be trapped beneath the eschar and cause deeper infection and abscess. Dakin's

antiseptic solution (diluted sodium hypochlorite) with gauze packs may be used to debride particularly dirty wounds or necrotic fat or fascia. Since Dakin's antiseptic solution may damage normal skin, its use should be reserved for patients with foot pulses. Dilute acetic acid solution 0.25% (vinegar) on gauze dressings three to four times a day is also effective in cleaning contaminated diabetic foot wounds, especially those with *Pseudomonas* species.

4. **Large heel ulcers** (>2 cm in diameter) often extend into subcutaneous fat and are extremely difficult to resolve. If possible, a clean dry eschar, which can be protected with a gauze pad, should be obtained. Vigorous debridement to bleeding subcutaneous fat frequently results first in deeper extension of the tissue necrosis and eventually in exposure of the calcaneus and osteomyelitis. These large heel ulcers may eventually lead to amputation, especially in diabetics with neuropathy.

5. **Foot cellulitis** is apparent by local swelling, erythema, tenderness, and warmth. Such infection may spread rapidly in diabetics. Optimum treatment includes strict bed rest, leg elevation, and administration of antibiotics. Before starting the patient on antibiotics, a Gram's stain and culture of foot ulcers should be done. An oral cephalosporin (e.g., cephalexin, 250–500 mg PO q6h) usually is effective for local cellulitis **without** diffuse forefoot involvement, lymphangitic spread, or fever. These signs of more extensive infection are an indication for parenteral therapy with broad-spectrum antibiotics. In general, antibiotics effective against anaerobes are unnecessary and probably should be withheld until specific anaerobes are identified. Foot soaks are not recommended, since they contribute nothing to the above therapy and only introduce more bacteria.

6. **Foot abscesses** require urgent and generous incision and drainage. In general, they require emergency hospitalization. Multiple small incisions with infected tunnels do not heal well. Gauze packing is preferable to rubber drains, since packing debrides better.

C. **Hospitalization.** Hospitalization obviously is indicated for foot lesions complicated by cellulitis, abscess, or sepsis. If conservative therapy has not begun to heal other minor foot ulcers after 3 weeks, the patient should be considered for an arteriogram and arterial reconstructive procedure or an amputation.

Selected Reading

Cina C et al. Utility of transcutaneous oxygen tension measurements in peripheral arterial occlusive disease. *J Vasc Surg* 1:362, 1984.

Dillon RS. Successful treatment of osteomyelitis and soft tissue infections in ischemic diabetic legs by local antibiotic injections and the end-diastolic pneumatic compression boot. *Ann Surg* 204:643, 1986.

Kozak GP et al. *Management of Diabetic Foot Problems* Philadelphia: Saunders, 1984.

Laing P. Diabetic foot ulcers. *Am J Surg* 167(Suppl 1A):31S, 1994.

Levin ME, and O'Neal LW (eds). *The Diabetic Foot* (3rd ed). St. Louis: Mosby, 1988.

Mueller MP, Wright J, Klein SR. Diabetes and Peripheral Vascular Disease. In FJ Veith, RW Hobson II, RA Williams, SE Wilson (eds), *Vascular Surgery* (2nd ed). New York: McGraw-Hill, 1994. Pp. 514–522.

Amputations

Amputation must be planned and conducted with the same meticulous care given to arterial reconstructions. Otherwise, the patient faces poor amputation healing and a long hospitalization. The therapeutic goals should be primary wound healing, minimal hospitalization, and rehabilitation so the patient can walk again.

This chapter is limited to amputations performed on patients with peripheral arterial occlusive disease and diabetes mellitus. Techniques for lower-extremity amputation for such patients are well described and illustrated in many textbooks.

I. Preoperative care

A. Patient acceptance. When the necessity of an amputation becomes apparent to the surgeon, he or she must help the patient accept the operation. If the patient is experiencing severe pain, he or she usually will accept amputation willingly. The surgeon must reassure the patient that every effort will be made to rehabilitate him or her so that walking will again be possible. It is especially important to discuss the need for amputation and the plan for rehabilitation with the patient's family. In addition, we ask the amputation rehabilitation service to evaluate the patient before operation. In most cases, upper-extremity and some lower-extremity strengthening exercises will be initiated before amputation is performed.

B. Medical stabilization. Except when an infection is life-threatening, we prefer a period of local wound care and administration of antibiotics prior to amputation for cases in which cellulitis has complicated tissue necrosis. Management of the infected foot is described in Chap. 14.

Occasionally, an elderly patient who is toxic from an ischemic, infected foot will present in diabetic coma, with severe dehydration and electrolyte imbalance, acute myocardial infarction, acute congestive heart failure, or digitalis toxication. Emergency amputation in such patients has a high mortality rate. Ideally, the medical condition of such patients must be stabilized before operation. A valuable adjunct in preparation of these critically ill patients for amputation has been a technique called **selective physiologic amputation.** It involves local hypothermia with tourniquet occlusion just above the level of necrosis or infection. The technique has been carefully investigated in a large number of patients and should be familiar to surgeons who treat such severely ill patients.

The following technique is recommended for selective physiologic amputation in patients who need urgent amputation but are so critically ill on admission that they could not tolerate immediate operation.

1. The extent of gangrene or infection is determined and the site for physiologic amputation is chosen. Generally, the physiologic amputation is done below

the knee and the subsequent definitive surgical amputation is performed above the knee. Recent experience, however, indicates that 70% of patients who are initially treated by cryoamputation of the foot can undergo a successful below-knee amputation.

2. Tissue distal to the selected site is wrapped in sheet wadding, and a soft rubber tourniquet is applied proximal to the infected or necrotic tissue to occlude arterial supply. Local infiltration anesthesia may be used at the tourniquet site. However, this area usually is already numb, and local anesthesia is unnecessary. This tourniquet must be secure, since accidental release could shower the systemic circulation with acidotic debris and bacteria.

3. One-inch thick blocks of dry ice are wrapped in towels and placed around the extremity no higher than 3 inches **below** the tourniquet. These dry ice packs may be held in place by a rubber sheet or pad. The dry ice is replaced every 8 hours.

4. The duration of physiologic amputation may be hours to several days; the average duration is approximately 3 days, with a range of 9 hours to 15 days.

5. Physiologic amputation should be reserved for patients who are desperately ill from both gangrene or infection and life-threatening medical problems. In our experience, this technique is seldom necessary but is highly effective in the rare patient who requires intensive medical stabilization before amputation.

II. **Amputation level.** Selecting a proper amputation level is based primarily on clinical examination and knowledge of the extent of arterial occlusive disease in the individual patient. Pulse volume recordings (PVRs), segmental limb pressures, and transcutaneous oxygen (TcO_2) tensions are helpful but not infallible (see Chap. 5). Our data also suggest that a TcO_2 tension value of at least 40 mm Hg measured on the skin flap of the proposed level of amputation is predictive of success (see Chap. 5). An amputation site-to-chest TcO_2 ratio greater than 0.59 is also associated with a high likelihood of healing. Final judgment must be based on the following clinical criteria:

A. Active infection controlled.

B. Good-looking skin at amputation site.

C. No dependent rubor proximal to the level of amputation.

D. Venous filling time of less than 20 seconds.

E. No pain proximal to the amputation level.

III. **Operative technique.** The following principles of operative technique are crucial to the success of single-digit amputations, transmetatarsal amputations (TMAs), below-knee amputations (BKAs), and above-knee amputations (AKAs). Gentle handling of tissues and careful hemostasis are the two critical prerequisites to primary healing.

A. **Single-digit amputation.** The skin incision for single-digit amputation should be made at a 90-degree angle to avoid beveling. The medial and lateral skin flaps should be left long and then trimmed if necessary. The proximal phalanx should be divided through the shaft of the bone and not through the joint. A single-layer closure is made with interrupted simple sutures. A soft, bulky dressing is applied.

B. **Transmetatarsal amputation** can provide excellent results, especially in diabetics who have neuropathic toe ulcers. A strongly positive forefoot PVR or TcO_2 tensions greater than 40 torr are the best noninvasive predictors of success. Several aspects of the technique warrant emphasis. The plantar flap should be cut 1 cm from the web space and not undercut. Likewise the dorsal flap should never be retracted. The cut should be carried directly through the tendons; small vessels nourishing the forefoot pass between the tendons. A single-layer closure is carried out with no subcutaneous stitches, and the forefoot is splinted for 3–5 days. A problem area of wound healing often is the mid-dorsal flap. If a small area of necrosis occurs here, the TMA may be salvaged by careful local debridement of the necrosis and placement of a small gauze wick.

C. **Below-knee amputation** is preferable to an AKA, since rehabilitation is easier when the knee joint is preserved. In addition to the above criteria for amputation level, a BKA generally will not be appropriate when either a temperature demarcation or ischemic lesions extend above the ankle or when a knee contracture is present. We prefer a long posterior myocutaneous flap, which is cut about 1 inch longer than the anterior-posterior diameter of the proximal calf. The anterior edge of the tibia should have a 45-degree bevel to keep it from protruding. The fibula is cut 1 inch shorter than the tibia. The muscle fascia and enveloping fascia of the calf are approximated with interrupted absorbable sutures, and the skin is closed with fine interrupted sutures of 4-0 nylon. The skin should not be handled with tissue forceps at any time. The stump is carefully padded with fluffed gauze bandages, and a rigid posterior plaster splint is applied and left undisturbed for 5 days. This period of immobilization prevents any disturbance of the incisional closure, reduces wound edema, and maintains the knee in extension so that knee contracture is minimized. We generally do not drain these amputations.

D. **Above-knee amputation** is seldom necessary if the below-the-knee skin condition is good and a good femoral pulse is present. As much thigh length as possible should be preserved when an AKA is done. The end of the femur will migrate to the lateral edge of the amputation stump unless some step is taken to fix it in the mid-portion of the stump. This can be accomplished by placing several large mattress sutures between the vastus lateralis and the biceps muscle just lateral to the femur. As in other amputation procedures, the skin must be closed with a gentle technique. Fluffed bandages are applied to the incision and are held in place with a stockinette secured by benzoin painted on the proximal thigh.

E. **Management of failed femorodistal grafts.** When synthetic bypass grafts to the knee or leg fail, a BKA or AKA is often necessary. The amputation frequently cuts across the thrombosed graft. If the graft is infected prior

**Table 15-1. Postamputation results,
rehabilitation, and energy expenditure[a]**

Primary healing	75%
Eventual healing	80%
Mortality	7–10%
Rehabilitation with prosthesis	
Conventional techniques[b]	65%
Immediate postoperative prosthesis	87%
Average time from amputation to rehabilitation	
Conventional techniques	133 days
Immediate postoperative prosthesis	31 days
Energy expenditure (% increase compared to controls)	
Below-knee amputation	9–25%
Above-knee amputation	25–100%
Bilateral below-knee amputation	40%

[a]These data are averages from a large number of surgical series.
[b]Conventional techniques include a delay of several weeks for primary wound
healing before fitting a prosthesis.
Source: Modified from JM Malone, J Goldstone. Lower Extremity Amputation.
In WS Moore (ed), *Vascular Surgery* (2nd ed). Orlando: Grune & Stratton, 1986.

to amputation, it must be completely removed to prevent
the persistence of a septic focus in the lower limb, especially if the graft is attached to a more proximal
aortofemoral graft. Likewise, an amputation site that
becomes infected and contains an old thrombosed graft
end is unlikely to heal until all the prosthetic material is
removed.

  F. Ischemic amputation sites. Occasionally, an AKA
stump will become ischemic with rest pain, necrotic
edges, or gangrene. Such ischemia prevents healing and
must be corrected by improving profunda femoris perfusion. Otherwise, the patient faces a higher AKA or hip
disarticulation. The attendant mortality rate of higher
amputation is nearly 30%.

IV. Postoperative care (Table 15-1). We have found that certain guidelines ensure primary wound healing and facilitate
early postoperative physiotherapy and eventual rehabilitation at an experienced rehabilitation center. The immediate
postsurgical prosthesis has been under investigation for more
than two decades and has been reported to be highly successful and to accelerate rehabilitation. This method has merits,
but we caution that it must be used by individuals who are
highly skilled in its use. Otherwise, the following principles of
postoperative care generally will give good results.

  A. Primary dressing and splint. The primary dressing
and splint are left intact for the first 5–7 days and are not
removed unless the patient has fever of unclear etiology.
At this point, the initial dressing is removed, and the
amputation site is inspected. If it is healing satisfactorily,
a new plaster pylon cast is applied and changed every
7–10 days. After about 3 weeks, the amputation stump is
ready for suture removal and progression toward a tem-

porary prosthesis.
B. Physiotherapy. A physical therapist should see the patient on the first postoperative day. Upper-extremity strengthening exercises can be continued at that time. If the condition of the patient allows, quadriceps-strengthening exercises are also initiated. Between the seventh and fourteenth postoperative days, the patient begins using a wheelchair. Crutch-walking usually is begun between the tenth and fourteenth day.
C. Suture removal. Sutures are left intact for at least 3 weeks.
D. Prosthesis fitting. Measurements and fitting for a prosthesis usually are done 4 weeks after operation, unless the immediate postoperative fit is being used.
E. Rehabilitation. During the first postoperative week, long-term rehabilitation plans are discussed with the patient and his or her family. They are assisted in selecting a rehabilitation center that is well qualified and convenient to their home. These arrangements must be initiated early, since they often require 7–14 days to confirm.

Selected Reading

Bodily KC, Burgess EM. Contralateral limb and patient survival after leg amputation. *Am J Surg* 146:280, 1983.

Bunt TJ. Gangrene of the immediate postoperative above-knee amputation stump: Role of emergency revascularization in preventing death. *J Vasc Surg* 2:874, 1985.

De Frang RD, Taylor LM Jr, Porter JM. Amputations. In JM Porter, LM Taylor Jr. (eds), *Basic Data Underlying Clinical Decision Making in Vascular Surgery*. St. Louis: Quality Medical Publishing, 1994. Pp. 153–158.

Humphrey LL et al. The contribution of non-insulin-dependent diabetes to lower-extremity amputation in the community. *Arch Intern Med* 154:885, 1994.

Hunsaker RH et al. Dry ice cryoamputation: A twelve-year experience. *J Vasc Surg* 2:812, 1985.

Malone JM. Lower Extremity Amputation. In WS Moore (ed), *Vascular Surgery* (4th ed). Philadelphia: Saunders, 1993. Pp. 809–854.

Messina LM, Zelenock GB. Lower Extremity Amputation. In LJ Greenfield (ed), *Surgery: Scientific Principles and Practice*. Philadelphia: Lippincott, 1993. Pp. 1668–1674.

Rubin JR et al. Management of infection of major amputation stumps after failed femorodistal grafts. *Surgery* 98:810, 1985.

Tunis SR, Bass EB, Steinberg EP. The use of angioplasty, bypass surgery, and amputation in the management of peripheral vascular disease. *N Engl J Med* 325:556, 1991.

Wheelock FC Jr, Rowbotham JL, Hoar CS Jr. Amputations. In GP Kozak et al. (eds), *Management of Diabetic Foot Problems*. Philadelphia: Saunders, 1984. Pp. 186–212.

Aneurysms

Optimum management of aneurysms of the aorta and the femoral and popliteal arteries requires an understanding of their natural history, a preoperative patient evaluation, and surgical treatment. The best results have followed carefully planned elective repair before complications of rupture, thrombosis, or emboli have threatened the life or limb of the patient. The contrast between operative mortalities for an unruptured (2–5%) versus a ruptured (50–70%) infrarenal abdominal aortic aneurysm (AAA) remains one of the most striking differences between elective and emergency surgical treatment of any disease. Consequently, we emphasize early recognition and correction of aneurysmal disease before the development of complications.

Although aneurysmal disease may involve nearly any artery, peripheral artery aneurysms occur most commonly in the abdominal aorta and the iliac, femoral, and popliteal arteries. This chapter focuses on the recognition and management of aneurysms in these locations. The hemodynamics of aneurysm disease are discussed in Chap. 1. Chapter 3 outlines the initial physical evaluation, and Chap. 6 describes appropriate radiologic tests.

Abdominal Aortic Aneurysm

I. **Epidemiology.** During the past 30 years, the incidence of AAAs has tripled. The rise in detection may be due to increased use of ultrasound and computed tomography (CT). The rising incidence has been tenfold for small AAAs (<5 cm), while the incidence for larger aneurysms has increased by only a factor of two. Small aneurysms now account for about 50% of all clinically recognized AAAs. This is an important epidemiologic finding because many physicians are uncertain about the appropriate management of small AAAs.

Although AAAs have been traditionally related to atherosclerosis, several reports have emphasized familial tendencies. Nearly 20% of patients with an AAA have a first-degree relative with an aneurysm.

II. **Natural history.** AAAs usually form and slowly expand over several years. Recent data from several population-based studies indicate that the median expansion rate is 2–3 mm per year. The rate increases as the aneurysm enlarges. Approximately 20% expand at a rate of more than 4 mm per year, while the remaining 80% grow at a slower pace.

Rupture remains the most threatening outcome of an AAA. Numerous studies have confirmed that this risk is related primarily to aneurysm diameter. Although this concept is not controversial, experts still debate the size at which an aneurysm should be repaired. For years, AAAs greater than 6 cm in diameter were considered appropriate

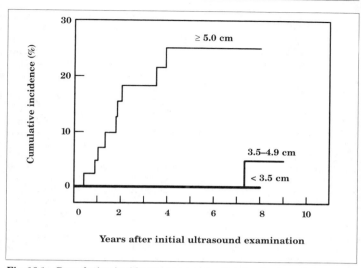

Fig. 16-1. Cumulative incidence of rupture of abdominal aortic aneurysms according to the diameter of the aneurysm at the initial ultrasound examination. (From MP Nevitt, DJ Ballard, JW Hallett Jr. Prognosis of abdominal aortic aneurysms: A population-based study. *N Engl J Med* 321:1009, 1989.)

for elective repair. Subsequently, autopsy data revealed that even small aneurysms (4–5 cm) could rupture, resulting in a more aggressive approach to smaller AAAs. These autopsy cases were selective for the entire general population and, of course, were measuring ruptured aneurysms that were no longer under arterial pressure. Consequently, they tended to underestimate the true AAA size. **More recent data from population-based studies of living patients have indicated that rupture risk escalates when the AAA exceeds 5 cm in size (Fig. 16-1).** Rupture risk for small AAAs is approximately 1% per year, 5% per year for medium-sized (5–7 cm) AAAs, and at least 10% per year for large (7 cm) AAAs. Approximately one-third of small AAAs will require elective repair over a 5-year follow-up. Nearly all small AAAs that eventually rupture have enlarged to over 5 cm in diameter.

Unfortunately, the frequency of AAA rupture remains high despite more elective aneurysm repairs. This discouraging outcome is due to the fact that at least 50% of patients with a ruptured AAA do not know of their aneurysm until the day of catastrophic hemorrhage. They obviously never had a chance for elective repair.

Other important adverse outcomes of abdominal aortic and femoropopliteal aneurysms include limb-threatening ischemia secondary to embolic debris shed from the lining of the aneurysm or thrombosis of the aneurysm occurring in association with occlusive disease. Occasionally, an AAA will rupture into the vena cava. The result may be a large aorto-caval fistula that may precipitate acute congestive heart failure. In a few cases, aneurysms may become infected, presenting as a pulsatile abdominal mass accompanied by unexplained fever and bacteremia. Another uncommon outcome of an AAA is erosion into the intestine, presenting as gastrointestinal bleeding from an aortoenteric fistula.

The natural history of thoracoabdominal aneurysms is not clearly defined since longitudinal follow-up based on serial CT scans has not been widely reported. Most surgeons extrapolate rupture risk data from AAAs and consider repair when the aneurysm enters the 5–7 cm range in low-risk patients.

Most of the natural history data on femoropopliteal aneurysms is based on retrospective reviews of patients who presented with thrombosed aneurysms or large ones that were easily detected on physical examination. Symptomatic thrombosed popliteal aneurysms result in limb-threatening ischemia in at least one-third of such cases and lead eventually to amputation if revascularization is not performed. In our review of clinically recognized popliteal aneurysms, the asymptomatic aneurysms at greatest risk of eventual thromboembolic events had three characteristics: (1) size greater than 2 cm, (2) intraluminal thrombus seen on ultrasound, and (3) decreased pedal pulses indicating compromised runoff from thromboembolism or atherosclerosis.

III. **Indications for operation**
  A. In low-risk patients, **an AAA approaching or entering the 5–6 cm diameter range is an indication for elective repair.** For higher-risk individuals, we generally defer operation until the aneurysm shows progressive enlargement, usually more than 6 cm, or until a smaller aneurysm becomes tender or symptomatic. Smaller aneurysms (4–5 cm) may need to be simultaneously repaired in patients who undergo aortofemoral bypass for aortoiliac occlusive disease.
  B. A less common but more urgent indication for surgical repair is evidence of **peripheral emboli** to the feet.
  C. Emergency operation is indicated for all patients with a known aneurysm that has become **acutely tender** or is associated **with abdominal pain or backache.** These patients should be hospitalized and considered to have a symptomatic aneurysm, although their abdominal symptoms may be nonspecific at first and their initial vital signs may be normal.
  D. Patients with **ruptured aneurysms** and shock should be taken directly to the operating room for resuscitation and operation.

IV. **Preoperative evaluation.** The preoperative evaluation for an elective AAA should define the size and extent of the aneurysm, the associated medical risks, and other vascular disease that needs operative correction. Diagnostic tests should be carefully selected so that information is not duplicated and costs are minimized.
  A. **Size and extent.** The reliability of abdominal examination to detect and size an AAA is poor enough that a more accurate diagnostic method is necessary. Currently the simplest

and least expensive test to diagnose and measure an AAA is ultrasound. It can reliably measure the aneurysm within 3–4 mm of its actual size. Technical features of ultrasound resolution make the measurement of the anterior-posterior diameter more reliable than the transverse measurement. More recently developed ultrasound equipment allows accurate assessment of the juxtarenal aorta and common iliac arteries in most patients.

Although some surgeons prefer routine CT or magnetic resonance imaging (MRI) scanning of a suspected AAA, these imaging modalities cost considerably more than ultrasound and should probably be used for specific indications. For example, CT imaging is particularly useful when searching for other causes of abdominal pain or mass. It is also essential when physical examination, chest x-ray, or ultrasound suggests a suprarenal or thoracoabdominal aneurysm. One must remember that a CT scan may overestimate the size of an aneurysm because the measurements are made perpendicular to the body axis and may be distorted if the aorta is tortuous.

B. Aortography. What is the role of arteriography in the evaluation of an AAA? It is certainly not reliable for size determination since intraluminal clot may obscure the outer limit of the wall. Some experts favor routine aortography to detect unrecognized multiple renal arteries, mesenteric artery stenoses, or important pelvic arterial occlusive disease. However, if certain clinical criteria are considered, aortography can be used more selectively. Such criteria include:

1. Decreased femoral or peripheral pulses and bruits indicating arterial occlusive disease.
2. Hypertension poorly controlled by medication or progressing renal insufficiency, indicating possible renal artery occlusive disease.
3. Juxtarenal, suprarenal, or thoracoabdominal aortic aneurysms that require clear delineation of the renal, intestinal, and intercostal arteries involved by the aneurysmal disease.
4. Symptoms of intestinal ischemia or a high-pitched epigastric bruit, indicating possible visceral artery disease that may predispose to postoperative colonic ischemia or intestinal angina.
5. A suspected horseshoe kidney on ultrasound, CT scan, or excretory urogram (usually associated with multiple renal arteries).

One or more of these criteria is present in 30–50% of patients with an AAA. The appropriate role of magnetic resonance aortography is currently under clinical investigation at many centers.

C. Medical risks. Most significant medical risks can be detected by a good history and physical examination. The majority of patients with AAAs are hypertensive, and at least 35–50% have obvious coronary artery disease. A cardiologist should evaluate all patients with a past history of myocardial infarction, angina pectoris, chronic congestive heart failure, chronic arrhythmias, severe hypertension, or significant heart murmurs. In our experience, preoperative stabilization of cardiac disease and careful operative and perioperative cardiac care contribute significantly to keeping elective operative mortality at a low level (2–3%). Preoperatively, pulmonary function tests are not done routinely. They are indicated for patients with known chronic obstructive pulmonary disease and for patients for whom the history and physical examination suggest significant dyspnea.

Several authors have encouraged a more aggressive approach to elective AAA repair for elderly patients and patients with increased cardiac or pulmonary risks. Obviously, these patients must be carefully selected and operated on by an experienced anesthetic and surgical team in excellent intensive care facilities. Under these conditions, aneurysm operations on high-risk patients can be accomplished with a fairly low operative mortality of 5–7%. If not operated on, about 30–50% of these higher-risk patients die of aneurysm rupture. Their operative mortality rate for surgery after rupture exceeds 80%.

Patients with significant coronary artery disease should undergo myocardial revascularization before elective aneurysm repair is attempted. About 5% of AAA patients will have significant angina requiring preoperative coronary revascularization before AAA repair. For 85% of such patients, surgical revascularization will be necessary while the remaining 15% can be adequately revascularized by percutaneous coronary angioplasty. Those patients who undergo coronary artery bypass grafting usually need 6–8 weeks of recovery before AAA repair, although earlier operation may be judicious for those individuals with huge (>8 cm) AAAs. In contrast, AAA repair can usually proceed within 7–10 days after coronary balloon angioplasty. Likewise, patients with severe obstructive pulmonary disease require intensive preoperative stabilization of pulmonary function before operation (see Chap. 7).

Nonresective treatment of an AAA by acute thrombosis and axillofemoral bypass has been recommended for high-risk patients with multiple medical problems. In our opinion, this approach seldom is indicated. Present anesthetic management and surgical technique allow a direct attack on the aneurysm in most high-risk patients (Fig. 16-2).

Another option is endovascular grafting introduced by Parodi et al. (Fig. 16-3), which involves the transfemoral passage of a collapsed synthetic graft into the aorta from the femoral artery with graft placement by expandable intraluminal stents. This relatively new technique faces several potential limitations: inability to pass the device up through diseased or tortuous iliac arteries, peripheral embolism of aneurysm plaque or thrombus, and inadequate anastomoses resulting in persistent perianastomotic leak into the aneurysm sac or graft migration. The future impact of this exciting innovation will require several years of investigation and long-term follow-up.

D. Associated vascular disease. In a small number of patients (10%), an asymptomatic carotid bruit will be

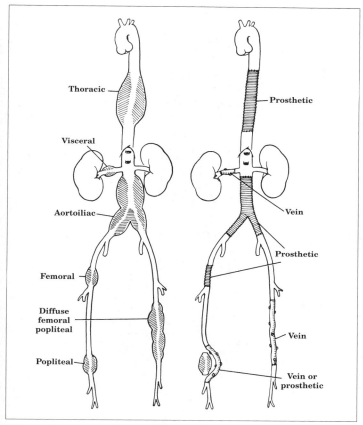

Fig. 16-2. The standard treatment for arterial aneurysms remains **surgical repair with either a synthetic prosthesis or autogenous vein graft.**

detected at the time of preoperative evaluation. In our practices, these patients undergo noninvasive carotid studies to ascertain the hemodynamic significance. Patients with bilateral high-grade (80–99%) carotid stenoses may undergo elective repair of one side before aneurysm repair. However, patients with symptomatic or large (>7 cm) aneurysms should undergo AAA repair without delay for cerebrovascular surgery. The risk of perioperative stroke with asymptomatic carotid disease is relatively low.

V. Preoperative preparation. The preoperative preparation for **elective** AAA repair is identical to the routine described previously for aortic reconstruction for occlusive disease (see Chap. 12). If autotransfusion is to be used, arrangements for the equipment and technician should be confirmed at least 24 hours before surgery. The routine use of rapid intraoperative

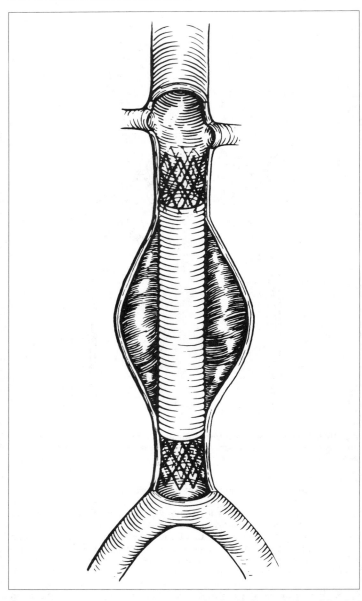

Fig. 16-3. Clinical trials are examining the feasibility, safety, and durability of stented intraluminal grafts passed retrograde from a femoral-
artery surgical exposure into abdominal aortic aneurysms and secured
by expandable metallic stents. (Modified from JC Parodi, JC Palmaz,
HD Barrone. Transfemoral intraluminal graft implantation for abdominal aortic aneurysms. *Ann Vasc Surg* 5:491, 1991.)

autotransfusion has allowed 70–80% of patients to undergo aneurysm repair without any bank homologous blood.

VI. **Management of a ruptured aneurysm**. The key factor underlying successful management of a ruptured AAA is expeditious movement of the patient to an operating room. There resuscitation can continue, the aorta can be exposed and clamped, and the aneurysm can be repaired. We emphasize early transport to the operating room, because delay in the emergency ward or radiologic department may result in further deterioration and death of the bleeding patient or the patient with imminent rupture.

Operative mortality for a ruptured AAA has remained essentially unchanged in the past 20 years. Only 50% of patients with a ruptured AAA who arrive at the hospital will be discharged alive. The most critical factors predicting death from rupture remain profound shock, preexisting cardiopulmonary or renal disease, and technical complications during operation. Several factors, however, can enhance the likelihood of survival for a patient with a ruptured AAA:

A. **Rapid transport.** Patients with suspected AAA rupture should be transported rapidly by helicopter or ambulance to a major hospital, where a surgical team should be waiting for initial assessment and resuscitation. An operating room should be ready as soon as the patient arrives.

B. **Resuscitation.** Initial resuscitation should include at least two large-bore (14- to 16-gauge) intravenous lines, a nasogastric tube, and a Foley bladder catheter. Blood should be typed and cross-matched for at least 6–8 units of packed red blood cells. If a rapid autotransfusion device is available, it should be set up immediately in the operating room. Ringer's lactated solution is the most cost-effective fluid for initial volume expansion. Prophylactic antibiotics should be administered. Arterial and central venous lines can be placed in the operating room.

C. **Accurate diagnosis.** If the diagnosis of ruptured AAA is in question and the patient is hemodynamically stable, an abdominal CT scan or ultrasound should be considered. An electrocardiogram (ECG) should be performed to rule out acute myocardial infarction.

D. **Immediate operation.** A patient with a known AAA and signs of rupture should be taken **directly** to the operating room without delay in the emergency ward.

E. **Temperature control. Cold kills!** Patients with a ruptured AAA and shock become hypothermic quickly. Those with a body temperature below 33°C develop a capillary leak syndrome necessitating massive fluid volumes, manifest a diffuse coagulopathy, and frequently slip suddenly into life-threatening cardiac arrhythmias. The two most useful means of preventing hypothermia are (1) warming the operating room to 70–80°F **before** the patient arrives and (2) using the Bair Hugger warming tent over the upper thorax and head.

F. **Aortic control.** Since blood pressure can crash with induction of anesthesia, the abdomen and groins should be prepped, and the operating team should be gowned and ready when the patient is anesthetized and intubated. A midline abdominal incision from xyphoid to symphysis pubis is the most direct approach. If the retroperitoneal hematoma if massive, initial aortic control should be gained by compression or clamping of the aorta at the diaphragm (Fig. 16-4). In many patients, however, the aorta can be safely clamped below the renal arteries. At this site care must be taken to avoid injury to the duodenum and left renal vein. Rarely, a patient with multiple prior abdominal operations may need a left thoracotomy for initial aortic clamping. Prior to clamping, mannitol (12.5–25.0 g) is administered as a diuretic and free-radical scavenger. Low-dose intravenous dopamine (2–3 μg/kg/minute) is also useful for its vasodilatory effect for both the renal and mesenteric circulations and may alleviate both acute renal failure and bowel ischemia.

G. **Anticoagulation.** Administration of heparin during repair of a ruptured AAA is controversial. If the patient has sustained profound shock and hypothermia, a coagulopathy may already exist and heparin may worsen the situation. On the other hand, distal iliofemoral or femoropopliteal thrombosis is not an uncommon problem during emergent AAA repair. Consequently small systemic (2,500–3,000 units) or distal irrigation doses of heparin may minimize lower-limb thrombotic complications.

H. **Assessing limb and vital organ perfusion.** Lower-extremity perfusion must be assured **before** leaving the operating room by palpation of pulses, Doppler signals at the feet, or calf plethysmographic pulse wave forms. If thrombosis is suspected, a Fogarty thromboembolectomy catheter should be passed immediately. Likewise, the left colon should be inspected for viability. If the appearance is questionable, intravenous fluoroscein (2 ampules) can be given intravenously and the bowel can be inspected with a Wood's lamp. When the abdomen is massively distended and a tight closure could compromise renal or colonic perfusion, a Silastic or polytetrafluoroethylene silo of the incision should be considered. This silo can be taken down when the massive abdominal swelling has subsided.

VII. **Principles of aneurysm repair.** The following technical principles underlie safe emergent or elective AAA repair and minimize both intraoperative and postoperative complications (Fig. 16-5).

A. **Aneurysm exposure** is best obtained through a long midline incision. We have found that, although transverse abdominal incisions or lateral extraperitoneal abdominal incisions may be used, they may make proximal aortic control of high aneurysms more difficult. Flank incisions also limit exposure of the right distal iliac arteries. For aneurysms that extend nearly to the renal arteries, exposure is facilitated by division of the left renal vein, leaving the adrenal and gonadal branches for venous outflow from the left kidney. Another alternative is leaving the main left renal vein intact but mobilizing it by ligation of the adrenal, gonadal, and left renal-lumbar branches. Thoracoabdominal aortic aneurysms obviously require a thoracoabdominal incision.

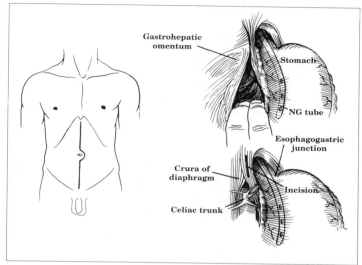

A

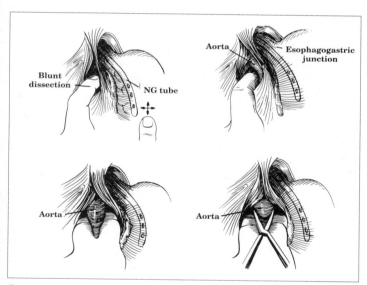

B

Fig. 16-4. Supraceliac aortic clamping is useful for large ruptured abdominal aortic aneurysms and huge retroperitoneal hematomas that obscure the proximal aneurysm neck at the renal level. (NG = nasogastric.) (By permission of the Mayo Foundation.)

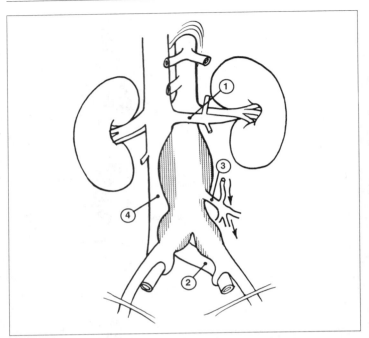

Fig. 16-5. Anatomic trouble spots in abdominal aortic aneurysm exposure. (1) The left renal vein or one of its branches (left renal lumbar,
gonadal, or adrenal) may be injured during exposure of the aneurysm
neck, especially with ruptured aneurysms. In 5% of cases, the left renal
vein lies posterior to the aorta and may be injured in any attempt to
encircle the proximal aorta for control. (2) The common iliac veins are
usually adherent to the iliac arteries and may be injured during dissection. (3) The inferior mesenteric artery should be ligated on or within
the aneurysm sac to avoid ligation of critical collateral vessels from the
marginal artery of Drummond. (4) Dissection of the aneurysm sac from
the vena cava is usually unnecessary.

B. **Limited dissection** of the lateral and posterior
aneurysm is done to minimize blood loss and operative
time. After proximal and distal clamping, the graft is
sutured inside the aneurysm sac after all aneurysm wall
thrombi have been removed (Creech technique). If the
duodenum is densely adherent to the aneurysm (inflammatory aneurysm), we do not dissect the duodenum free
from the aneurysm but attempt to work around it. If
aneurysm infection is suspected clinically by aneurysm
tenderness and unexplained fevers, the aneurysm should
be cultured and completely excised. Maintaining adequate blood flow to the left colon via the inferior mesenteric artery or hypogastric arteries is essential to preventing colonic ischemia following abdominal aortic
reconstruction.

C. **Retroperitoneal coverage** of the graft must be complete. If it is not, the intestine, especially the duodenum, may adhere to the graft and eventually cause an aortoenteric fistula. Leaving the original aneurysm sac in place provides extra tissue with which to wrap the graft and separate it from the intestine.

VIII. **Concurrent intraabdominal disease**. In general, we prefer not to combine elective aneurysm surgery with other intraabdominal procedures that could be safely postponed. However, certain circumstances have led us to combine aneurysm repair with other procedures.

A. Asymptomatic gallstones usually are left alone. Cholecystectomy is performed when **gallbladder disease** is apparent—that is, when the patient has had recent symptoms of cholecystitis, the gallbladder appears chronically inflamed, multiple small stones are present, or common duct stones are palpable. The rationale for cholecystectomy in the latter group is prevention of postoperative cholecystitis, which is associated with a high mortality rate.

B. **Severe peptic ulcer disease** that is not well controlled by medication may be an indication for a highly selective vagotomy that does not open the gastrointestinal tract.

C. **Severe reflux esophagitis** that is not controlled medically may be managed by some type of fundoplication.

D. **Renal tumors** may require nephrectomy at the time of aneurysm repair.

E. **Colon or bladder tumors** present the dilemma of whether they should be resected before or after aneurysm repair. If a tumor is found incidentally during elective aneurysm repair, we manage the aneurysm first and return 3–6 weeks later to resect the tumor. If both the tumor and the aneurysm are known preoperatively, we address the more pressing problem first. For example, an obstructing colonic tumor would be relieved before repair of a smaller (4–6 cm) aneurysm. Occasionally, we encounter the combination of a tender aneurysm and a nearly totally obstructive colonic tumor, such that both diseases may require correction at the same operation. Normally, graft contamination can be avoided if the retroperitoneum is completely closed before the bowel resection.

F. **Benign prostatic hypertrophy** (BPH) requiring transurethral prostatic resection (TURP) or **prostatic cancer** requiring prostatectomy plus iliac node dissection is a common problem in patients with aortoiliac aneurysms. If the BPH has caused urinary retention and/or infection, a TURP should be considered before AAA repair. When a prostatectomy for cancer is indicated, we tend to repair aortoiliac aneurysms first if they are 5 cm or larger and do the iliac node sampling simultaneously. The radical prostatectomy is delayed until the patient has recovered from the AAA repair.

IX. **Postoperative care.** General principles of cardiorespiratory and multiorgan support after operation are summarized in Chap. 10. Specific principles of postoperative care for aortic surgery are discussed in Chap. 12.

X. **Postoperative complications.** Chapters 10 and 12 outli
the recognition of general and specific complications followi
major aortic surgery. General problems include cardiorespi
tory dysfunction, bleeding, stress ulceration of the gastro
testinal tract, renal failure, and postoperative psychosis (s
Chap. 10). Graft-related problems include anastomotic he
orrhage, graft thrombosis, colonic ischemia, aortoenteric f
tula, graft infection, and sexual dysfunction (see Chap. 12

XI. **Long-term follow-up.** The key determinant of late survi
is coronary heart disease. Patients with clinically evide
heart disease have a significantly impaired late survival r
(50% at 5 years and only 30–40% at 10 years). In encouragi
contrast, patients without evident coronary disease have
70–80% 5-year survival rate and a 50% 10-year survival ra
Although less common than cardiac morbidity, stroke affe
5% of AAA patients at 5 years and 10% by 10 yea
Hypertension appears to be a significant factor for both c
diac and cerebral events. Late graft complications (e.
thrombosis, infection, anastomotic aneurysms) affect 3–5
Although these problems can occur any time, they tend
appear relatively late (i.e., 5–15 years after graft placemer
Finally, about 5–10% of AAA patients will eventually devel
another aortic aneurysm in the chest or upper abdomen.

After the initial postoperative evaluation, patients shou
be examined at least yearly. Besides checking for graft pate
cy and anastomotic pseudoaneurysm, the surgeon shou
look carefully for other peripheral femoral or poplite
aneurysms. Since coronary artery disease is a leading cau
of late death in these patients, we recommend that tho
with severe angina pectoris be referred to a cardiologist
evaluation and intense medical therapy or, in selected cas
for coronary revascularization.

Femoral Artery Aneurysm

Arteriosclerotic femoral artery aneurysms (FAAs) genera
are found in patients who have diffuse aneurysmal disease
the abdominal aorta and the femoral and popliteal arteri
The primary dangers of femoral artery aneurysms are acu
and chronic thrombosis, distal embolization, and ruptu
Approximately 30% of such aneurysms present as a surgi
emergency. Therefore, elective surgical repair is warran
for most cases.

I. **Preoperative evaluation.** Because numerous patie
with FAAs will have an associated AAA or popliteal art
aneurysm, the preoperative evaluation must include care
palpation of the abdominal aorta and popliteal arteri
Ultrasound of the abdominal aorta and the popliteal sp
will help substantiate physical findings. An arteriogram
the involved femoral artery and distal runoff should be d
to delineate involvement of the profunda femoris and sup
ficial femoral arteries.

II. **Operative principles.** Three factors govern the choice
operation for common FAAs: (1) location of the origin of

profunda femoris artery, (2) patency of the superficial
femoral artery, and (3) patency of the aneurysm itself.

A. In **type 1** FAAs in which the profunda femoris orifice is
distal to the aneurysm and all vessels are patent, the simplest and most successful repair is a vein or synthetic
graft interposition for the resected aneurysm.

B. In **type 2** aneurysms, the profunda femoris arises from
the aneurysmal sac. We cannot overemphasize the
**importance of maintaining patency of the profunda
femoris when such aneurysms are repaired.** In most
instances, such aneurysms are resected and an interposition graft is carried out to the superficial femoral artery.
A small side-arm graft then is constructed to the profunda femoris artery.

C. When the superficial femoral artery is **chronically
occluded**, it is ligated and an end-to-end anastomosis of
the graft to the profunda femoris artery is performed.

III. Postoperative follow-up. After FAA repair, patients must
be followed at least yearly. Duplex ultrasound is an ideal
method to monitor grafts and to discover other aneurysms.
Newly discovered aneurysms of the abdominal aorta or
popliteal arteries should be corrected as indicated.

Popliteal Artery Aneurysms

Popliteal artery aneurysms (PAAs) threaten limb survival
because of thrombosis of the aneurysm or embolization from
it to the distal tibial vessels. These aneurysms seldom rupture, and when they do, the hemorrhage is confined to the
popliteal space. They may present as a painful mass behind
the knee, as an occlusion of the popliteal vein, or with compression of the posterior tibial nerve. In over 50% of patients
with PAAs, either acute or chronic ischemia will be the primary threat to the involved limb. Amputation is more common (30–35%) when acute thrombosis of the PAA is associated with embolization, thrombosis, or chronic arteriosclerosis
of the entire tibial outflow tract.

I. Preoperative evaluation. Like patients with FAAs, these
patients must be carefully examined for other aneurysms,
especially in the aortoiliac location. Preoperative angiography should show not only the location of the PAA but also
delineate the below-the-knee runoff. The presence of a patent
distal popliteal artery or an adequate posterior or anterior
tibial artery is the most important determinant of successful
repair for PAAs.

II. Operative principles. The preferred surgical treatment for
a smaller (3 cm) PAA is proximal and distal ligation of the
aneurysm combined with a reverse saphenous vein bypass.
The aneurysm is exposed through a medial knee incision.
When possible, the aneurysm should not be resected, since
this dissection can injure the popliteal vein. Larger
aneurysms should be opened, the thrombus removed, and a
portion of the sac resected to prevent compressive symptoms
from the mass effect of the aneurysm.

When thromboembolism has occluded the infrapopliteal
outflow acutely, two methods may help reestablish distal
flow. One is regional thrombolytic therapy used preoperatively or smaller regional doses (250,000–500,000 units of
urokinase) instilled directly into the tibial arteries at the
operating table. The second is retrieval of thrombus by a
Fogarty thromboembolectomy catheter.

Occasionally chronic infrapopliteal thromboembolism
and/or atherosclerosis will have occluded the tibial runoff
and left an unfavorable anatomic situation for a bypass. If
the ankle-brachial index is 0.35 or higher and the only symptom is rest pain, a lumbar sympathectomy may help avert
the need for amputation.

III. **Postoperative follow-up.** Patients surgically treated for
PAAs should be reevaluated at least yearly. Ultrasound is the
ideal test to monitor any popliteal graft and to check for associated aneurysms of the aortic, femoral, and opposite
popliteal artery.

Selected Reading

Cronenwett JL et al. Variables that affect the expansion rate and
outcome of small abdominal aortic aneurysms. *J Vasc Surg*
11:260, 1990.

Darling RC III et al. Are familiar abdominal aortic aneurysms
different? *J Vasc Surg* 10:39, 1989.

Gloviczki P et al. Ruptured abdominal aortic aneurysms: Repair
should not be denied. *J Vasc Surg* 15:851, 1992.

Hallett JW Jr, Naessens JM, Ballard DJ. Early and late outcome
of surgical repair for small abdominal aortic aneurysms: A
population-based analysis. *J Vasc Surg* 18:684, 1993.

Hollier LH, Taylor LM, Ochsner J. Recommended indications for
operative treatment of abdominal aortic aneurysms. *J Vasc
Surg* 15:1046, 1992.

Johnston KW, Scobie TK. Multicenter prospective study of nonruptured abdominal aortic aneurysms. I. Population and operative management. *J Vasc Surg* 7:69, 1988.

Johnston KW. Multicenter prospective study of nonruptured
abdominal aortic aneurysm. Part II. Variables predicting morbidity and mortality. *J Vasc Surg* 9:437, 1989.

Lowell RC, Gloviczki P, Hallett JW Jr. Popliteal artery
aneurysms: The risk of nonoperative management. *Ann Vasc
Surg* 8:14, 1994.

Nevitt MP, Ballard DJ, Hallett JW Jr: Prognosis of abdominal
aortic aneurysms. *N Engl J Med* 321:1009, 1042, 1989.

Parodi JC, Palmaz JC, Barone HD. Transfemoral intraluminal
graft implantation for abdominal aortic aneurysms. *Ann Vasc
Surg* 5:491, 1991.

Roger VL, Ballard DJ, Hallett JW Jr, et al. Influence of coronary
artery disease on morbidity and mortality after abdominal
aortic aneurysmectomy: A population-based study, 1971–1987.
JACC 14:1245, 1989.

Svensson LG et al. Experience with 1509 patients undergoing
thoracoabdominal aortic operations. *J Vasc Surg* 17:357, 1993.

Renovascular Hypertension

Renal artery reconstruction can be one of the most technically difficult of all vascular operations. In most cases, such procedures are performed to correct a renal artery stenosis causing renovascular hypertension or chronic renal insufficiency. Other less common lesions include aneurysms, emboli, traumatic lesions, and arteriovenous fistulas. This chapter summarizes general principles of diagnostic evaluation, indications for angioplasty or operation, surgical options, operative techniques, and perioperative care associated with renal artery reconstruction.

The options for managing renovascular disease continue to expand. Advances have recently been made in medical, radiologic, and surgical management. Newer antihypertensive medications such as angiotensin-converting enzyme (ACE) inhibitors and calcium-entry blockers are allowing better control of severe hypertension caused by renal artery stenosis. Radiologists have become active in performing percutaneous transluminal balloon dilatation of renal artery lesions. Surgical options also have increased. Ex vivo renal reconstruction, renal autotransplantation, and finer anastomotic technique done under magnification have allowed the vascular surgeon to correct difficult renal artery problems that previously resulted in nephrectomy.

I. **Renin-angiotensin system.** To logically manage renovascular hypertension, one must review the relationship of the kidney to blood pressure control. By adjusting sodium and water retention, the kidney helps maintain normal blood pressure by regulation of the extracellular fluid volume. A decrease in blood volume or an obstruction of a renal artery lowers renal blood flow. Baroreceptors in the juxtaglomerular apparatus detect the fall in renal blood flow. Their response to renal hypoperfusion is increased release of the enzyme **renin**. Renin stimulates conversion of a circulating plasma globulin, angiotensin I, to a powerful vasopressor, angiotensin II. Angiotensin II increases blood pressure by stimulating adrenal release of aldosterone, by causing arteriolar constriction, and by exerting an antidiuretic, antinatriuretic action on the kidney. The result is renal sodium and water retention. Extracellular fluid volume expands to increase blood pressure. Recent research has identified a complementary hormone, atrial natriuretic hormone, a natriuretic and vasorelaxant peptide secreted by the atria. This atrial peptide inhibits renal renin secretion and adrenocortical secretion of aldosterone, and opposes the vasoconstrictive action of angiotensin II.

II. **Diagnostic evaluation.** Approximately 5–15% of patients with arterial hypertension have a treatable renal artery stenosis. This association occurs more often in hypertensive children, who more commonly have abdominal aortic coarctations and associated renal artery stenoses. Nonetheless, history, physical examination, and routine laboratory tests do not usually allow differentiation between renovascular and essential hypertension.

A. **Screening tests.** Traditionally the test for renovascular hypertension was an intravenous pyelogram (IVP) showing delayed function in the affected kidney. However, the IVP has a sensitivity of approximately 75% and consequently may miss some patients with significant renal artery stenosis. Two newer functional tests for renovascular hypertension may be better: the **captopril test** and **captopril renal scanning**. The captopril test involves oral administration of captopril, an ACE inhibitor, after baseline measurement of plasma renin activity and blood pressure. Renovascular hypertension should be suspected when the post-captopril plasma renin level is excessively high. Some studies indicate that the sensitivity of this test approaches 100% with a specificity of 90%. However, the test is less accurate in the presence of renal failure. Criteria for a positive captopril renal scan include a reduction in glomerular filtration rate and a delay in the time to peak clearing of the radionuclide. Complementing these tests are two other imaging modalities: duplex ultrasonography and magnetic resonance imaging (MRI) angiography. Ultrasound requires a fasting patient, a skilled ultrasonographer, and a dedicated period of time (usually 1–2 hours). MR angiograms provide limited clarity in some patients, are relatively expensive, and are not always technically possible.

B. **Arteriography**. The cornerstone of diagnosis remains arteriographic demonstration of stenotic lesions in one or both renal arteries. We generally recommend an arteriogram when one or more of the following indications exist in a hypertensive patient:

1. Hypertension poorly controlled by adequate medical therapy.
2. Hypertension of recent origin with recent progression.
3. Hypertension in a child, adolescent, or young adult.
4. Hypertension associated with a localized epigastric bruit.
5. Possible renovascular etiology suggested by the IVP, duplex scan, renal scan, or MR angiogram.
6. Rising serum creatinine.

C. **Renin determination.** The presence of a renal artery stenosis on an arteriogram does not establish its functional importance. A comparison of renin determinations of venous samples taken from each renal vein and the inferior vena cava above and below the renal veins is required. Since an ischemic kidney will produce more renin, a renal vein ratio of at least 1.5:1.0 should be present if the stenosis is to be considered hemodynamically significant. One exception to this rule occurs when definite collateral vessels have developed.

Certain aspects of renal vein renin determination must be emphasized if meaningful results are to be obtained. Antihypertensive medications and unrestricted sodium intake are two factors that may affect renal vein renin assay. For example, beta blockers can suppress renin output. The result is false nonlateralization of the renal vein renins. Likewise, sodium intake may also reduce renin output.

Probably the most practical current method to stimulate a difference in renal vein renins is captopril administration (25 mg PO) after baseline renins are collected. Renal renin levels are recollected 30 minutes after captopril. A 30-minute post-captopril renal venous ratio of 3 or greater enhances the likelihood that hypertension will respond to surgical or angioplastic treatment or a renal artery stenosis.

The arteriogram should include (1) an abdominal aortogram, (2) selective renal artery injections in different planes, and (3) a celiac artery injection if the splenic or hepatic arteries are to be used for either a splenorenal or hepatorenal bypass.

III. **Indications for operation.** There are four main indications for reconstruction of a renal artery.

A. **Renovascular hypertension** is by far the most common indication for operation. A renal vein renin ratio of 1.5 with laterality to the affected kidney is predictive of improvement or cure in about 75% of cases. Success also depends on the etiology of the renal artery disease and the age of the patient. The best surgical results have been reported in younger patients (<50 years old) with fibromuscular dysplasia or focal atherosclerotic lesions. Long-term relief or cure of hypertension occurs in at least 90% of such patients. In contrast, patients with renal artery disease and generalized atherosclerosis may have less satisfactory surgical improvement. Although most patients with advanced renal atherosclerosis will not be cured, their blood pressure can usually be controlled with less medication. Consequently, 70–80% of such patients will be clinically improved (i.e., diastolic pressures <90 mm Hg).

Despite nonlateralizing renins, operation may be indicated if the clinical picture and arteriographic lesion suggest a high likelihood of renovascular hypertension.

In certain situations, initial treatment should be angioplasty. The primary example is the patient with fibromuscular renal disease of the main renal artery. Percutaneous transluminal balloon angioplasy is initially successful in 80–90% of these patients. Angioplasty also provides satisfactory dilation in some patients where the fibromuscular dysplasia extends into the first renal artery branches.

Finally, controversy continues over whether patients with renovascular hypertension should be managed medically until hypertension can no longer be easily controlled by antihypertensives. Recent evidence indicates that renal function continues to deteriorate in about 40% of patients with atherosclerotic renal artery stenosis under good medical control of hypertension. Consequently, medically treated patients must have their blood pressure, serum creatinine, and glomerular filtration rate followed every 3–6 months.

B. **The preservation of renal function** by renal artery reconstruction is receiving increased attention. Patients who are most likely to benefit from surgery to preserve renal function often are difficult to select. Certainly, consideration for operation should be given to patients with severe bilateral renal stenoses or a severe stenosis of a solitary functioning kidney (prior nephrectomy, nonfunctioning contralateral kidney, or total renal artery occlusions). Progressive renal deterioration may be indicated by decreasing kidney size, despite little angiographic change in the appearance of the renal artery stenoses and minimal change in serum creatinine.

Several surgeons have encouraged a more aggressive approach to revascularization of functioning kidneys with proximal renal artery occlusion. Such kidneys may retain significant function by collateral blood flow. No single factor predicts salvage of a kidney with a chronic renal artery occlusion. Although kidneys less than 9.0–9.5 cm in size have poorer results, successful revascularization has been achieved in smaller kidneys. Other predictors of renal salvage have been rich perihilar collateral circulation, distal renal artery reconstitution, and biopsy evidence of intact viable glomeruli. However, biopsy is subject to random sampling. In experienced hands, the best approach to such patients appears to be surgical exploration with either renal artery reconstruction if a viable kidney is present or nephrectomy if salvage is not possible.

C. **Surgical correction** of aneurysmal or occlusive disease of the aorta may necessitate preservation of a main or accessory renal artery. Accessory renal arteries less than 2 mm in size can usually be ligated without significant loss of renal function.

D. **Other renal artery problems** requiring renal artery reconstruction include aneurysms, emboli, dissections, traumatic lesions, and arteriovenous fistulas. Renal artery aneurysms generally should be repaired when they are associated with hypertension and they appear causative. Other indications for repair may be distal emboli arising from an aneurysm thrombus, increasing diameter size greater than 1.5–2.0 cm, and actual rupture. Rupture of a renal artery aneurysm appears more likely during pregnancy. Therefore, women with renal aneurysms in the childbearing period should be considered for elective aneurysm repair. A renal artery embolus should be suspected in any patient with conditions predisposing to arterial emboli who develops acute flank pain. Renal arteriovenous fistulas are difficult surgical problems, especially when they are in the renal parenchyma. Intrarenal arteriovenous fistulas may be treated by transcatheter steel coil occlusion accomplished under fluoroscopic control by a vascular radiologist.

IV. **Surgical options.** Preservation of a functioning kidney is the primary goal of any renal operative procedure. Nephrectomy is done only when no other method of saving a good kidney appears possible. A wide variety of autogenous

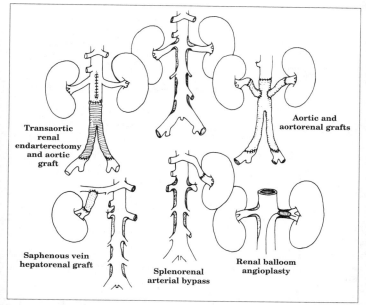

Fig. 17-1. Options for renal revascularization for atherosclerotic disease.

and synthetic graft materials are available for renal artery reconstruction. Endarterectomy is another alternative. Figures 17-1 and 17-2 illustrate our preferred methods of renal artery revascularization. Autogenous grafts, such as those from the saphenous vein or another artery, are preferable to synthetic materials. Factors that generally increase the risk of operative morbidity and mortality are azotemia (creatinine ≥3 mg/dl), complex or bilateral renal revascularizations, past myocardial infarction, compromised ventricular function, aortic aneurysm repair, and diffuse vascular disease.

V. Preoperative preparation. Before any renal artery revascularization, blood pressure and renal function must be stabilized as much as possible.

    A. Blood pressure. Most of these patients have significant hypertension, which increases the risk of myocardial and cerebrovascular events. Generally, blood pressure will improve with hospitalization and bed rest, sometimes allowing a reduction in antihypertensive medications. We try to stop diuretic therapy 24–48 hours prior to the operation so that chronically contracted intravascular volume can expand. Beta blockers should not be abruptly stopped since discontinuation may result in tachycardia and myocardial ischemia.

    B. Renal function. About one-third of patients undergoing renovascular surgery have chronic renal insufficiency

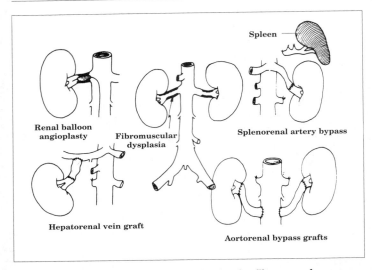

Fig. 17-2. Options for renal revascularization for fibromuscular disease.

(creatinine >2 mg/dl). Several factors can cause deterioration in their creatinine clearance prior to hospitalization and during preoperative evaluation.

1. Vigorous diuretic therapy can cause intravascular volume contraction and prerenal azotemia.

2. **ACE inhibitors** must be administered cautiously, if at all, in patients with bilateral renal artery stenoses or a solitary kidney with a high-grade stenosis. ACE inhibitors disturb renal blood flow autoregulation, probably by decreasing efferent arteriolar resistance, which must be maintained to provide an adequate perfusion gradient to the glomerulus. Worsening serum creatinine is frequently due to these drugs, which are being used increasingly for hypertension and congestive heart failure. We stop them in all patients with elevated serum creatinine. Generally creatinine will return to lower levels in 5–7 days.

3. Another frequent cause for an acute rise in serum creatinine is **angiographic contrast nephrotoxicity**. Multiple consecutive studies such as an intravenous digital subtraction arteriogram followed by a standard transfemoral renal, carotid, or coronary arteriogram can quickly worsen renal function. One must keep in mind that many computed tomography (CT) scans are also done with intravenous contrast. After all contrast studies are completed, we generally observe the serum creatinine level for at least 24 hours before proceeding with any renal surgery. If creatinine rises, we delay operation until the azotemia has resolved for at least 1–2 days.

VI. Operative principles

- **A. Incisions**. Proper operative exposure is one of the most difficult aspects of renal artery surgery. A midline xiphoid-to-pubic bone incision provides good access. An upper transverse or subcostal incision may be used but does not provide as good exposure of the distal aorta or iliac system. A left splenorenal arterial anastomosis can be constructed through a low, left thoracoabdominal incision (bed of the tenth rib) or a left subcostal incision.
- **B. Proximal renal lesions.** For central lesions, the midline retroperitoneum is opened over the aorta. On the left side, the left renal vein can be mobilized by ligation and division of the adrenal, gonadal, and left reno-lumbar branches. On the right side, the vena cava must be mobilized and retracted to expose the proximal right renal artery.
- **C. Middle or distal lesions.** For middle or distal lesions, on the right side, the duodenum must be reflected by a Kocher maneuver to expose the distal right renal artery. On the left side, the splenic flexure of the colon can be mobilized in a similar fashion.
- **D. Renal protection.** Several steps must be taken for renal protection:
    1. Intravenous hydration with a balanced salt solution (e.g., Ringer's lactated solution, 100–125 ml/hour) is started 8–10 hours before surgery.
    2. Heparin (5,000 units) is given intravenously before clamping the renal artery.
    3. Mannitol (12.5–25.0 g) is administered early in the procedure. If a good diuresis is not achieved, 20–40 mg of furosemide is used.
    4. The kidney may be cooled with 200–300 ml of a renal perfusate if anticipated renal ischemic time is greater than 45 minutes. We use a combination of 1 liter of Ringer's lactated solution, 18 g mannitol, 20 mg heparin, and 500 mg methylprednisolone (Solu-Medrol), chilled to 3°C in saline slush.
    5. Low-dose (2–3 µg/kg/minute) dopamine causes renal vasodilatation, which may help minimize vasomotor nephropathy. We start dopamine intravenously in the operating room before renal artery clamping and continue it for at least 12–24 hours.
- **E. Type of anastomosis**. The proximal anastomosis is constructed first. Then, the distal anastomosis is made end-to-end by the spatulation technique. The suture material usually is 6-0 or 7-0 polypropylene. For an especially difficult anastomosis, the suture line is interrupted. Low-power magnifying loops and a high-intensity headlight are essential in most renal artery reconstructions.
- **F. Intraoperative assessment of graft patency.** The simplest method to ascertain blood flow is the examination of the graft or renal artery with a sterile continuous-wave Doppler. Biphasic signals should be present. Recently, intraoperative duplex ultrasonography has provided a relatively quick and reliable method to detect technical problems after renal artery grafting or endarterectomy. Significant problems are detected in about 10% of recon-

structed arteries. Most of these problems are correctable and lead to results similar to those of patients with normal intraoperative ultrasound studies.

VII. Postoperative care. In the immediate postoperative period, intravascular volume must be carefully maintained to ensure adequate urine output. It may require use of a Swan-Ganz pulmonary artery line to monitor filling pressures in patients with significant cardiac disease. Low-dose dopamine is continued for renal vasodilation, and dobutamine is administered to patients with marginal cardiac output (<3 liters/m^2). Generally, we strive to maintain a urine output of 1 ml/kg/hour. Some patients have a massive diuresis (>200 ml/hour) and require urinary replacement (0.5 ml of crystalloid per ml of urine) for 12–24 hours. Diuretics are usually not necessary in the first 24 hours. When a question arises about the early patency of the reconstruction, we obtain a renal scan. Before discharging the patient from the hospital, the surgeon should consider ordering a renal scan or an arteriogram to document the patency of the reconstruction at that point. Any subsequent recurrence of hypertension or deterioration of renal function requires a repeat angiographic study. Percutaneous transluminal angioplasty may be performed on an anastomotic stenosis in an attempt to salvage a failing graft. Reoperation of stenotic or thrombosed renal grafts can achieve a successful result in more than 50% of patients.

VIII. Renal balloon angioplasty. Chapter 6 discusses the results of balloon angioplasty for selected renal artery stenoses caused by fibromuscular dysplasia and atherosclerosis. Surgeons must be informed about this technique and understand which patients are the optimal candidates.

IX. Quality of life. A major issue in treating renovascular hypertension and renal insufficiency is whether the side effects of medical therapy or the risks of surgical revascularization are worse than the disease itself. Certain antihypertensives (e.g., certain beta blockers) cause enough lethargy, sexual dysfunction, and sleep disorders for 15–20% of patients to withdraw themselves from therapy. Likewise, patients with renovascular-related renal failure that leads to chronic dialysis have only a 50–60% chance of normal activity and work. These discouraging results compare to a 75–90% chance of improved blood pressure and 90% chance of avoiding chronic dialysis after properly conducted renovascular operations. Operative risk ranges from 2–3% for patients without azotemia to 5–7% for those with a serum creatinine level greater than 2 mg/dl.

Selected Reading

Cambria RP et al. The durability of different reconstructive techniques for atherosclerotic renal artery disease. *J Vasc Surg* 20:76, 1994.

Canzanello VJ, Textor SC. Noninvasive diagnosis of renovascular disease. *Mayo Clin Proc* 69:1172, 1994.

Chaikof EL et al. Ischemic nephropathy and concomitant aortic disease: A ten-year experience. *J Vasc Surg* 19:135, 1994.

Dean RM et al. Evolution of renal insufficiency in ischemic nephropathy. *Ann Surg* 213:446, 1991.

Hallett JW Jr et al. Renovascular operations in patients with chronic renal insufficiency: Do the benefits justify the risks? *J Vasc Surg* 5:622, 1987.

Hanson KJ et al. Contemporary surgical management of renovascular disease. *J Vasc Surg* 16:319, 1992.

Izzo JL Jr, Black HR (eds). *Hypertension Primer.* Dallas: American Heart Association, 1993.

Novick AC et al. Trends in surgical revascularization for renal artery disease. *JAMA* 257:498, 1987.

Stanley JC. Renal Artery Occlusive Disease. In LJ Greenfield (ed), *Surgery: Scientific Principles and Practice.* Philadelphia: Lippincott, 1993. Pp. 1629–1643.

Stanley JC. The evolution of surgery for renovascular occlusive disease. *Cardiovasc Surg* 2:195, 1994.

Weibull H et al. Percutaneous transluminal renal angioplasty versus surgical reconstruction of atherosclerotic renal artery stenosis: A prospective randomized study. *J Vasc Surg* 18:841, 1993.

Zierler RE, Bergelin RO, Isaacson JA, Strandness DE Jr. Natural history of atherosclerotic renal artery stenosis: A prospective study with duplex ultrasonography. *J Vasc Surg* 19:250, 1994.

Intestinal Ischemia

Intestinal ischemia comprises a small portion of all peripheral vascular problems. Although aortic atherosclerosis may involve the origins of the mesenteric arteries, intestinal collateral blood flow usually is adequate enough to prevent symptomatic, chronic intestinal ischemia. Likewise, arterial emboli can obstruct mesenteric arteries, but more commonly they flow by the visceral vessels and lodge in the leg arteries. Consequently, these anatomic and hemodynamic features make intestinal ischemia less common than chronic claudication or acute ischemia of the lower extremities.

For several reasons, acute or chronic intestinal ischemia remains one of the most challenging problems of peripheral vascular surgery. Failure to recognize that a patient has some form of intestinal ischemia is one of the main reasons for poor results. Patients often are operated on too late to salvage the ischemic intestine or, many times, to save the patient's life. Even when intestinal ischemia is recognized and treated expediently, many patients still succumb because of serious underlying medical problems. The best surgical results have been achieved in patients with chronic intestinal angina who undergo intestinal revascularization before severe weight loss or acute thrombosis occurs.

In this chapter, we emphasize **early recognition** of intestinal ischemia. **Delay in diagnosis represents one of the primary failings in the care of these patients.**

Mesenteric Artery Anatomy

Certain anatomic features of the mesenteric circulation determine symptoms and influence management of intestinal ischemia (Fig. 18-1). Although the three major mesenteric arteries supply specific territories, they normally intercommunicate by excellent collateral channels. These collaterals enlarge when a proximal mesenteric artery is stenotic or occluded. The primary collateral pathways between the celiac and superior mesenteric arteries are via the gastroduodenal artery to the pancreaticoduodenal arteries that connect with the superior mesenteric artery. The inferior mesenteric artery has two main sources of collateral flow when it is obstructed (Fig. 18-2). The middle colic branch of the superior mesenteric artery connects around the transverse colon to the marginal artery of Drummond, a continuation of the left colic branch of the inferior mesenteric artery. The inferior mesenteric artery also receives collateral flow via the middle hemorrhoidal artery, a branch of the internal iliac artery. These abundant collateral channels for mesenteric circulation explain the clinical observation that **intestinal angina usually does not occur until at least two of the three main mesenteric arteries have severe occlusive disease.**

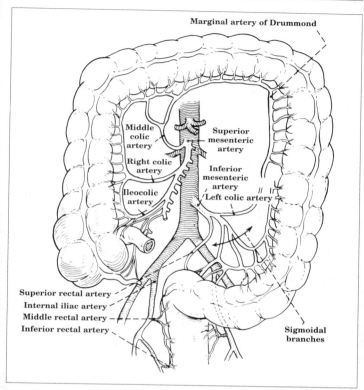

Fig. 18-1. Anatomy of the colonic arterial supply. When the inferior mesenteric artery is diseased or occluded by atherosclerosis, viability of the left colon may depend on collateral flow from the superior mesenteric artery via the marginal artery of Drummond. (Modified from CB Ernst. Intestinal Ischemia Following Abdominal Aortic Reconstruction. In VM Bernhard, JB Towne (eds), *Complications in Vascular Surgery*. Orlando: Grune & Stratton, 1985. Pp 325–350.)

Clinical Presentation

Intestinal ischemia is classified as either chronic or acute. However, the presentations may overlap, since chronic intestinal stenosis can progress to acute thrombosis and intestinal infarction.

I. **Chronic intestinal ischemia** often eludes early diagnosis because the chronic abdominal pain is attributed to some more common gastrointestinal (GI) disorder. Frequently, the patient has undergone a negative diagnostic evaluation of the gallbladder, liver, and entire GI tract. Because of progressive weight loss, some patients are mistakenly thought to have cancer. Certain clinical features, however, should raise suspicion of chronic intestinal ischemia.

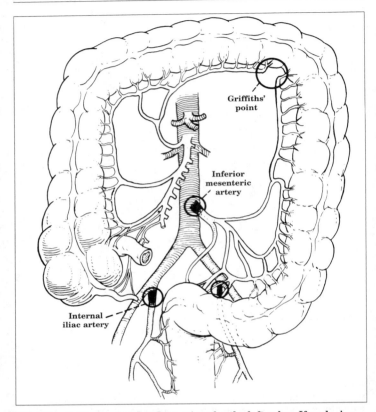

Fig. 18-2. Critical arterial inflow points for the left colon. If occlusive disease or operative reconstruction obliterates flow through both internal iliac arteries and the inferior mesenteric artery, the colon may become severely ischemic. Colonic ischemia is more than likely in this situation if the superior mesenteric-inferior mesenteric collateral connections are not developed or injured at Griffiths' point. (From CB Ernst. Intestinal Ischemia Following Abdominal Aortic Reconstruction. In VM Bernhard, JB Towne (eds), *Complications in Vascular Surgery.* Orlando: Grune & Stratton, 1985. Pp 325–350.)

A. Classically, the **chronic abdominal pain** is intermittent and postprandial. It usually is localized to the epigastrium and is a dull ache or colic that begins 30–60 minutes after eating and may persist for a few hours. Patients may have associated abdominal bloating or diarrhea.

B. **Involuntary weight loss** eventually occurs because the patient associates eating with pain. Consequently, a "food fear" develops. Oral intake often is modified until liquids become the primary nutrient.

C. Physical findings of chronic intestinal ischemia are limited primarily to **weight loss** and an **abdominal bruit.** Since the weight loss usually is insidious over several months and many patients with atherosclerosis have abdominal bruits, the significance of these nonspecific findings often is overlooked when the patient initially presents.

D. Chronic intestinal ischemia should be suspected in any adult who has chronic abdominal pain, progressive weight loss, other signs of generalized cardiovascular disease, and a negative work-up for more common GI disorders.

II. **Acute intestinal ischemia** has three main etiologies: thrombosis of an arterial stenosis, embolism, and nonocclusive small-vessel insufficiency. Although the initial symptom for all these etiologies is abdominal pain, the clinical setting often suggests the most likely underlying cause. The frequency of each etiology may vary among medical centers, but generally acute intestinal ischemia is caused by thrombosis in 40% of cases, embolism in another 40%, and intestinal hypoperfusion in 20% of cases.

A. **Severe generalized abdominal pain** that is disproportionate to the physical findings remains the classic presentation of acute intestinal ischemia. Nausea, vomiting, or diarrhea may follow shortly after the onset of symptoms. Although the abdomen may have diffuse tenderness, bowel sounds may be heard and peritoneal signs usually are absent. The only early laboratory abnormality may be an elevated white blood cell count. When these findings are made, the clinician must suspect acute mesenteric ischemia and undertake steps to alleviate it. Aggressive radiologic and surgical intervention at this point can salvage about 50% of such patients.

If intestinal ischemia remains unrecognized, physical findings will change as intestinal necrosis develops. Bloody diarrhea may occur, although often it is not present. Hypovolemia becomes evident as fluids are sequestered in the ischemic intestinal wall and surrounding tissues. Fever, peritoneal signs, and shock occur as sepsis becomes established. When intestinal ischemia has advanced to this point, the likelihood of salvaging the ischemic intestine and the critically ill patient is less than 15–20%.

B. The **clinical setting** and the patient's past medical history usually suggest the probable etiology of acute intestinal ischemia. If chronic intestinal angina preceded acute symptoms, mesenteric artery thrombosis is the most likely etiology. Emboli should be suspected when atrial fibrillation is present or if the patient has had previous cerebral or lower-extremity thromboembolism. Nonocclusive, mesenteric ischemia occurs in the setting of low cardiac output. The most common predisposing conditions for nonocclusive, mesenteric ischemia are myocardial infarction, congestive heart failure, renal or hepatic disease, or any major operation that leads to hypovolemia or hypotension in a patient with atherosclerosis. This type of nonocclusive, acute mesenteric ischemia is being recognized more commonly.

Diagnostic Tests

When acute or chronic intestinal ischemia is suspected, the most reliable diagnostic method is arteriography. **Early**

angiographic diagnosis is the most important principle of successful management of acute intestinal ischemia. An arteriogram with lateral views of the aorta to show the mesenteric artery origins is the definitive method. The angiographic catheter also has become an important route for delivering vasodilating drugs and thrombolytic agents to the mesenteric circulation.

The evaluation of possible chronic mesenteric ischemia usually includes other diagnostic tests before angiography is done—commonly, barium studies of the upper and lower GI tract. Abdominal ultrasound and computed tomography (CT) scanning may also reveal hepatobiliary disease or occult tumors such as cancer of the pancreas or lymphoma of the retroperitoneum. Duplex scanning can scan mesenteric blood flow patterns, allowing noninvasive determination of stenosis and changes in flow before and after a test meal. The use of velocity wave form parameters that can discriminate between normal subjects and those with visceral artery stenosis should reduce both the incidence of missed diagnosis and unnecessary angiography. The extent of diagnostic work-up for patients presenting with chronic abdominal pain obviously must be individualized.

Management

Treatment of intestinal ischemia also can be organized into the two broad categories of chronic and acute ischemia.

I. **Chronic intestinal ischemia** can be relieved only by correction of the occlusive lesions. There is no effective medical therapy. Surgical correction has been the most common technique, although balloon angioplasty has been successful in a few patients.

A. One aspect of preoperative preparation, **nutritional repletion**, deserves special emphasis. Since chronic intestinal ischemia leads to progressive weight loss, some patients are chronically malnourished and have no nutritional reserves for a major abdominal operation. We strongly recommend that such catabolic patients undergo a period of total parenteral nutrition before elective surgery. This nutritional repletion may prolong hospitalization but should enhance perioperative wound healing and the patient's ability to fight infection.

B. **There are two basic surgical options** for mesenteric revascularization: bypass grafting or endarterectomy. Over the years, different authors have preferred one technique to the other. Either supraceliac or infrarenal aortomesenteric bypass grafting is the procedure of choice for most patients. The optimum method of mesenteric revascularization, however, depends highly on the number of vessel occlusions and the condition of the abdominal aorta in each patient. Transaortic endarterectomy has also been successful for multiple visceral occlusive lesions at the origins of the mesenteric arteries. Combined infrarenal aortic replacement and Dacron bypasses to mesenteric arteries appears to be the technique of choice when severely symptomatic infrarenal aortic occlusive or aneurysmal disease coexists with chronic intestinal ischemia. However, combining mesenteric revascularization and aortic replacement carries a high mortality rate (10–20%) in these cachectic patients. In contrast, limiting the operation to some type of aortomesenteric grafting or endarterectomy alone minimizes mortality (3–5%).

Regardless of which method of revascularization is selected, early relief of intestinal angina is achieved in about 90% of patients. In our reported experience, the best long-term results have been obtained by revascularization of at least two occluded or stenotic vessels. In most patients this combination has included both the celiac and superior mesenteric arteries. Symptoms recurred in 10% of patients who underwent complete revascularization, in 25% who had two of three occlusive lesions corrected, and in 50% who had a single vessel revascularized. Since revascularization of a single mesenteric occlusion offers relief to most patients, complete revascularization must be weighed against the patient's overall condition, prognosis, and other technical factors.

Chronic or acute intestinal ischemia also may be the iatrogenic result of sacrificing the inferior mesenteric artery at the time of infrarenal aortic grafting. Revascularization of the inferior mesenteric should be performed when the superior mesenteric artery is occluded and a large (>3.5–4.0 mm) inferior mesenteric artery is present.

Another less common form of chronic mesenteric ischemia is median arcuate compressions and stenosis of the celiac axis. Some extrinsic compression of the celiac axis by the median arcuate ligament is common in women, but most experts question its functional importance. Certainly, a celiac stenosis may be critical when occlusive disease of the superior mesenteric and inferior mesenteric arteries is present also. Division of the median arcuate ligament with either patch angioplasty of the celiac stenosis or an interposition graft may alleviate symptoms.

II. Successful management of **acute intestinal ischemia** must begin with arteriography to define the mesenteric anatomy. Optimal therapy for acute mesenteric ischemia cannot be determined unless the clinician knows whether the problem is thrombotic, embolic, or hypoperfusion-related.

    A. Thrombosis usually is apparent on the arteriogram by obstruction of the superior mesenteric artery at its origin from the aorta. Systemic heparin is indicated to prevent clot propagation.

    Emergency abdominal exploration should be undertaken to assess bowel viability and to revascularize the obstructed artery. Resection of a nonviable intestine without revascularization of the remaining small bowel is associated with a high incidence of further intestinal infarction and death. Generally the bowel should be revascularized before intestinal resection. An exception to this rule is resection before revascularization when a segment of intestine is grossly gangrenous or perforated. A single aortomesenteric bypass is sufficient in these seriously ill patients. When bowel contamination is present, a vein graft is preferable to a synthetic material.

Clinical judgment of intestinal viability may be enhanced by fluorescein examination of the GI tract. The test is performed by injection of 2 ampules (1,000 mg) of sodium fluorescein through a peripheral vein and immediate examination of the bowel under an ultraviolet Wood's light in a darkened operating room. A viable bowel has a smooth or uniform fluorescence. A nonviable bowel has decreased, patchy, or no fluorescence. When it appears that the bowel may survive, it may be left alone and a second-look operation should be performed within 24 hours to reassess the intestinal viability. Doppler flow analysis has been used also to check intestinal perfusion, but it appears to be less reliable than fluorescein examination.

B. Emboli usually lodge a few centimeters beyond the origin of the mesenteric artery at the level of the first jejunal branches. Standard therapy remains identical to the management of thrombosis, except the embolus usually is removed by a mesenteric artery arteriotomy and Fogarty catheter thromboembolectomy. Sometimes a vein patch or a bypass graft is needed if significant arterial stenosis is present also.

C. Nonocclusive mesenteric ischemia generally is seen in critically ill patients who have low cardiac output. They often are poor risks for any surgery and many times are so labile that transport to the angiographic suite is a major undertaking in itself. Their arteriograms show peripheral mesenteric vasoconstrictions but no large-vessel occlusions. Noninvasive ischemic colitis appears to be mediated primarily by a remarkable sensitivity of the colonic vasculature to the renin-angiotensin axis.

The best results with this group of patients have been achieved by measures to improve cardiovascular hemodynamics and to vasodilate the peripherally constricted mesenteric vasculature. The recommended splanchnic vasodilator therapy is a papaverine infusion of 30–60 mg/hour through an angiographic catheter positioned in the superior mesenteric artery. If a vasopressor is needed to increase blood pressure, dopamine would be the drug of choice, since it reduces renal and mesenteric vascular resistance.

Selected Reading

Cormier JM et al. Atherosclerotic occlusive disease of the superior mesenteric artery: Late results of reconstructive surgery. *Ann Vasc Surg* 5:510, 1991.

Cunningham CG et al. Chronic visceral ischemia: Three decades of progress. *Ann Surg* 214:276, 1991.

Hallett JW et al. Recent trends in the diagnosis and management of chronic intestinal ischemia. *Ann Vasc Surg* 4:126, 1990.

McAfee MK et al. Influence of complete revascularization on chronic mesenteric ischemia. *Am J Surg* 164:220, 1992.

Moneta GL et al. Mesenteric duplex scanning: A blinded prospective study. *J Vasc Surg* 17:79, 1993.

Murray SP, Stoney RJ. Chronic visceral ischemia. *Cardiovasc Surg* 2:176, 1994.

Taylor LM, Moneta GL. Intestinal ischemia (basic data underlying clinical decision-making in vascular surgery). *Ann Vasc Surg* 5:403, 1991.

Zelenock GB. Visceral Occlusive Disease. In LJ Greenfield (ed), *Surgery: Scientific Principles and Practice.* Philadelphia: Lippincott, 1993. Pp. 1614–1629.

Upper-Extremity Arterial Disease and Vasospastic Disorders

In the spectrum of peripheral vascular diseases, upper-extremity arterial problems, including vasospastic disorders, are relatively uncommon. When pain, numbness, coldness, or ulcers involve the fingers or hand, patients generally seek early medical attention. Such symptoms restrict many normal activities and quickly raise the patient's fear of permanent loss of hand function.

The underlying causes of arm ischemia and vasospastic disorders are diverse. For simplicity, they may be organized into the broad groups of emboli, atherosclerotic or aneurysmal occlusions, trauma, and small-vessel arterial occlusive disease. In the initial patient evaluation, the clinician must determine which broad group the patient fits into (see Chap. 3). Then diagnostic tests can be selected to define the specific underlying etiology. This chapter emphasizes principles of management after a clinical diagnosis is established.

Common Clinical Presentations

Although the etiologies for upper-extremity arterial ischemia, including vasospastic disorders, are multiple, the clinical presentations are relatively few.

I. **Raynaud's phenomenon** is simply a description of a clinical presentation or syndrome that suggests vasospasm. The underlying causes are numerous (Table 19-1). Certain clinical features help differentiate Raynaud's phenomenon from other vasospastic disorders, such as acrocyanosis and livedo reticularis (Table 19-2).

   A. Raynaud's phenomenon defines an **episodic** constriction of the small arteries and arterioles of the extremities. The episodes generally are initiated by cold exposure or emotional stimuli. The symptoms of acrocyanosis and livedo reticularis are constant, although they increase with cold exposure.

   B. The phenomenon usually follows a definite **sequence of color** in the digits and hand: pallor, cyanosis, and rubor. The pallor occurs when small arterioles close and skin perfusion is minimal. As cutaneous flow begins to resume, it is sluggish, and blood desaturation leads to cyanosis. Finally, cutaneous flow resumes with a hyperemic phase causing skin rubor. Some patients will not demonstrate all these color changes. Attacks usually are accompanied by numb discomfort of the fingers. Pain generally is not severe unless ulcerations are present. In contrast, acrocyanosis occurs mainly in women and is characterized by

Table 19-1. Diverse etiologies of Raynaud's phenomenon

Systemic diseases or conditions
  Collagen vascular diseases (e.g., scleroderma)
  Cold hemagglutination or cryoglobulinemia
  Myxedema
  Ergotism
  Macroglobulinemia
Nerve compressions
  Carpal tunnel syndrome
  Thoracic outlet syndrome
Occupational trauma
  Pneumatic hammer operation
  Chain saw operation
  Piano playing
  Typing
Arterial occlusive disease

Table 19-2. Differentiation of vasospastic disorders

Characteristics	Raynaud's phenomenon	Acrocyanosis	Livedo reticularis
Sex	Primarily women (70–80%)	Primarily women (90%)	Men or women
Age	Young adults (15–35)	Young adults (15–35)	Any age
Color change	Pallor, cyanosis, rubor	Diffuse cyanosis	Mottled cyanosis or rubor
Location	Fingers, toes, sometimes face	Usually hands, sometimes feet	Usually legs, sometimes arms
Duration	Intermittent	Continuous	Continuous
Effect of cold exposure	Increased symptoms	Increased symptoms	Increased symptoms
Skin ulceration	Occurs when collagen vascular disease (e.g., scleroderma) is present	None	Rare

continuous bluish discoloration of the hands and occasionally of the lower extremities. Livedo reticularis also is a continuous vasospastic condition consisting of a mottled or reticulated reddish blue discoloration of the lower extremities and occasionally of the hands.

C. The phenomenon is **localized** to the fingers, toes, and occasionally nose and ears. Attacks are limited most commonly to the upper extremities and rarely involve only the toes.

D. The chance of ulceration or gangrene of the tips of the digits depends on the underlying etiology.

  1. Raynaud's disease is the term applied to Raynaud's phenomenon that has no clear association with any systemic disease. It rarely results in tissue necrosis. Raynaud's disease usually occurs in young females (70% of cases). It has been suggested that, before the diagnosis of Raynaud's disease is made, the following strict criteria should be met:

   a. Bilateral, symmetric Raynaud's phenomenon is present.

   b. No large arterial occlusions are evident.

   c. Slight or no gangrene or trophic changes apparent.

   d. Symptoms present for a long period, usually 2 years, without evidence of any other systemic disease associated with Raynaud's phenomenon.

2. **Raynaud's phenomenon** is the term applied when a local or systemic disease appears to be the precipitating factor. Gangrene or ulceration of digits is more common in these patients, especially when they have scleroderma. Scleroderma is the most common collagen vascular disease associated with Raynaud's phenomenon. Raynaud's phenomenon is the initial symptom in 30% of cases and eventually affects 80% of patients with scleroderma. The other common rheumatic diseases associated with Raynaud's phenomenon include mixed collagen vascular disease (80%), systemic lupus erythematosus (30%), dermatomyositis/polymyositis (20%), and rheumatoid arthritis (10%). It must be remembered that Raynaud's phenomenon may exist for years before some underlying systemic collagen vascular or immunologic disease is diagnosed.

3. **Acrocyanosis** is not associated with skin ulceration. **Livedo reticularis** may occur with ulcerations, generally when some systemic disease (e.g., periarteritis nodosa) is present or atherosclerotic microembolism is evident.

II. **Tissue necrosis** includes gangrene and nonhealing ulcerations. It is not uncommon for patients to mistake microemboli or small ulcers of the fingers for inconsequential bruises or sores of the finger, not recognizing their more serious etiology. If Raynaud's phenomenon precedes the onset of tissue necrosis, other symptoms and signs of underlying systemic disease should be sought. In the absence of Raynaud's phenomenon, evidence of large-vessel occlusive disease, emboli, or small-vessel arterial occlusive disease associated with occupational trauma must be sought.

A. **Large-vessel occlusive disease** of the arm usually is localized to the subclavian or axillary arteries. Usually these lesions are arteriosclerotic, and, most commonly, the origin of the left subclavian artery is involved. A less common etiology of proximal upper-extremity arterial occlusion is thrombosis of an axillary artery aneurysm caused by years of crutch use (e.g., by patients with poliomyelitis). Chronic subclavian artery trauma related to thoracic outlet syndrome also may eventually lead to vessel occlusion. Extensive acute deep venous thrombosis of the arm can cause venous gangrene, which may be initially mistaken for arterial insufficiency. Finally, postmastectomy irradiation of the axillary area can result eventually (10–20 years later) in radiation-induced axillary-subclavian arterial stenosis.

B. Emboli to the digits may originate from the heart or the subclavian artery. In severe arm ischemia secondary to emboli, the heart is the place of origin in about 50% of cases, while the other 50% of emboli are shed from the subclavian or axillary arteries. The proximal upper-extremity arteries may develop atherosclerotic ulcerative plaques or aneurysms that shed emboli. Poststenotic subclavian aneurysms associated with thoracic outlet compression or axillary aneurysms caused by prolonged crutch use also may cause embolism to the hand. Embolic or acute arterial ischemia can also be caused by thrombus shed from the anastomotic site of an occluded axillo-femoral bypass graft.

C. Small-vessel arterial disease associated with occupational hand trauma may cause severe hand ischemia. Occupations involving repetitive vibration or percussion of the fingers or hand predispose some individuals to spasm, thrombosis, or aneurysms of the ulnar, radial, palmar, or digital arteries. The ulnar artery is especially susceptible to local trauma over the hypothenar eminence, where it is fairly superficial and easily compressed against the underlying pisiform and hamate bones. The term **hypothenar hammer syndrome** has been applied to this form of posttraumatic digital ischemia. Activities that may lead to hand ischemia are pneumatic hammer, lathe, or chain saw operation; riveting; and less strenuous activities such as piano playing and typing. In industry, the term **vibration-induced white finger** has been applied to posttraumatic digital ischemia.

Rapid onset of hand ischemia has also been seen with small-vessel occlusion caused by hypersensitivity angiitis. This etiology should be suspected when no large-vessel occlusion is present and no systemic diseases are identified.

III. Arm claudication is an unusual presentation of arm ischemia in our experience. In general, exertional arm fatigue is more commonly caused by neurologic compression at the cervical spine or thoracic outlet. Because of excellent collateral channels around the shoulder, subclavian occlusive disease often is asymptomatic or mildly symptomatic (Fig. 19-1). However, active adults, especially manual laborers, may experience forearm claudication from subclavian or brachial artery stenosis.

Diagnostic Tests

Patient history and physical examination provide most of the information necessary to diagnose the general type of upper-extremity arterial disease (see Chap. 3). The following tests may be done to confirm the clinical impression, to identify underlying etiologies, and to monitor therapy.

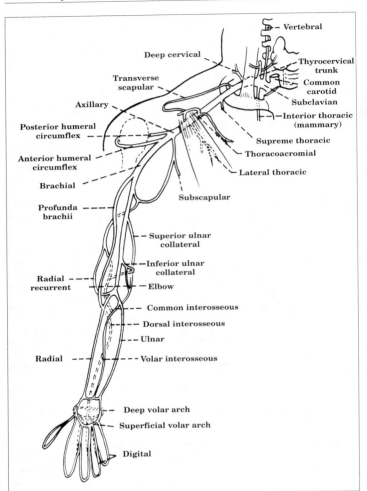

Fig. 19-1. Arterial anatomy of the upper extremity. The collateral circulation of the arm is well developed, and consequently proximal large-vessel occlusion seldom results in distal extremity necrosis and amputation.

I. **Doppler velocity flow detection**. The Doppler system is a simple means for auscultating arm arterial flow when pulses are not palpable. The axillary, brachial, radial, ulnar, palmar, and digital arteries can easily be checked for flow. Biphasic or triphasic arterial sounds are normal, while monophasic dampened signals suggest significant obstruction. Upper-arm and forearm blood pressures can be measured with a routine blood pressure cuff and the Doppler unit. In cases of suspected arm claudication, baseline brachial pressures should be obtained and then a drop in pressure after arm exercise for 2–5 minutes should be observed.

II. **Digital plethysmography** may be helpful in the evaluation of digital ischemia and vasospastic disorders. Flat or severely diminished (<5 mm) pulse volume recordings (PVRs) confirm severe digital flow reduction and are predictive of poor healing when ulcers are present. The digital PVRs can be repeated to assess digital blood flow improvement after treatment, especially after alphablockade or sympathectomy.

III. **Arteriography**. Arteriography is most helpful when large-vessel occlusion is obvious. In such cases, arteriography defines the location of the occlusion and shows the runoff to the forearm and hand. Transfemoral arteriography is recommended, since the catheter can be positioned to demonstrate the origin of the subclavian artery or be manipulated into the arm when distal runoff is of greatest interest. Arteriography is not necessary to diagnose vasospastic disorders but may be necessary to rule out any large-vessel ulcerative lesions when Raynaud's phenomenon is complicated by finger ulcers. Arteriography must show the entire upper-extremity vasculature from its origin (innominate on the right and subclavian on the left) to the digital arteries. Failure to obtain complete upper-extemity arteriography is a common reason for a missed diagnosis (e.g., digital occlusions due to an ulcerated atheroma in the proximal subclavian artery).

IV. **Digital temperature recovery time** can help establish the diagnosis of Raynaud's phenomenon. The physiologic principle behind the test is simple, and the technique of the test also is fairly easy. Digital cutaneous blood flow is linearly related to digital skin temperature over a wide range. Normally, digital skin temperature recovers to normal within 10–15 minutes after cold exposure. In contrast, digital skin temperature in patients with Raynaud's phenomenon does not recover for at least 20–25 minutes after cold stimulus. The accuracy of the test is improved when the following guidelines are followed for measuring the digital temperature recovery time:

A. The patient should sit in a warm (24°C ± 2°), quiet room for at least 30 minutes before the test.

B. Baseline digital pulp temperatures are taken with a thermistor probe.

C. The hand is immersed in an ice-water mixture for 20 seconds, removed, and dried.

D. Digital temperatures are checked every 5 minutes for 30–45 minutes.

E. A temperature-time graph can be constructed to show the digital temperature versus recovery time.

F. Controls for a particular laboratory should be established for comparison.

V. **Systemic disease work-up**. Since systemic diseases so often underlie vasospastic disorders and upper-extremity ischemia, a number of screening laboratory tests should be considered. A platelet count should be done, since thrombocytosis can mimic Raynaud's phenomenon. An elevated sedimentation rate should raise suspicion of a systemic illness. Since serum protein abnormalities may be associated with vasospasm, a serum protein electrophoresis should be performed and cryoglobulins, macroglobulins, and cold agglutinins should be checked. Basic immunologic tests should include antinuclear antibody, rheumatoid factor, and lupus erythematosus tests. If scleroderma is suspected, a skin biopsy in an affected area may confirm the diagnosis or a barium esophagogram may reveal characteristic esophageal dysfunctions.

Management

In our experience, these guidelines have provided the best assurance of relieving upper-extremity ischemia, including vasospastic disorders. Where there are areas of controversy, we offer several different points of view.

I. **Vasospastic disorders**

   A. **Raynaud's disease** usually can be satisfactorily managed by nonoperative methods. Tissue necrosis rarely is a problem; consequently, the patient needs assurance that loss of fingers or their function is not likely to occur if the following guidelines are observed.

   1. **Avoidance of any tobacco use and protection from cold exposure** are the fundamentals of initial treatment. Tobacco leads to vasoconstriction, a fact that can be documented by comparing baseline digital PVRs to tracings taken immediately after the patient smokes several cigarettes. The basics of protection from cold exposure include warm gloves and footwear during cold weather and gloves when working with the refrigerator. Maintaining core body temperature by wearing warm clothing over the trunk also helps. For many patients, these simple measures are enough.

   2. When vasospasm is not satisfactorily relieved by these simple measures, several **medical options** are available and are usually effective. The best results are obtained with drugs that diminish sympathetic neuromuscular transmission and new calcium-entry–blocking agents. Recently the drug of choice has been nifedipine, 10 mg PO tid. For some patients the long-acting nifedipine (XL tablets, 30–90 mg daily) causes fewer side effects. The most common side effects include headache, dizziness, palpitations, flushing, and edema. Our second choice of drugs has been the alpha-adrenergic blocker phenoxybenzamine (Dibenzyline), 10–30 mg PO daily. The dosage should be increased slowly; otherwise, dizziness from postural hypotension may be a bothersome side effect. Another effective drug is guanethidine, 10–30 mg PO daily. In some patients, the best result will be obtained by a combination of these two drugs. Although our experience is limited to the above drugs, others have reported success with oral prazosin and reserpine.

3. **Thermal biofeedback** has demonstrated excellent results in patients in whom anxiety and stress play a major role in the initiation of vasospastic attacks. After biofeedback training, 80–90% of patients can avert an attack of Raynaud's phenomenon, and some can actually increase skin temperature as much as 4°C.

4. The role of **surgical sympathectomy** for Raynaud's disease is limited. Few patients should need sympathectomy, since conservative management controls symptoms in at least 80% of patients. Reasonable candidates for sympathectomy are those patients whose vasospastic attacks are becoming progressively debilitating, especially when trophic or ulcerative changes have occurred. Approximately 50–60% of such patients with primary Raynaud's phenomenon and no underlying systemic collagen vascular or immunologic disease will have improvement after sympathectomy, although the initial results may not last more than 3–6 months. For reasons that are not clear, sympathectomy for lower-extremity symptoms is more effective than that for arm symptoms.

B. **Raynaud's phenomenon** secondary to underlying systemic disease often is a more difficult problem to manage than Raynaud's disease. Tissue necrosis with exceptionally painful digital ulcers can be a chronic problem. The fundamentals of therapy remain avoidance of tobacco, protection from cold, and calcium channel blockers. Sympathectomy is far less effective than it is for Raynaud's disease. In fact, only 20–30% of patients with scleroderma and Raynaud's phenomenon improve after sympathectomy, so we rarely recommend sympathectomy in these patients. Good results for digital ulceration have been reported with upper-extremity digit sympathectomy performed with an operating microscope. This procedure should be done by an experienced hand surgeon.

C. **Acrocyanosis** does not lead to tissue loss, so treatment is directed at relieving cold-induced symptoms. The conservative management described for Raynaud's disease usually is sufficient.

D. **Livedo reticularis** also is manageable in most cases by conservative treatment. Digital ulceration may occur when livedo reticularis is associated with periarteritis nodosa, lupus erythematosus, or cholesterol embolization. In such cases, sympathectomy should be considered, although results have been variable.

E. **Cold hypersensitivity** may be seen after recovery from frostbite. The affected area may become bluish and have an associated burning pain with even mild cold exposure. The problem seems to be a variant of reflex sympathetic dystrophy (sympathetically maintained pain). Initially, the medical treatment described for Raynaud's disease should be undertaken. For severe cases, regional sympathectomy may provide lasting relief, especially if it is done before pain becomes chronic.

II. **Threatened limb loss.** Although vasospastic disorders may cause ulcerations of the tips of the digits, the hand and arm seldom become ischemic. Severe hand ischemia usually is associated with large-artery occlusions, emboli, or trauma.

A. **Acute ischemia** generally requires emergency surgical intervention. The history and physical examination usually will identify the probable cause. If there is a delay for medical stabilization and arteriography, we administer heparin systematically to the patient to prevent thrombus propagation. Patients who develop brachial artery occlusion after cardiac catheterization should undergo immediate brachial thrombectomy and repair under local anesthesia. Although the patient's hand may initially be relatively asymptomatic, a chronic brachial artery occlusion can cause bothersome arm claudication in active individuals. Thus, early brachial thrombectomy and repair are preferable to delayed surgery, can be accomplished at minimal risk under local anesthesia, and achieve return of distal pulses in 98% of patients.

B. **Emboli** usually can be successfully extracted with Fogarty embolectomy catheters. Thromboemboli lodged in the subclavian axillary segment generally are approached through an infraclavicular pectoral muscle-splitting incision. More distal forearm clots are more completely removed by brachial artery cutdown. Although distal digital and small-vessel clots have been irretrievable by Fogarty catheters, adjuvant thrombolytic agents may be helpful in selected patients with recent thrombosis. In many such cases, however, the distal thrombosis is relatively chronic. Thrombolytic therapy does not help much when the clots are older than a few days. Emboli originating from proximal subclavian ulcerative lesions will require endarterectomy or grafting to remove the source of the emboli.

C. **Large-artery occlusion** generally will require bypass grafting, replacement, or reimplantation. Proximal subclavian obstructions may be bypassed by vein, autogenous artery (e.g., hypogastric), or synthetic grafts. A carotid-to-subclavian bypass and reimplantation of the subclavian artery into the common carotid artery are two options. Subclavian artery thrombosis secondary to thoracic outlet syndrome will require resection of the first rib and any cervical rib in conjunction with arterial repair. However, axillary and subclavian **vein thrombosis** secondary to thoracic outlet compression can be alleviated by thrombolytic infusions and anticoagulation followed by first rib resection in 2–3 months. Thrombosed axillary aneurysms usually are replaced with saphenous vein grafts. Saphenous vein also is the best graft material for brachial, radial, and ulnar revascularization.

III. **Arm claudication.** As discussed above, incapacitating arm claudication is fairly uncommon because of the rich collateral blood flow to the arm. For the few patients who need revascularization, the surgical options described for threatened limb loss (see sec. **II**) also are applicable to relieve claudication. Success also may be achieved by balloon angioplasty of proximal subclavian and axillary stenoses.

Long-Term Prognosis

The long-term prognosis for most arterial problems of the upper extremity is good. Nonoperative treatment is successful in many patients. Therefore, unless the viability of the extremity is acutely threatened, a period of conservative treatment and observation should be followed. The patients with the worst prognosis generally are those with Raynaud's phenomenon secondary to progressive collagen vascular disease or those with extensive distal small-vessel occlusion secondary to recurrent emboli or thrombosis.

Selected Reading

Austin EH, Wolfe WG. Aneurysm of aberrant subclavian artery with a review of the literature. *J Vasc Surg* 2:571, 1985.

Fugitani RM, Mills JL. Acute and chronic upper extremity ischemia. I. Large vessel arterial occlusive disease. In JM Porter, LM Taylor (eds), *Basic Data Underlying Clinical Decision Making in Vascular Surgery*. St. Louis: Quality Medical Publishing, 1994. Pp. 159–165.

Gloviczki P, Kazmier FJ, Hollier LH. Axillary-subclavian venous occlusion: The morbidity of a nonlethal disease. *J Vasc Surg* 4:333, 1986.

Machleder HI. Vascular Disease of the Upper Extremity and the Thoracic Outlet Syndromes. In WS Moore (ed), *Vascular Surgery: A Comprehensive Review* (4th ed). Philadelphia: Saunders, 1993. Pp. 592–605.

Machleder HI (ed). *Vascular Disorders of the Upper Extremity*. New York: Futura, 1989.

Mills JL, Fugitani RM. Acute and Chronic Upper Extremity Ischemia. II. Small Vessel Arterial Occlusive Disease. In JM Porter, LM Taylor (eds), *Basic Data Underlying Clinical Decision Making in Vascular Surgery*. St. Louis: Quality Medical Publishing, 1994. Pp. 166–170.

Specific Venous Problems

Varicose Veins

Varicose veins are one of the most common vascular problems seen in office practice. They affect about 15% of the adult population. Most varicose veins are the result of a congenital or familial predisposition that leads to loss of elasticity in the vein wall and the absence or incompetence of venous valves. These primary varicosities generally progress downward in the greater saphenous system. Secondary or acquired varicosities occur when the venous valves have been damaged by trauma, deep venous thrombosis, or inflammation. Prolonged standing and obesity make all leg varicosities more symptomatic. The basic pathophysiology and natural history of varicose veins are summarized in Chap. 2. A description of the initial lower-extremity venous examination is found in Chap. 4. This chapter focuses on the principles of medical and surgical therapy.

I. **Clinical presentation.** The most common complaints of patients with varicose veins are their unsightly appearance and aching or heaviness of the legs after prolonged standing. Symptoms may not correlate well with the degree of anatomic defect. Occasionally, a patient will abrade a varicosity, which may cause a rather impressive hemorrhage. A more common complication of varicose veins is superficial thrombophlebitis, which may cause considerable pain and disability but rarely leads to pulmonary embolism. Longstanding varicose veins may also result in chronic ankle induration, stasis dermatitis, and occasionally leg ulcerations.

   A. For the **initial history**, patients should be asked specifically about prior leg trauma, bone fractures, phlebitis, and bleeding or ulceration of the varicosities. In addition, they should be asked about previous treatment, including vein stripping, injection therapy, and support stockings.

   B. On **physical examination**, both legs should be inspected with the patient standing in good lighting. The clinician should palpate for fascial defects that indicate sites of incompetent communicating veins with the deep venous system. The varicosities and perforators should be accurately recorded on a drawing of the leg. The femoral triangle and the lower abdomen should be palpated to rule out any masses compressing the leg veins. Patency of the deep venous system and incompetent valves with reflux can be determined accurately with the Doppler ultrasonic velocity flow detector (see Chap. 5).

   C. One unusual variant of varicose veins occurs with the **Klippel-Trenaunay syndrome**, which appears to be a fetal developmental abnormality. The result is maintenance of microscopic arteriovenous communications in the upper or lower limb. The classic clinical triad includes (1) hemangiomas, (2) hypertrophy of soft tissue and bone with overgrowth of the extremity, and (3) varicose veins. Because of the benign course of this disease, the majority of these patients do not have surgery and do well with conservative therapy. Occasionally, a more aggressive operative approach may be necessary in patients with large, symptomatic varicosities, especially if hemorrhage or ulceration has occurred.

II. Medical treatment

A. The majority of patients with varicose veins can be managed initially by nonoperative treatment. The patient should be instructed to **avoid (1) prolonged standing, (2) prolonged sitting, (3) obesity, and (4) constricting garments.** They also are instructed to:

   1. Shower or bathe in the evening.

   2. Apply well-fitted, below-the-knees support stockings (20–40 mm Hg) before ambulating in the morning. Above-the-knee heavy support stockings generally are not necessary, since the majority of symptoms from varicose veins occur below the knee, where venous pressure is highest. Women with varicose veins may receive adequate support from a variety of high-quality sheer panty hose with graduated pressure from the ankle to waist. Several companies that specialize in venous hosiery currently offer such panty hose (e.g., Sigvaris and Futuro).

   3. Elevate the feet 10–15 minutes, 3–4 times daily.

   4. Walk to improve the musculovenous pump of the calf.

   5. Avoid trauma to varicose veins.
   These simple measures will alleviate the heavy, aching leg feelings that bother most patients with varicose veins.

B. Sclerotherapy is the injection of a sclerosing agent into the varicose vein to damage its endothelium and thus cause an aseptic thrombosis, which organizes and closes the vein. We use sclerotherapy as primary treatment for less extensive varicose veins and spider vein clusters. In contrast, sclerotherapy is not durable treatment for large (8–12 mm) varicosities that cascade down the entire lower extremity from a completely incompetent greater saphenous vein. The reaction from sclerotherapy may make subsequent surgical stripping of large varicosities more difficult. Sclerotherapy probably is also useful to obliterate small residual varicosities that persist after great saphenous stripping and ligation of perforating veins. Over a long follow-up period, surgery improves or cures about 80% of patients with varicose veins, while injection therapy succeeds in one-third of patients followed to 5 years.

   The essentials of safe and effective sclerotherapy are as follows:

   1. Veins that should **not be injected** include those in the lower one-third of the leg and ankle, particularly those arising from incompetent ankle perforators; veins on the foot; veins in fat legs where perivenous reactions may cause painful fat necrosis; and veins in the areas of postphlebitic stasis dermatitis.

   2. No more than 0.5 ml of the sclerosant (sodium tetradecyl sulfate 3%, hypertonic saline, or morrhuate sodium) should be used in any one injection site. A small-gauge (size 25 or 26) needle is used to inject four to six locations at one injection session.

3. The injection is done while the patient is reclining, not standing. The sclerosant is retained in the vein segment by compressing it above and below the injection site for about 1 minute. The injection is stopped if the patient complains of severe local pain, since this suggests extravasation of the sclerosant outside the vein.

4. A compressive elastic bandage is applied and the patient is actively ambulated immediately. This ambulation helps the musculovenous pump of the calf wash out any sclerosant that may have leaked into the deep venous system. The exact time the compressive bandage remains in place is variable, but usually 1 week is sufficient for an average injection in the small vein.

III. **Surgical treatment.** Varicose veins of the great and small saphenous systems can be cured by proper stripping and ligation of incompetent communicating veins.

   A. **Indications for operation.** The best surgical candidates are active, healthy patients who are not overweight. Severe aching varicosities, varicose vein hemorrhage, or superficial thrombophlebitis are indications for operation. Some patients simply desire removal of the varicose veins for cosmetic reasons. Occasionally, primary varicose veins lead to leg ulcers.

   B. **Preoperative preparation.** The area of skin preparation includes the groin as well as the lower extremity. Before operation, the varicose veins are marked with an indelible felt-tipped pen or other nontoxic dye while the patient stands. The sites of suspected perforators are marked with an X. The surgeon should do this marking and be sure that the patient agrees with the veins to be removed. The best time for marking is immediately before operation. After being marked, the patient should wear pajama pants or have a sheet placed between the lower extremities to prevent ink marks rubbing off onto the opposite leg. Unless the patient has had a history of thrombophlebitis, prophylactic low-dose heparin is not used.

   C. **Operative technique.** Several technical features of varicose vein surgery deserve emphasis. The operation is, in part, a cosmetic procedure; therefore, skin incisions should be small (0.5–1 cm). At the ankle, the great saphenous vein should be exposed medially and slightly inferior to the medial malleolus, so that the branches extending onto the foot can be ligated accurately or removed. Each tributary at the proximal saphenofemoral junction (usually five or six) should be ligated carefully. A meticulous search must be made for accessory greater saphenous veins, which are not uncommon. Perforators are ligated at the fascial level (Fig. 20-1). Finally, skin incisions are closed with fine, interrupted sutures (e.g., 4–0 nylon). Some surgeons prefer interrupted absorbable subcuticular sutures. Steri-Strips may be applied to complete this plastic closure. Compressive gauze bandages are applied with an elastic wrap from the toes to the groin. Some sur-

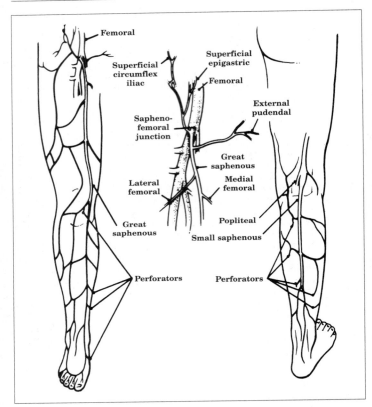

Fig. 20-1. Anatomy of the great and small saphenous veins and perforators. The enlarged vein of the saphenofemoral region demonstrates the major proximal branches of the saphenous vein that should be ligated and divided during ligation and stripping of the great saphenous veins.

geons strip only the evident varicose veins and preserve the greater saphenous trunk. This approach is reasonable if the greater saphenous vein is competent. However, most patients with large, symptomatic lower-limb varicose veins have a diffusely incompetent greater saphenous vein from the groin to the leg.

D. Postoperative care. For the first postoperative night, the patient is kept at bed rest with the operated leg elevated. On the next morning, the dressings are removed and a new below-the-knee elastic bandage is applied. The patient should ambulate every 2 hours for 5–10 minutes beginning on the first postoperative day. At the surgeon's discretion, the patient is discharged on the day of operation or the next morning, depending on the extent of groin and lower-limb dissection and early postoperative pain.

In general, these patients do not have much postoperative pain. Below-the-knee elastic support is continued until the patient is rechecked in the office in 1 week. For some patients, this support is continued for several more weeks to alleviate mild leg swelling and dependent heaviness that may follow lower-extremity venous surgery.

Selected Reading

Baskerville PA, Ackroyd JS, Browse NL. The etiology of the Klippel-Trenaunay syndrome. *Ann Surg* 202:624, 1985.

Bergan JJ. New developments in the surgical treatment of venous disease. *Cardiovasc Surg* 1:624, 1993.

Bergan JJ, Yao JST (eds). *Venous Disorders*. Philadelphia: Saunders, 1991.

Lange J. Surgical treatment of saphenous varices with preservation of the main great saphenous trunk. *J Vasc Surg* 2:886, 1985.

Lindenauer SM. Venous Physiology and Disorders of the Superficial Veins. In LJ Greenfield (ed), Surgery: Scientific Principles and Practice. Philadelphia: Lippincott, 1993. Pp. 1757–1764.

Servelle M. Klippel and Trenaunay's syndrome: 768 operated cases. *Ann Surg* 201:365, 1985.

Venous Thromboembolism

The current clinical approach to venous thromboembolism is remarkable for recent progress in prevention, diagnosis, and treatment. A better understanding of the pathophysiology of acute deep venous thrombosis (DVT) and pulmonary embolism (PE) has resulted in more aggressive preventive measures. The limitations of the physical examination in accurate diagnosis of venous thromboembolism have culminated in the development of noninvasive methods to detect DVT and document PE. Finally, clinical trials continue to define optimal treatment regimens. The details of prevention, diagnosis, and treatment are still debated. However, certain principles of care are generally accepted. These fundamental concepts are the focus of this chapter.

I. **Prevention.** Several prophylactic measures may decrease the incidence of venous thromboembolism, especially in sick patients at bed rest. These preventive measures may be organized conveniently around Virchow's etiologic triad for venous thrombosis: stasis, hypercoagulability, and vein injury.

A. **Stasis.** Prolonged immobilization of the lower extremities is perhaps the single most important event that precedes acute DVT. At bed rest, blood tends to pool in large, valveless venous sinuses of the calf muscles. The soleus venous plexus normally drains anteriorly into the tibial veins. Consequently, if the body is supine, blood pools in the calf muscles unless these muscles contract to empty the calf veins. ^{125}I-labeled fibrinogen studies show that calf vein thrombosis often begins while the patient is supine on the operating table.

Venous stasis in the calf may be prevented by elevation and intermittent or continuous mechanical compression of the leg. Simply elevating the leg 15–20 degrees improves emptying of major leg veins but may not completely empty the soleus venous sinuses. Likewise, graduated compression stockings may hasten flow in the tibial veins but not completely empty the soleus plexus, where clots often begin. Generally we do not use them in patients with arterial occlusive disease since the compression may worsen ischemic skin. Several studies have confirmed that intermittent pneumatic leg compression reduces postoperative DVT, especially in urologic and neurosurgical patients. Although effective, pneumatic boots are somewhat cumbersome and expensive. Finally, one of the simplest, yet most effective, methods of preventing calf vein stasis is to have the patient exercise the legs (plantar flexion) against a footboard for 5 minutes every hour. This exercise not only promotes venous flow but actually may enhance fibrinolytic activity, which clears small clots.

We generally take the following approach to mechanical prevention of venous stasis in patients undergoing major vascular operations. At the time of operation, the operating table is placed at 15 degrees of the Trendelenburg position to hasten deep venous emptying. After surgery, patients do footboard exercises for at least 5 minutes every waking hour and are encouraged to exercise more frequently if they can. Some physicians question whether patients will comply with this exercise program; we have found that patients will exercise regularly when the importance of these exercises is explained to them and encouragement is given after the operation. These calf exercises also help maintain muscle tone when several days of bed rest are necessary. We do not routinely use elastic antiphlebitic hose, pneumatic compressive boots, or low-dose heparin for patients who undergo vascular procedures. However, patients at higher risk for thromboembolism generally receive pneumatic compression devices on the lower extremities and/or some type of anticoagulant therapy, either with low-dose heparin or warfarin sodium (Coumadin).

B. Hypercoagulability. Acute DVT is more likely to occur in patients with some abnormality of coagulation. Low levels of antithrombin III have been found in women taking oral contraceptives. Antithrombin III activity also diminishes with soft-tissue trauma and operative wounding. Increased platelet adhesiveness may be another problem that predisposes certain patients to recurrent DVT. Recurrent venous thromboembolism has also been correlated with congenital deficiencies of protein C and protein S, the presence of antiphospholipid antibodies (e.g., lupus anticoagulant and anticardiolipin antibodies), and abnormal levels of fibrinogen and plasminogen. These findings of hypercoagulability support anticoagulation as another method of preventing DVT, especially when thromboembolism is most likely to complicate patient recovery.

Certain patients are at increased risk of DVT and PE. They usually are referred to **as high-risk patients** and include those who have experienced (1) previous venous thromboembolism; (2) lower-extremity trauma (e.g., hip fracture) and other orthopedic surgery of the hip, knee, or lower limb; (3) major pelvic operations (e.g., open prostatectomy or gynecologic operations); (4) prolonged bed rest or extremity immobility (e.g., stroke or back surgery); (5) acute myocardial infarction; (6) chronic congestive heart failure; and (7) malignancies (e.g., pancreatic cancer), as well as those on oral contraceptives. Prophylactic anticoagulation does offer these patients significant protection against venous thromboembolism. Several anticoagulative agents are available: warfarin, low-dose heparin, low-molecular-weight (LMW) heparin, dextrans, and antiplatelet drugs. Of course, a major hazard of anticoagulant therapy in surgical patients is bleeding, but major bleeding complications are rare if therapy is properly delivered and monitored and certain contraindications are observed. These contraindications include an active peptic ulcer, intracranial or visceral injury, hemorrhagic diathesis, gastrointestinal bleeding, severe hypertension, and gross hematuria or hemoptysis.

1. **Adjusted-dose warfarin** can be an effective prophylaxis for thromboembolism. However, there is not widespread acceptance of warfarin for prophylaxis. The dosage may be difficult to regulate and an excessively prolonged prothrombin time (PT) is associated with increased bleeding complications. Still, we have found adjusted-dose warfarin to be effective and safe when PT is maintained in the 16–20 second range (control = 12 seconds) or preferably at an international normalized ratio (INR) between 2.0–2.7.

   To standardize the PT for oral anticoagulation, the World Health Organization (WHO) has developed an international reference thromboplastin from human brain tissue and has recommended that the PT be expressed as the INR. With the past conventional use of rabbit brain thromboplastin reagents, a PT ratio of 1.3–1.5 (16–20 seconds) corresponds to an INR of 2.0–3.0. Recent clinical trials support less intense oral warfarin therapy (INR of 2.0–3.0) for most clinical conditions.

   Generally, warfarin anticoagulation should be reserved for patients with hip fractures, major hip surgery, open prostatectomy, and major gynecologic pelvic procedures. Low-dose heparin has not been uniformly effective in this group of high-risk patients. Patients who are chronic users of warfarin for prosthetic heart valves or because of a past thromboembolism may remain on warfarin during other major operations, provided the PT or INR is adjusted to lower levels. Another alternative in such patients is discontinuance of warfarin and coverage with low-dose heparin (5,000 units q8h) during the perioperative period.

2. **Low-dose unfractionated heparin** has received widespread attention for its use in the prevention of fatal postoperative PE. A meta-analysis of 78 randomized trials with over 15,000 patients confirms its benefit. Compared to those who receive no prophylaxis, heparin-treated patients experience a 40% reduction in nonfatal and a 64% reduction in fatal PE. The usual dosage schedule has been a loading dose of 5,000 units given subcutaneously 2 hours before operation and then 5,000 units q8–12h until the patient is fully ambulatory. This low-dose heparin apparently enhances antithrombin III activity with minimal to no change in coagulation tests. However, bleeding and wound complications may be more common in patients on low-dose heparin, although the absolute excess in bleeding is only about 2–3%. Therefore, the use of low-dose heparin probably should be reserved for those individuals at increased risk of thromboembolism, including patients with prior venous thromboembolism, those immobilized for long periods, and those subjected to major procedures involving extensive extremity or pelvic dissection or soft-tissue trauma.

3. **LMW heparins** have three potential advantages over unfractionated heparin: (1) effective prophylaxis with

once-daily administration, (2) improved efficacy, and (3) a lower frequency of bleeding. The LMW heparins have higher bioavailability and extended half-life compared to unfractionated heparin. Several randomized clinical trials have demonstrated that LMW heparin is as effective and as safe as unfractionated heparin in the management of proximal DVT. In addition, it does not require monitoring or dose adjustment. A meta-analysis of the literature from 1984–1991 has concluded that the relative risk of DVT with LMW heparin compared with standard heparin was 0.74, the risk of pulmonary embolism was 0.43, and the risk of major bleeding was essentially the same (0.98). Consequently, LMW heparin is still finding its niche in prophylaxis for venous thromboembolism.

4. **Dextrans and antiplatelet drugs** appear to have some merit in thromboembolism prophylaxis, but the data are equivocal. **Low-molecular-weight dextran** (LMD) is a glucose polymer that impairs platelet function by causing decreased platelet aggregability. An effective dosage regimen for LMD is 500 ml of a 10% solution started as a 100-ml IV bolus in the operating room and continued at 20 ml/hour until the patient is ambulatory. Bleeding complications of dextran therapy are similar to those of oral anticoagulants. Other potential problems include volume overload in patients with heart failure, allergic reactions, and renal tubular damage. Dextran also is more expensive than other anticoagulative agents. Its role in prophylaxis may be treating patients who cannot receive heparin because of heparin-associated thrombocytopenia.

5. **Aspirin** inhibits platelet function and has proved effective only for males in thromboembolism prophylaxis after total hip replacement. The final place of aspirin in prophylactic therapy for other patients remains to be established. **Dipyridamole** appears to be ineffective in preventing venous thromboembolism. However, neither of these agents is currently a first-line choice in patients at high risk of venous thromboembolism.

6. Many questions about the **optimum methods of thromboembolism prophylaxis** remain unanswered. In our practice, we continue to limit warfarin or low-dose heparin prophylaxis to high-risk patients. Other patients receive simple mechanical prophylaxis with leg elevation and footboard exercises. This approach has resulted in a low (1–2%) incidence of clinically apparent and significant venous thromboembolism in patients hospitalized with peripheral arterial or venous disease.

C. **Vein injury.** During elective operations, meticulous attention must be given to the gentle dissection and handling of veins. Large-vein injuries should be repaired by fine lateral suture technique, and ligation should be avoided. The surgeon also must avoid prolonged compression of the vena cava or other large veins with retractors or packs. Experimental studies have also documented endothelial tears that occur in extremity veins remote from an elective operative site. These endothelial lesions may become the focus of DVT.

II. **Diagnosis.** Patient history and physical examination frequently are unreliable in establishing an accurate diagnosis of either acute DVT or PE. Since either condition requires systemic anticoagulation, with its potential complications, we recommend the following approach to ensure that an accurate diagnosis is established.

A. **Superficial thrombophlebitis** generally is recognized by the physical findings of a tender superficial venous cord. Usually, there is no deep vein involvement. If the process extends to the groin, extension into the deep femoral system may be present. Duplex ultrasound is the best method to ascertain thrombotic involvement of the common femoral vein.

B. **Deep venous thrombosis** is suggested by leg pain, swelling, and tenderness. Since these findings are not specific for venous thrombosis, treatment generally should not be started without further noninvasive studies or a venogram to confirm the diagnosis. If the patient has had no previous DVT, our initial diagnostic test is a duplex ultrasound examination in high-risk patients or venous plethysmography in low-risk patients (see Chap. 5). Noninvasive studies, however, have definite limitations, especially in the pelvic veins, below the knee, and in the profunda femoris vein. Also, Doppler examination may be difficult to interpret if the patient has had previous DVT that has not recanalized. If the results of noninvasive tests are normal, other etiologies for the leg symptoms are investigated. Venography is reserved for patients with equivocal noninvasive results and an elevated clinical suspicion of DVT. Most experts now agree that positive noninvasive studies without a venogram are sufficient evidence to begin therapy in most patients.

C. **Pulmonary embolism** may present with chest pain, dyspnea, and occasionally hemoptysis. The source of the emboli is nearly always the leg or pelvic veins. Similar symptoms may occur with myocardial ischemia, bronchitis, pneumonia, or pleurisy, so PE must be confirmed by other tests.

1. Although hypoxia demonstrated on **arterial blood gas testing** is common with PE, a low arterial PO_2 is not diagnostic. Other laboratory tests may be abnormal but often are inconclusive also. Electrocardiographic abnormalities may include a rhythm disturbance and ST segment depression or T wave inversion, particularly in leads III, aVF, V_1, V_4, and V_5. These findings are indicative of myocardial ischemia associated with acute PE. The electrocardiogram (ECG) can also rule out an acute myocardial infarction as the cause of chest pain. The chest x-ray may look normal. In seriously ill patients, the x-ray may show infiltrates from pneumonitis or atelectasis.

2. **New plasma markers (D-Dimer test)** are being evaluated in the diagnostic work-up of suspected DVT and PE. A positive D-Dimer test, however, needs confirmation by some anatomic test.

3. **Radioisotope lung perfusion scanning** has become the primary screening test for PE. False-positive tests, however, may occur in many patients due to preexisting lung pathology such as asthma, emphysema, chronic bronchitis, pneumonitis, or neoplasm. Consequently, the chest x-ray should be checked before a lung scan to identify any disease process that may affect the scan. **In properly performed and interpreted scans, normal results essentially exclude a significant pulmonary embolus.** High-probability scans predict the presence of PE in about 90% of patients. If other alternative diagnoses appear unlikely, a positive ventilation-perfusion scan with a large $\dot{V}/\dot{Q}$ mismatch or multiple moderate areas of $\dot{V}/\dot{Q}$ mismatch is definitive. In cases of intermediate probability of PE, we recommend a pulmonary angiogram. In our recent experience, about 30% of patients can be treated after a lung scan alone, while the remainder need a pulmonary angiogram for definitive diagnosis and treatment.

4. **Pulmonary arteriography** remains the definitive diagnostic test for pulmonary thromboembolism if lung scanning cannot define the diagnosis. One must remember that most pulmonary emboli resolve in days to several weeks, and consequently, a pulmonary arteriogram may look normal after a while.

D. **Recurrent pulmonary embolism** from lower-extremity clots that occur while the patient is on adequate anticoagulation is indication for a vena cava filter. In addition, we consider a vena cava filter in patients with a documented extensive iliofemoral thrombosis or PE who cannot be safely anticoagulated (e.g., because of a recent brain tumor resection). Candidates for a vena cava filter usually have a pulmonary arteriogram to establish the diagnosis and a venacavogram to define the anatomy. The surgeon and interventional radiologist must know whether the patient has any major vena cava anomalies and where the renal veins are located before attempting placement of a filter.

E. **Subclavian-axillary venous thrombosis** is usually associated with thoracic outlet syndrome or central venous catheters. Acute diffuse upper limb swelling and a tight discomfort or pain are the most common manifestations. Thrombolytic drugs can recanalize the vein and quickly alleviate symptoms. Of course, definitive treatment requires surgical correction of the thoracic outlet compression. To prevent propagation of clot into the superior vena cava or retrograde into the arm, we favor removing all central venous lines that precipitate thrombosis. Anticoagulation with heparin is continued until acute symptoms resolve. Some patients are continued on coumarin anticoagulants for 2–3 months while the veins have a chance to recanalize and heal. Thoracic outlet surgical decompression is delayed for 2–3 months. This period of time generally allows the subclavian vein to recanalize in some patients and is associated with maximum development of collateral venous pathways that reduce edema.

III. Treatment. In Chap. 2, we emphasized that the natural history of DVT and PE may be altered by anticoagulation. In certain situations, surgical intervention also may help the patient. Thrombolytic therapy has also added another important alternative to managing serious DVT and PE.

   A. Treatment of **superficial thrombophlebitis** depends on the extent of the phlebitis and the general health of the patient. Elastic support, local heat, and an antiinflammatory medication (e.g., aspirin or a nonsteroidal antiinflammatory agent) may relieve localized superficial phlebitis. Resolution may take 7–14 days. If the phlebitis involves most of the greater saphenous vein and the leg is swollen, rest and elevation may hasten recovery. Anticoagulation is reserved for patients in whom deep venous thrombophlebitis is documented or in whom the phlebitis extends to the saphenofemoral junction and deep venous extension seems likely. If the thrombophlebitis is confined to superficial veins and the patient is a good operative risk, excision of the thrombosed vein and ligation and stripping of the greater saphenous vein may be curative and may shorten the time of disability.

   B. For **established DVT**, the patient is systemically heparinized with an intravenous bolus of 5,000–10,000 units followed by a continuous infusion of 1,000–1,500 units/hour.

   1. Continuous heparin infusion has been associated with fewer bleeding complications than has intermittent intravenous therapy. A solution sufficient for 6–8 hours of therapy should be used to avoid accidental heparin overdose. Ideally, continuous heparin therapy should be administered by an infusion pump. Although the ideal method of monitoring heparin therapy is debatable, an activated partial thromboplastin time test (APTT) is the standard in most hospitals. Anticoagulation is considered adequate when these test values are at least 1.5–2.0 times the pretreatment values. There is a common misconception that an APTT greater than twice normal (usually >100 seconds) is associated with more bleeding complications. On the contrary, clinical trials demonstrate a lack of association between a supratherapeutic APTT (ratio of 2.5 or greater) and the risk of clinically important hemorrhage. Platelet counts should also be checked at least every other day, since heparin may induce thrombocytopenia, intravascular thrombosis, or hemorrhage. Heparin-induced thrombocytopenia generally is recognized at least 3 days after onset of therapy, appears more commonly in patients with prior heparin therapy, and may be reversed by stopping heparin. **Recent clinical trials indicate that the length of heparin therapy can be shortened to 5 days without loss**

**Table 21-1. Dosages for common anticoagulants
and thrombolytic agents for venous thromboembolism**

Drug	Initial dose	Maintenance dose	Coagulation monitoring tests
Heparin	5,000–10,000 units IV bolus	1,000–1,500 units/hr continuous IV infusion	PTT Platelet count[*]
Warfarin sodium (Coumadin)	10–15 mg PO qd	5–10 mg PO qd	PT
10% dextran 40 (low-molecular-weight)	100–500 ml during operation	20 ml/hr (500 ml/day)	PT PTT
Streptokinase	250,000 units IV over 30 min	100,000 units/hr up to 72 hr	Thrombin time (2–3 times control)
Urokinase	2,000 units/lb body weight IV over 30 min	2,000 units/lb body weight	Euglobulin lysis time (15–20 min) PTT, fibrinogen

PT = prothrombin time; PTT = partial thromboplastin time.
[*]Heparin therapy may be associated with thrombocytopenia and disseminated intravascular coagulopathy. Therefore, platelet count should be followed during therapy.
Source: Some dosages were taken from AG Gilman, TW Rull, AS Nies, P Taylor (eds). *The Pharmacological Basis of Therapeutics* (7th ed). New York: Pergamon, 1990; and AV Persson. Fibrinolytic Therapy. In VM Bernhard, JB Towne (eds), *Complications in Vascular Surgery* (2nd ed). Orlando: Grune & Stratton, 1986.

    **of effectiveness or safety if oral anticoagulants
are started on the first or second day of treatment for DVT or PE.**

2. **Oral anticoagulants** are started during heparin therapy and are continued for 3–6 months. During this
period, the deep veins usually recanalize slowly. Since
warfarin inhibits blood clotting by interference with
liver synthesis of vitamin K–dependent clotting factors
(II, VII, IX, X), adequate anticoagulation with oral
agents requires several days of therapy. The appropriate dosages of the common anticoagulants are provided
in Table 21-1. The safest method of instituting warfarin
therapy is the nonloading technique, giving 10–15 mg
orally each day until prothrombin time is in the therapeutic range. An INR of 2.0–3.0 is therapeutic. A more
prolonged INR places the patient at increased risk of
bleeding complications. Such doses are just as effective
and less likely to cause bleeding complications than
maintaining a higher dosage.

    The target INR for warfarin should be **at least
2.0–3.0** for at least 1–2 days before stopping the
heparin. When oral anticoagulation is started, the

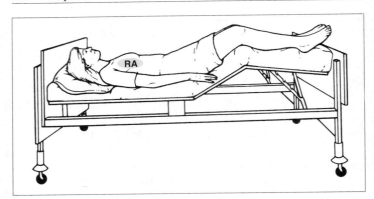

Fig. 21-1. Bed position for patients with lower-extremity venous thromboembolism. (RA = right atrium.)

level of protein C may decline and result in a thrombogenic potential. By overlapping the heparin and warfarin therapy for 4–5 days, this potential procoagulant effect of warfarin can be counteracted.

Oral anticoagulation is usually continued for **at least 3–6 months.** It may be continued longer or indefinitely in patients with underlying risk factors for venous thromboembolism. For patients who cannot take warfarin (e.g., pregnant women), adjusted-dose heparin is an alternative. A subcutaneous dose of heparin is administered twice a day to maintain a prolonged APTT, which is initially regulated by measuring the APTT just prior to the next dose.

3. **Leg pain and swelling** may be alleviated by bed rest, leg elevation, local heat, and analgesics. Figure 21-1 illustrates the proper bed position. Bed rest not only alleviates leg pain and edema but also allows the thrombus to organize and adhere to the vessel wall, a process that generally requires 24–72 hours. Bed rest is continued until leg swelling and tenderness resolve. For calf thrombosis, this usually takes 3–5 days. For iliofemoral thrombosis, 5–7 days may be required. When ambulation is begun, we have the patient use a below-the-knee elastic support (30–40 mm Hg) to reduce pain and swelling. This elastic support is continued for a minimum of 2–3 months. If the thrombosis involved the popliteal and femoral veins, we recommend that the patient wear lifelong 30–40 mm Hg below-the-knee compression hose to alleviate postphlebitic syndrome.

4. The final role of **thrombolytic therapy** in acute DVT has not been established. Streptokinase and urokinase promote dissolution of clots by stimulating the conversion of plasminogen to plasmin, an enzyme that breaks down fibrin. Complete lysis of iliofemoral thrombosis with maintenance of valve integrity has been accomplished with combined thrombolytic agents and heparin therapy. Thrombolytic therapy also may offer improved

results in patients with extensive iliofemoral thrombosis and cutaneous gangrene (phlegmasia cerulea dolens). Thrombolytic therapy is expensive and may be associated with major bleeding complications or allergic reactions. It is contraindicated in patients with active internal bleeding and recent (within 2 months) cerebrovascular accidents or other active intracranial disease. It also may cause serious hemorrhage after recent (<10 days) major surgery, obstetric delivery, organ biopsy, and previous puncture of a noncompressible vessel. Therefore, thrombolytic therapy must be used only by physicians who are completely familiar with its dosage and contraindications and in a setting in which therapy can be continuously monitored (see Chap. 6).

5. **Surgical therapy** of acute DVT has had less than spectacular results over the years. Late evaluation indicates that one-third of patients undergoing iliofemoral venous thrombectomy have good to excellent results, another one-third are improved, and one-third are not changed by operation. However, more recent experience with venous thrombectomy with a temporary arteriovenous fistula demonstrated that less than 10% of anticoagulated patients with iliofemoral venous thrombosis were completely free of postthrombotic symptoms compared to 40–45% of operated patients. Late venography has shown a 60–65% patency rate. Venous thrombectomy plus temporary arteriovenous fistula may be recommended for young patients with acute iliofemoral venous thrombosis to avoid development of incapacitating postphlebitic syndrome. In our experience, however, the role of venous thrombectomy for acute DVT remains very limited.

C. **Pulmonary embolism** (Table 21-2) also requires systemic heparinization followed by long-term oral anticoagulation. The dosages, methods of administration, and duration of therapy are the same as those used for acute DVT (see Table 21-1). Heparin and warfarin are intended to prevent further thromboembolism or clot propagation in the lung. They do little to resolve an existing thrombus. In contrast, thrombolytic therapy appears to allow more complete resolution of thromboemboli than do heparin and oral anticoagulants. Thrombolytic therapy also appears to improve capillary perfusion and diffusion, which may decrease the incidence of late pulmonary hypertension. Emergency pulmonary embolectomy, either by percutaneous suction catheter or surgery, is indicated for salvageable patients who have documented massive PE and persistent refractory hypotension despite maximum medical therapy. Chronic pulmonary embolectomy also may improve chronic hypoxia and respiratory disability in selected patients with recurrent PE and chronic organized pulmonary thrombi.

D. **Recurrent pulmonary embolism** after adequate anticoagulation or in situations where anticoagulation is contraindicated generally is considered an indication for a vena cava filter. Contraindications usually include gas-

Table 21-2. Classification of pulmonary thromboembolism

Class	Signs	Pulmonary artery occlusion (%)	Pulmonary artery pressure (mm Hg)	Management
I	None	<20	Normal	Anticoagulation
II	Tachypnea	20–30	<20	Anticoagulation
III	Collapse, hypoxemia	30–50	>20	Anticoagulation, thrombolytic therapy, vena cava filter
IV	Shock, hypoxemia	>50	>25–30	Pulmonary catheter embolectomy, vena cava filter
V	Cor pulmonale	>50	>40	Anticoagulation, vena cava filter

Source: Modified from LJ Greenfield. Pulmonary Embolectomy and Vena Caval Interruption. In JJ Bergan, JST Yao (eds), *Vascular Surgical Emergencies*. Orlando: Grune and Stratton, 1987. Pp 453–460.

trointestinal hemorrhage, recent stroke or neurosurgery, or hemorrhage requiring transfusion after anticoagulation was started. It must be remembered that small pulmonary emboli may continue during anticoagulation as lower-extremity or pelvic vein thrombi lyse. Such small emboli may go unrecognized or cause minimal physiologic problems and consequently would not be considered adequate indications for vena cava interruption.

Vena cava filtering prevents further PE in at least 90% of patients. Approximately 25% of patients who have a vena cava filter will develop chronic leg swelling. Vena cava filtering may be accomplished by a variety of percutaneously placed devices. Operative caval clipping or ligation is performed rarely anymore. We currently prefer a Greenfield filter or bird nest filter, which can be placed percutaneously via the jugular or femoral vein. We recommend that, before vena cava filtering is attempted, a pulmonary arteriogram be done to document embolism and an inferior venacavogram be done to delineate the level of the renal veins and any anomalous venous patterns, such as a double vena cava.

Vena cava filters and associated caval thrombosis may cause acute leg swelling. Bed rest and leg elevation usually is helpful after the procedure. When ambulation resumes, below-the-knee elastic support hose (30–40 mm Hg) should be worn to prevent postphlebitic syndrome. A few patients will have edema to their groins and may be more comfortable with full-length panty-type elastic support hose. If anticoagulation can be continued, it appears to improve the postphlebitic syndrome in about 80% of patients compared to only 50% of patients who have anticoagulation discontinued after filter placement.

Selected Reading

Goldhaber SZ, Morpurgo M, for the World Health Organization Task Force on Pulmonary Embolism. Diagnosis, treatment, and prevention of pulmonary embolism. *JAMA* 268:1727, 1992.

Greenfield LJ. Venous Thrombosis and Pulmonary Thromboembolism. In LJ Greenfield (ed), *Surgery: Scientific Principles and Practice.* Philadelphia: Lippincott, 1993. Pp. 1764–1778.

Hirsh J et al. Oral anticoagulants: Mechanism of action, clinical effectiveness, and optimal therapeutic range. *Chest* 102(4):313s, 1992.

Hull RH, Raskob GE, Rosenbloom D. Optimal therapeutic level of heparin therapy in patients with venous thrombosis. *Arch Intern Med* 152:1589, 1992.

Lofgren EP, Lofgren KA. The surgical treatment of superficial thrombophlebitis. *Surgery* 90:49, 1981.

Plate G et al. Thrombectomy with temporary arteriovenous fistula: The treatment of choice in acute iliofemoral venous thrombosis. *J Vasc Surg* 1:867, 1984.

Silver D. Heparin-Related Coagulation Complications. In CB Ernst, JC Stanley (eds), *Current Therapy in Vascular Surgery* (2nd ed.). Philadelphia: B.C. Decker, 1990. Pp. 576–579.

Postphlebitic Syndrome and Chronic Venous Insufficiency

Most patients who have had femoropopliteal deep vein thrombosis will develop some degree of postphlebitic syndrome. However, in 20–50% of patients with symptoms and signs of chronic venous insufficiency, no history of deep venous thrombosis (DVT) is obtainable. The classic physical findings are a chronically indurated ankle, dark stasis pigmentation around the ankle, and skin ulceration in some patients. Postphlebitic syndrome or primary deep valvular incompetence can be especially disabling for active ambulatory workers, since leg dependency increases pain and swelling and impedes ulcer healing. Fortunately, proper elastic leg support, skin care, and, in some situations, surgery can alleviate chronic venous insufficiency enough that patients can remain comfortable and active.

Management of postphlebitic syndrome is based on our present understanding of its pathophysiology (see Chap. 2). Thrombophlebitis damages deep venous valves and often leaves them incompetent. The musculovenous pump can no longer reduce ambulatory venous pressures. Consequently, the patient has chronic venous hypertension in the lower leg when he or she stands. These high venous pressures are transmitted through communicating veins from the deep to superficial venous system. The exact means by which this chronic venous hypertension causes stasis skin changes and ulceration is still unclear. The most recent evidence suggests that local capillaries leak fibrinous protein that is not adequately removed by fibrinolysis. A liposclerosis occurs and local tissue oxygen diffusion may be impeded. The result is tissue necrosis and skin ulceration. **Skin ulceration seldom occurs unless the popliteal vein valves are incompetent.**

In patients with chronic iliofemoral venous obstruction, venous capacitance is increased at rest and cannot compensate during exercise. The result is severe thigh pain and sensation of tightness with vigorous exercise **(venous claudication).** Symptoms are apparently more common in patients with chronic venous obstruction than in those who have recanalized veins with incompetent valves. A surprising observation is that 5–10 years after lower-extremity DVT, 80% of patients will have symptoms of chronic venous insufficiency **regardless** of the initial site of the thrombosis.

I. **Prevention.** Proper elastic leg support can alleviate the symptoms of leg pain and swelling. In addition, skin ulceration is less likely to occur in patients who routinely wear elastic leg support. To be effective, elastic leg support must be combined with a program of leg elevation at intervals throughout the day and proper skin care.

   A. In postphlebitic syndrome, ambulatory ankle venous pressures seldom drop more than 20–30% during leg exercise. Normally, ankle venous pressures would drop about 70% with exercise. The greatest venous pressure is found at the ankle, where most postphlebitic changes occur. This chronic venous hypertension **cannot be corrected by elastic leg support.** However, elastic leg support can prevent some of the leg edema caused by the elevated venous pressures.

Experience has demonstrated that the leg support should provide at least 30–40 mm Hg pressure at the ankle to prevent postphlebitic edema. This amount of pressure can be provided by either an elastic bandage or an elastic support hose. The most commonly used 30–40 mm Hg support hose are the Jobst graduated pressure hose, the Futuro elastic hosiery, and the Sigvaris graduated compression support. We generally recommend that the support hose be fitted below the knee and not carried above the popliteal space. There are several reasons for recommending below-the-knee support only. First, postphlebitic problems nearly always occur below the knee, where venous pressures are highest. Thigh swelling seldom is a problem after acute DVT has resolved. Second, support hose that comes above the knee often binds or constricts the popliteal space, especially if the hose slip down the leg. Third, patients generally do not like a heavy support hose that covers the entire leg. Many patients who are given full-length or panty-type heavy support hose will wear them only when visiting their physician for a check-up. However, some patients with vena cava occlusion and severe leg swelling to the waist will need full-leg heavy support hose and will wear them without complaint.

Several suggestions should be offered to the patient to ensure the proper and comfortable use of heavy support hose. First, the hose should be put on immediately on arising in the morning. Otherwise, early leg swelling may begin before the elastic support can control it. This routine usually requires that the patient bathe or shower before going to bed at night. Second, because these heavy hose may be difficult to slide on the leg, the patient may need a special stocking application device. A preferable method is to wear a knee-length light nylon hose beneath the heavy support sock. Some companies provide a silky slipper that can be removed after the heavy support hose is in place.

Elastic support hose must be properly fitted or the patient will not wear them. We encourage patients to contact the fitting shop for adjustments if their new hose do not fit satisfactorily. We also periodically recheck patients in the outpatient clinic to ensure that their hose fit properly. In general, most heavy elastic support hose will need to be replaced every 6–12 months.

B. **Leg elevation** remains a simple and effective method of alleviating ankle edema. Patients with postphlebitic syndrome should elevate their legs above the level of the heart for 10–15 minutes every 2–4 hours while they are ambulatory. This recommendation may seem impractical for the working individual. However, most workers are allowed several breaks during their normal work hours, when this elevation can be done. Periodic leg elevation allows most patients to remain comfortable during work. An explanatory note from the physician to the patient's employer often avoids any problem that the patient may encounter by periodically sitting down on the job.

C. **Skin care** is important if dermatitis, local infections, and ulcerations are to be prevented. Scaly pruritic skin of the foot or ankle may indicate fungal infection, which is managed by a topical fungicide such as Desenex or clotrimazole 1% solution (Lotrimin). Eczematous stasis dermatitis may be alleviated by a topical steroid cream, such as hydrocortisone cream 1%. Routine leg washing should be done with warm water and a mild soap. We discourage soaking the leg, since this may macerate friable skin and increase swelling due to dependency of the extremity.

D. **Diagnostic evaluation.** The anatomy and hemodynamics of the postphlebitic lower limb can be defined by descending venography, duplex scanning, Doppler signal analysis, and various types of plethysmography (see Chap. 5). For initial evaluation, we generally perform the Doppler analysis to assess valvular incompetency and impedance plethysmography to determine obstruction. Photoplethysmography is a good method to noninvasively examine ambulatory venous pressure and venous recovery time. Recently, duplex ultrasound has become an excellent method to image superficial and deep veins for both patency and reflux.

II. **Venous ulcers** classically occur on the medial side of the ankle at either the upper internal ankle perforator or the middle internal ankle perforator (Fig. 22-1). Less commonly, they occur on the lateral or posterior calf at the site of the lateral ankle perforator or the mid-posterior calf perforator (see Fig. 22-1). In our experience, ulcers may also present adjacent to the medial malleolus.

The oldest, most widely used, and most successful method of healing venous ulcers is use of a compression bandage. This bandage simply controls local ankle edema until the ulcer heals. The same result could be obtained by putting the patient on strict bed rest; however, such treatment incapacitates active individuals and may be attended with recurrent DVT.

Adherence to certain principles of compression therapy for venous ulcers will ensure success:

A. **Control infection.** If the ulcer appears infected, a culture should be taken and the wound washed with soap and water. Local cellulitis usually responds to a 5- to 7-day course of an oral antibiotic, such as a cephalosporin, 250–500 mg q6h. Local infection should be controlled by leg elevation and antibiotics before a compression bandage is applied. In general, topical antibiotics should not be applied beneath an Unna's paste boot, since topical allergic reactions are common. Generally, a sterile petroleum jelly is adequate to prevent the adherence of bandages.

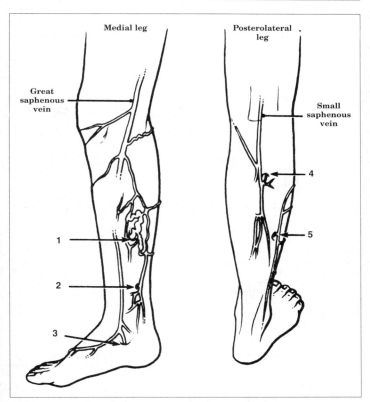

Fig. 22-1. Location of major lower-leg venous perforators. The perforating vein sites (numbered) on the medial leg, especially 1, 2, and 3, are common locations for postphlebitic venous ulcers. Ulcers seldom occur at the posterior and lateral venous perforators (4 and 5).

    B. Apply compression. The compressive bandage must be strong enough to counteract the very high venous pressures (80–100 mm Hg) that cause these ulcers (Fig. 22-2). Such compression can be accomplished with removable elastic bandages or an Unna's paste boot covered with a firm elastic wrap from the level of the toes to below the knee. This bandage can be left in place for 7–10 days before being changed. The commercially available Unna's boot bandages usually contain zinc oxide.

III. Recurrent or nonhealing venous ulcers. Proper elastic compression, leg elevation, and control of local infection will heal at least 85% of venous ulcers. A few patients will continue to have recurrent venous ulcers despite routine compression therapy. These patients often must stand for very long periods at work or do not routinely wear their support hose. When a suspected venous ulcer is not healing despite routine care, the physician must question whether some

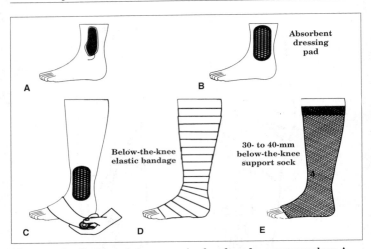

Fig. 22-2. Application of a compressive bandage for a venous ulcer. A. The ulcer should be washed with warm water and a mild soap. In general, topical antibiotics should be avoided since they may cause topical allergic reactions. For grossly infected ulcers, the infection should be controlled before the bandage is applied. B. A soft absorbent pad should be placed over the ulcer. C–D. The leg from the foot to the knee is wrapped with a compressive dressing: an Unna's paste boot bandage, an Ace wrap, or a 30- to 40-mm below-the-knee support stocking.

other factor is retarding healing. Other coexistent problems may be arterial ischemia, steroid-impaired healing, collagen vasculitis, or skin cancer.

If other etiologies have been excluded, several options are available for management of recurrent venous ulcerations. Some authors recommend continued nonoperative compressive therapy, sometimes with more leg elevation or bed rest. Certainly this approach eventually succeeds in many patients. Nonetheless, some active patients continue to have incapacitating leg swelling, pain, and recurrent ulceration. A surgical procedure may help such patients.

A. **Subfascial ligation of perforating veins.** In our experience, the healthy active patient with recurrent venous ulceration despite compression therapy is a candidate for a surgical approach to alleviating chronic venous hypertension. This operation may require stripping of the great and small saphenous veins as well as subfascial ligation of all incompetent communicating veins of the lower leg. Subfascial ligation of perforating veins can be performed through a variety of incisions and by using laparoscopic instruments. We have found properly performed subfascial ligation of perforating veins to be highly successful, although others report a 50% recurrence of ulcerations. Success with subfascial ligation requires **meticulous attention to the details of surgical technique and postoperative care**. Several principles of perforating vein ligation must be emphasized:

1. Although subfascial ligation of perforators may be accomplished through open ulcers, we generally heal ulcers by compression therapy and schedule the operation for at least 3–4 weeks after healing is complete.

2. Postoperative complications and ulcer recurrence are reduced if the patient loses excess weight before undergoing operation.

3. Patients should be otherwise healthy, active individuals. Chronically debilitated patients should be managed by nonoperative methods.

4. After surgery, the operated leg should be protected for a minimum of 7 days in a compressive bandage.

5. The patient usually remains at bed rest until the initial bandage is changed. Bed rest prevents leg edema that occurs with this procedure. Either low-dose heparin, 5,000 units SQ q8–12h, or oral warfarin sodium (Coumadin) should be considered to prevent DVT. The unoperated leg should be exercised against a footboard for 5 minutes every hour while the patient is awake.

6. If wound healing appears satisfactory at the first dressing change, a compressive Unna's paste boot or an elastic Ace wrap are reapplied from the toes to below the knee. This bandage is essential until the sutures are removed on or after the twenty-first postoperative day. Nylon sutures are used and generally cause minimal reaction.

7. On the first postoperative day, the patient should begin to dangle the leg over the bedside for short periods of time (3–5 minutes). This routine allows the leg to become gradually accustomed to a dependent position again before full ambulation.

8. Depending on the extent of surgery and postoperative pain, ambulation begins between the first and third postoperative days for 5–10 minutes every 2–4 hours. At first, the ankle may be stiff and crutches or a walker may be used to assist the patient. A normal walking pattern returns in 5–7 days.

9. Wound healing problems are best managed by bed rest and delayed ambulation. Skin grafting may be necessary.

10. Patients who undergo subfascial venous interruption must understand that they must continue to wear below-the-knee elastic support hose following operation, as the procedure does not correct the deep venous hypertension due to valvular incompetence and reflux.

B. Other operations. Direct transvenous repair of incompetent femoral vein valves has successfully alleviated severe chronic venous insufficiency in selected patients. Crossover femorofemoral or direct iliofemoral vein bypass grafts for iliofemoral venous occlusion can also relieve severe leg swelling, incapacitating venous claudication, and recurrent venous ulceration. However, these direct surgical attacks on the deep veins and valves can be technically difficult procedures, so there has not been widespread acceptance of direct venous reconstruction for most patients with postphlebitic syndrome or primary valvular imcompetence.

Selected Reading

Bergan JJ, Yao JST (eds). *Venous Disorders*. Philadelphia: Saunders, 1991.

Greenfield LJ. Chronic Venous Insufficiency. In LJ Greenfield (ed), *Surgery: Scientific Principles and Practice*. Philadelphia: Lippincott, 1993. Pp. 1778–1784.

Greenfield LJ. Lymphatic System Disorders. In LJ Greenfield (ed), *Surgery: Scientific Principles and Practice*. Philadelphia: Lippincott, 1983. Pp. 1784-1789.

Kistner RL. Valve Repair and Segment Transposition in Primary Valvular Insufficiency. In JJ Bergan, JST Yao (eds), *Venous Disorders*. Philadelphia: Saunders, 1991. Pp. 261–272.

Linton RR. John Homan's impact on diseases of the veins of the lower extremity, with special reference to deep thrombophlebitis and the post-thrombotic syndrome with ulceration. *Surgery* 81:1, 1977.

Moore DJ, Himmel PD, Sumner DS. Distribution of venous valvular incompetence in patients with the postphlebitic syndrome. *J Vasc Surg* 3:49, 1986.

Raju S. Venous Reconstruction for Chronic Venous Insufficiency of the Leg. In CB Ernst, JC Stanley (eds), *Current Therapy in Vascular Surgery* (2nd ed). Philadelphia: B.C. Decker, 1991. Pp. 977–980.

Miscellaneous Problems

Hemodialysis Access

In 1972 an amendment to the Social Security Act provided Medicare coverage for all patients suffering from end-stage renal disease. This legislation opened the way for thousands of patients to undergo chronic hemodialysis. The magnitude of this expenditure is impressive. In 1991, Medicare spent $6 billion dollars per year for this program. Although dialysis was initially limited to patients less than 45 years of age and was denied to patients with diabetes mellitus, these groups are no longer excluded. In fact, the average age of patients on chronic dialysis is increasing. More than 52% of patients who currently receive chronic dialysis in the United States are older then 55 years of age. They often have significant medical comorbidity.

In most medical centers, surgical residents and fellows play a primary role in the surgical placement of hemodialysis access. One of the most predictable aspects of chronic hemodialysis is the need for access revision. Access failure is especially common for prosthetic arteriovenous (AV) shunts. Consequently, this chapter focuses on essentials in the initial evaluation, placement, and revision of hemodialysis accesses.

Indications for Dialysis

Dialysis for acute or chronic renal failure is indicated when one or more of the following clinical problems are present.
  I. **Uremic signs and symptoms** are the most common indication for chronic dialysis. They become prominent as the blood-urea-nitrogen (BUN) and creatinine levels rise. Mortality and morbidity may be reduced if the BUN level is maintained below 100 mg/dl. Neurologic symptoms that require dialysis include lethargy, seizures, myoclonus, asterixis, and peripheral polyneuropathies. Uremic pericarditis is another manifestation.
 II. **Hyperkalemia (>6 mEq/liter)**, especially when accompanied by electrocardiogram (ECG) or neuromuscular abnormalities, requires immediate dialysis. Dietary restriction and potassium-bonding resins may suffice for lower levels of hyperkalemia.
III. **Fluid overload** is another indication for both acute and chronic dialysis. This includes patients who have not responded satisfactorily to fluid restriction and diuretics.
 IV. **Drug overdose** is a less common indication for hemodialysis but one that occasionally arises in a busy emergency room or critical care practice.

Choices of Access for Hemodialysis

Several techniques can be used to establish dialysis (Fig. 23-1). Selection of the appropriate technique for an individual patient depends on several clinical factors. Does the patient

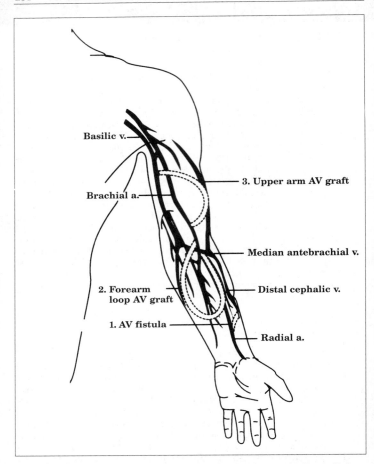

Basilic v.

3. Upper arm AV graft

Brachial a.

Median antebrachial v.

2. Forearm loop AV graft

Distal cephalic v.

1. AV fistula

Radial a.

Fig. 23-1. The three most common types of upper-extremity hemodialysis accesses include (1) a primary radiocephalic arteriovenous (AV) fistula, (2) a forearm polytetrafluorethylene AV shunt graft, or (3) an upper arm AV graft.

need immediate dialysis or will dialysis will be started in a number of days or weeks? Does the patient need temporary or permanent access? Does the patient have satisfactory extremity arterial inflow and suitable venous outflow veins for construction of an access? If peritoneal dialysis is selected, is the patient's abdominal cavity suitable for such a technique?

I. A variety of **dialysis catheters** are currently available for acute hemodialysis. These catheters provide quick access and are generally placed percutaneously or by surgical cutdown in the internal jugular or subclavian veins. They may be used for days to weeks. Infection or central venous thrombosis, however, are ever-present dangers for this form of hemodialysis.

A. The most common dialysis catheters (Shiley, VasCath, or Quinton catheters) are **noncuffed, dual-lumen catheters** placed pericutaneously using the Seldinger method.

B. **Cuffed dialysis catheters** (PermCath or VasCath) are generally placed by a venous cutdown. These catheters are relatively soft and well-tolerated by patients and will often function for weeks or even a few months. Again, central venous thrombosis and catheter infection are the major complications and generally necessitate catheter removal.

II. An **autologous AV fistula** of the upper extremity is the most durable and complication-free chronic dialysis access. The most common type of primary AV fistula is constructed between the cephalic vein and the radial artery at the wrist **(Brescia-Cimino fistula).** The three-year patency rate for an autologous AV fistula is 80–90% compared to 60–70% for prosthetic AV grafts. A Cimino-Brescia fistula, however, takes about 6–8 weeks to mature. Consequently, it cannot be used as soon as a prosthetic AV shunt. Other types of autologous AV dialysis fistulas include an antecubital anastomosis made between the basilic or cephalic veins and the brachial artery.

III. **Synthetic AV shunt grafts** are the most common type of access for chronic dialysis. Our first choice is a loop polytetra-fluoroethylene (PTFE) AV shunt placed in the nondominant forearm of the patient. In our experience, this type of access has been preferable to a straight forearm graft in the radial artery to an antecubital vein. Such straight forearm grafts have a very limited area for puncture, may be difficult to perform to heavily calcified radial artery and appear to have decreased patency rates compared to forearm loop grafts. Our second choice for an upper-extremity AV graft is an upper-arm loop graft between the brachial artery and the axillary vein. When the nondominant upper extremity has been expended for dialysis access, we then move to the opposite upper extremity. The lower extremity is used only when the upper extremities can no longer accept some type of hemodialysis access. Although grafts can be placed in the groin area, infection is a greater problem than it is in the upper extremity.

IV. **Chronic peritoneal dialysis** is another alternative preferred by some patients. Peritoneal dialysis can be performed at home and generally at a lower cost than hemodialysis. The major long-term disadvantage is the possibility of recurrent peritonitis. For patients with difficult upper-extremity access for hemodialysis, chronic peritoneal dialysis becomes an important option.

Patient Assessment

History and physical examination provide critical information in determining the suitability and type of dialysis access. The following factors should be considered in each patient.

I. One must ascertain whether the dialysis is intended to be **temporary** or **permanent**. If patients develop acute renal failure in the setting of previously normal renal function, many of them will recover from the acute renal failure over a period of days to weeks. In contrast, patients who develop acute renal insufficiency in the setting of chronic renal failure are likely to need chronic dialysis.

II. Several aspects of the **history** influence the type and outcome of dialysis access procedures. First, one must assess whether the patient has other medical comorbidities (e.g., poor cardiac function that may make hemodialysis more difficult.) Diabetics also have worse results with long-term dialysis and are particularly susceptible to hand ischemia due to vascular steal from their AV access. Second, one must ascertain whether the patient is right- or left-handed. Generally, access should be placed in the nondominant upper extremity. Third, any prior or current arterial or venous problems of the upper extremity must be identified. Such abnormalities will often affect the suitability or placement of an AV access. Fourth, any prior hemodialysis access procedures must be identified, including their prior locations and any problems associated with the previous fistula. Likewise, prior abdominal operations may affect the suitability for peritoneal dialysis. Finally, anticoagulation problems must be identified, including tendencies to both thrombosis or hemorrhage.

III. The **physical examination** is the primary determinant of the hemodialysis access site.

   A. **Skin condition** must be checked for any signs of infection or other dermatologic disorders that would impair healing.

   B. The extremities should be examined for any acute **swelling** or chronic edema. Chronic swelling may indicate past subclavian or axillary vein thrombosis or lymphedema due to other operations (e.g., past mastectomy).

   C. The **cephalic and basilic veins** should be inspected for patency. They should be palpated carefully for compressibility (normal vein) and for firm cords (chronic thrombosis). Application of an upper arm tourniquet may be helpful in delineating suitable veins in some patients.

   D. The axillary brachial, radial, and ulnar **pulses** should be palpated. Decreased pulses obviously indicate possible proximal chronic arterial occlusive disease or local arterial thrombosis from prior procedures.

   E. **Blood pressure** should be recorded in both arms. A difference of greater then 5–10 mm Hg indicates a chronic arterial stenosis in that extremity.

   F. The proximal subclavian arteries in the area of the supraclavicular fossa should be auscultated. Any **bruits** in this area indicate underlying arterial stenosis. The proximal left subclavian artery is one of the sites most susceptible to chronic atherosclerotic disease.

   G. Perfusion of the hand should be checked with an **Allen's test**. With the patient's hand making a tight fist, the examiner should compress the radial and ulnar arteries. Separately, the radial and then the ulnar artery should be released as the examiner looks at the opened hand for return of capillary refill. Most hands are ulnar dominant. This fact indicates that obliteration of the radial artery or diversion of flow from the radial artery into the AV fistula will not compromise perfusion to the hand.

H. The abdomen should be carefully examined for prior **surgical scars**. Multiple prior abdominal operations may compromise the placement of a chronic peritoneal catheter.

Selection of Access

I. The best access for **acute dialysis** is a subclavian or jugular vein percutaneous catheter. These catheters can be used immediately. Occasionally, one may need to construct an external Scribner AV shunt at the wrist or ankle.

II. The type of access for **chronic dialysis** depends on the timing for dialysis.

  A. If dialysis is scheduled for the future (several weeks to a few months), an autogenous AV fistula is the best choice.

  B. Dialysis that is already underway or will be needed in less than 1 month generally requires a prosthetic AV shunt graft for hemodialysis. Peritoneal dialysis is another option. Prosthetic grafts generally take 5–10 days to achieve good tissue incorporation. Puncturing the grafts prior to tissue incorporation can result in large subcutaneous hematomas and poor healing of the graft. New quick-sealing prosthetic grafts (i.e., specialized PTFE) may allow puncture of hemodialysis AV shunt grafts within 24 hours.

Preoperative Preparation

I. The indication for dialysis, the type of dialysis, and potential complication should be discussed with the patient and any family members. In particular, infection, thrombosis, and ischemic steal syndrome of the hand should be explained.

II. **Prophylactic antibiotics** (e.g., vancomycin, 500 mg on call to the operating room) have been shown to reduce the risk of infection.

Intraoperative Technique

The details of surgical construction of the hemodialysis access are beyond the scope of this handbook. However, a few technical concepts and tips should be mentioned.

I. Most extremity hemodialysis access procedures can be performed under **local anesthesia**. A supplemental axillary block may be helpful in some individuals.

II. Although **anticoagulation** is not mandatory, a small dose of heparin (e.g., 2,000–3,000 units) may alleviate early thrombosis in synthetic grafts where venous vasoconstriction may initially cause slower flow rates.

III. Skin incisions should be constructed so that the graft has **good tissue coverage** at the end of the procedure. Whenever possible, skin incisions should **not** be placed directly over the course of the synthetic graft.

IV. When the access has been completed, it is essential to check the **presence of pulses** at the wrist. In addition, it is helpful to auscultate flow in the palmar arch of the hand with a sterile continuous-wave Doppler. The loss or severe diminution of wrist pulses and the absence of Doppler flow in the palmar arch are harbingers of postoperative hand ischemia.

Postoperative Care

The period of greatest risk for early postoperative thrombotic or ischemic complications is the first 12–24 hours.

I. The extremity with the new dialysis access should be placed at a **position of comfort**. Generally, it does not need to be elevated. In fact, elevation may exacerbate hand ischemia in patients who have marginal perfusion following placement of an AV shunt. Tight, constrictive bandages should obviously be avoided.

II. The access should be checked for patency within 6 hours of placement. The two most reliable signs of patency are **palpable thrills** over the venous anastomosis and distal vein. In addition, a loud **machinery murmur** heard with the stethoscope is indicative of shunt or fistula patency.

III. The hand must be checked for any symptoms or signs of **ischemic steal syndrome**. The earliest symptom is numbness of the fingers. With severe ischemic steal, progressive paresis of the intrinsic muscles of the hands will evolve over 24 hours. An absent radial pulse that was previously present is the key physical finding in such patients. In addition, patients with a hand ischemia will generally have monophasic or no Doppler flow over the radial, ulnar, and palmar arteries. **If ischemic steal syndrome of the hand is present and progressive, the AV access must be revised immediately**. One technique is to decrease flow in the shunt by "banding," which involves narrowing the flow in the graft by a variety of techniques. One technique that has worked well for us has been reduction of a 6-mm graft to a 4-mm size by the lateral application of small Weck clips along the side of the proximal graft for approximately 1 cm. With adequate banding, the wrist pulses will usually increase and the Doppler signals of the wrist arteries and palmar arch will improve from monophasic to biphasic signals.

IV. Generally, a synthetic AV graft can be punctured in 7–10 days. An autogenous AV fistula will generally need to mature for 6–8 weeks before use. Development of an autologous AV fistula is assisted in some patients by daily exercise of the hand by squeezing a soft, spongy rubber ball.

Late Complications

A variety of complications can occur any time with a hemodialysis access. The most important complications are thrombosis, infection, chronic ischemic hand ischemia, or pseudoaneurysms along the graft.

I. **Infection** is uncommon with an autogenous AV fistula. Synthetic grafts are more susceptible. Generally, physical findings of local erythema, induration, tenderness, and purulent drainage from incisional sites are pathognomonic. Occasionally, a patient will present with a fever of unknown origin and minimal signs of local graft infection. Positive blood cultures may be present. An Indium-labeled white blood cell scan may localize infection to the synthetic graft. An infected synthetic graft must be removed entirely. A localized infected graft segment can occasionally be resected with a new segmental bypass around the infected area.

II. **Thrombosis** is most common with synthetic AV shunt grafts. In fact, 30–40% of such grafts will have acute occlusion within 3 years. Most of these occlusions occur suddenly with no warning. However, a few grafts will begin to show a decreased flow rate on dialysis. A flow rate of less than 250–300 ml/minute and a recirculation rate greater than 15% or venous pressures in excess of 150 mm Hg indicate a failing graft. In such cases, a **fistulogram** or a **duplex ultrasound** may identify a site of stenosis. Most synthetic grafts fail at the venous anastomosis where intimal hyperplasia occurs. Such failing grafts should be revised before acute occlusion. Subclavian or internal jugular hemodialysis catheters have a propensity for thrombosis. In many cases, the catheter can be salvaged by injecting 5,000–10,000 units of urokinase into each catheter port.

III. **Pseudoaneurysm** is another relatively common problem of chronic synthetic AV shunt grafts. These false aneurysms generally occur at puncture sites where subcutaneous hematomas have accumulated. They can gradually erode through the skin and lead to serious hemorrhage. Consequently, pseudoaneurysms should be repaired by resection of the pseudoaneurysm site and an interposition or bypass graft around the area.

Selected Reading

Bennion RS, Wilson SE. Hemodialysis and Vascular Access. In WS Moore (ed), *Vascular Surgery: A Comprehensive Review* (4th ed). Philadelphia: Saunders, 1993. Pp. 606–625.

Bennion RS, Kumpe DA. Arteriovenous Access. In D Eugene Straudness Jr, A van Breda (eds), *Vascular Disease: Surgical and Interventional Therapy*. New York: Churchill Livingstone, 1994. Pp 1045–1106.

Byrne C, Vernon P, Cohen JJ. Effects of age and diagnosis on survival of older patients beginning chronic dialysis. *JAMA* 271:24, 1994.

Vascular Trauma

Significant arterial and venous injuries are a relatively small problem in **all** types of trauma. However, when arterial or venous injuries are present, they become pivotal in mortality (i.e., exsanguinating hemorrhage) and morbidity (i.e., limb loss or stroke). Blood vessel injuries are an important contributor to more than 100,000 accidental deaths that occur each year in the United States.

The spectrum of vascular trauma is broad since any area of the head and neck, torso, or extremities can be involved. Vascular trauma is most commonly the result of violent crimes, motor vehicle accidents, and interventional arteriograms and angioplasties. In busy emergency departments, gunshot wounds account for 55% of vascular injuries, while knives cause 35% and blunt trauma the remaining 10%. The vast majority (75%) occur in an extremity. Neck wounds account for 15%, while arterial injuries of the visceral arteries (5%) and aorta (5%) are less frequent.

The scope of vascular trauma is so large that entire books have been written about it. This brief chapter, however, focuses on the initial recognition and management principles of arterial and venous injuries. It is a primer and not a treatise.

Mechanisms of Injury

Management of arterial and venous injuries is determined by the mechanism and severity of the injury.

I. **Penetrating wounds** from knives and low-velocity missiles (i.e., pistol bullets) cause localized damage to blood vessels. In contrast, high-velocity bullets (1,500–3,000 feet/second; e.g., hunting rifle) create a wide area of explosive **cavitation damage** around the missile tract. This damage zone extends for an area 30–40 times the size of the missile. The violence of the blast expansion disrupts surrounding muscle, may rupture blood vessels and nerves, and may fracture bone at distances removed from the missile path. As the blast cavity collapses, debris (i.e., clothing, dirt, skin) may be sucked into the depths of the wound. Likewise, close-range shotgun blasts scatter multiple pellets into the wound and often propel fragments of the shotgun wadding and clothing into the body.

II. **Blunt trauma** is more likely to cause vascular injury by several mechanisms. First, fracture fragments may directly injure vessels. Fracture-dislocations can cause excessive sudden stretch contusions of arteries. The result is intimal and media disruption with thrombosis. For example, posterior fracture-dislocation of the knee is a notorious cause of acute popliteal artery trauma. Bilateral first rib fractures are also commonly associated with subclavian artery injuries. Second, sudden flailing of an extremity or the neck may simply cause an excessive stretch of an artery against an adjacent bony prominence. The result is intimal-media disruption and sometimes dissection. Traumatic carotid artery dissection is classically associated with a sudden hyperextension of the neck. Finally, crushing force can contuse or disrupt an artery or vein. Blunt renal artery trauma secondary to a motor vehicle accident is a good example.

Recognition

The early diagnosis and repair of a vascular injury is essential to preventing serious hemorrhage and to preserving limb or organ function. In the setting of multiple injuries, recognition may be difficult. More pressing head, chest, or abdominal injuries may divert attention from occult vascular trauma. Poor extremity pulses may be attributed initially to hemorrhagic shock, hypothermic vasoconstriction, crush injury, or vasospasm.

However, the following symptoms and signs should raise suspicion of arterial or venous damage.

I. **External hemorrhage** from a penetrating wound, especially in proximity to a large artery or vein, is pathognomonic for a major vascular injury.

II. A pale, cool, and **pulseless extremity** may or may not be due to arterial injury. However, absent pulses mandate further observation and objective evaluation (i.e., Doppler ultrasound examination and/or arteriography).

III. **A penetrating wound adjacent to a major vessel** requires attention to be certain that no underlying vascular injury is present.

IV. Likewise, signs of a **major nerve injury** (i.e., paralysis and analgesia), especially associated with a penetrating wound, should lead to a search for associated vascular trauma.

V. **Fractures or dislocations** (i.e., knee or elbow) are commonly associated with vascular injuries. Moreover, presence of a distal pulse does not rule out a vascular injury. An intimal tear or flap may have occurred, but distal pulses may remain present as long as the artery does not completely thrombose. An arteriogram or other imaging modality (e.g., ultrasound) must settle the issue.

VI. A large-extremity, neck, or abdominal **hematoma** should raise suspicion of a major arterial or venous disruption.

VII. A **bruit** or **machinery murmur** at or near an injury site suggests disturbed blood flow from an arterial stenosis or arteriovenous fistula.

Initial Care

When a vascular injury is recognized or suspected, certain principles should guide early management. These principles (Fig. 24-1) apply to all vascular trauma, regardless of cause. Of course, greater emphasis may be placed on specific guide-

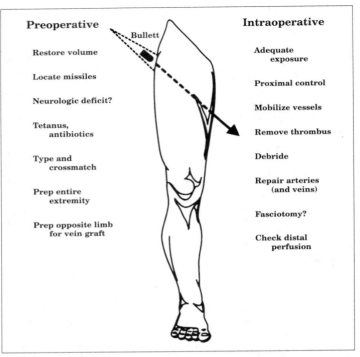

Fig. 24-1. Principles of preoperative and intraoperative management of vascular injuries. (Adapted from RJ Freeark, WH Baker, JJ Klosak. Arterial Injuries. In DC Sabiston Jr [ed], *Textbook of Surgery*. Philadelphia: Saunders, 1991.)

lines, depending on the mechanism and severity of injury. **Time from vascular injury to repair is a critical ingredient in successful outcome.** Advanced ischemia becomes established within 6–8 hours after arterial disruption or occlusion.

I. **Hypotension** is evidence that significant blood loss has occurred. Trauma victims should be completely uncovered and inspected on the front and back of the body for entrance and exit sites when penetrating trauma is suspected. Overt bleeding from penetrating wounds can usually be controlled by point pressure while the remaining examination is completed.

II. The initial management of arterial trauma includes the general principles of trauma **resuscitation**, including the "ABCs" (*a*irway, *b*reathing, and *c*irculation). Intravenous lines are inserted, crystalloid solutions are infused, and blood should be typed and cross-matched.

III. **Fractures** should be splinted and dislocations should be reduced as soon as possible.

IV. **Tetanus prophylaxis** and **intravenous antibiotics** should be administered.

V. Appropriate **radiographs** in search of fractures should be ordered.

VI. When a localized penetrating injury is associated with hemorrhage, expanding hematoma, or absence of distal pulses, no specific diagnostic tests are necessary. The patient needs an expeditious trip to the **operating room**.

VII. If a hematoma is present at the site of injury, **duplex ultrasound** can ascertain whether a false aneurysm or arteriovenous fistula is present.

VIII. **Arteriography** is generally recommended for patients who are at high risk of arterial injury, including those with bilateral first rib fracture (subclavian), deceleration chest injuries with sternal or rib fractures (torn thoracic aorta), and fracture dislocations of the knee (popliteal artery).

IX. If the penetrating injury is not associated with ongoing hemorrhage or expanded hematoma and is accompanied by a normal duplex ultrasound at the site of injury, the patient in general would be observed unless distal pulses subsequently disappear.

Operative Principles

Although the exact operative approach varies with the specific site of trauma, certain principles apply to the intraoperative management of all arterial or venous injuries.

I. **A wide operative field** should be prepared. For a neck or upper-extremity wound, the prepped area should include the adjacent chest in case median sternotomy or thoracotomy is necessary. When the wound involves the abdomen, the patient should be prepped from nipples to knees. Both lower extremities should be prepared when the wound involves one leg.

II. An uninvolved lower extremity for ready access to a **saphenous vein** should be prepped. Saphenous vein remains the best arterial substitute for all but the largest injured arteries and veins.

III. **Proximal control** of the injured artery should be gained before entering any large hematomas.

V. **Damaged arteries and veins** should be resected. Most injuries will involve a 1- to 2-cm segment of blood vessel. One must be certain that all of the damaged vessel has been removed before a reanastomosis or graft is placed.

V. The distal circulation should be checked for accumulation of **thrombus**. Generally, a Fogarty balloon catheter should be passed distally, gently inflated, and drawn back to retrieve any distal clot.

VI. In general, 1–2 cm of artery may be resected and reconstituted by a **primary anastomosis**. Larger areas of injury require a **graft**. Saphenous vein is appropriate for vessels measuring up to 6 mm. Larger vessels will usually require a synthetic graft (i.e., Dacron or polytetrafluoroethylene).

VII. Concomitant **venous injuries** should be repaired whenever possible. Ligation of major peripheral veins often results in long-term disabling venous stasis of the extremity. If the vein cannot be repaired by lateral suture, an autologous vein graft should be used. Patency for even 24–72 hours may be sufficient to allow the establishment of additional collateral venous return.

VIII. **All devitalized tissue** in the area of injury should be debrided. Such debridement is especially important in patients with high-velocity missile wounds. These wounds are generally associated with extensive, explosive cavitation destruction.

IX. After arterial repair, adequate **soft-tissue coverage** of the affected artery is imperative. An exposed arterial repair may dehisce due to desiccation or infection. Muscle is the preferable coverage and can often be secured by transposition of adjacent muscle. When extensive muscle and soft tissue have been destroyed by the injury, it may be necessary to use a **myocutaneous flap** for coverage.

X. **Displaced fractures** and **dislocations** must be stabilized to prevent tension on a vascular repair. Whether the fracture or dislocation should be managed first or after the vascular repair will vary from patient to patient. Because ischemia has often been prolonged, repair of damaged arteries or veins is often done first. External skeletal traction or fixation is then performed. Generally, internal fixation of a fracture is avoided because of the increased risk of infection from wound contamination. If a fracture or dislocation must be treated to allow adequate exposure for an arterial repair, a shunt can often be placed from the proximal injured artery to the distal injured artery to restore circulation while the fracture is being treated.

XI. **Concomitant nerve injuries** are usually identified and tagged with identifying sutures for delayed repair. Generally, disrupted nerves are not repaired at the time of the initial operation.

XII. Prolonged ischemia is often present with arterial injuries. Muscle swelling, especially after reperfusion, can create a **compartment syndrome**. Fasciotomy (Fig. 24-2) should be seriously considered at the time of initial arterial repair for (1) popliteal artery and vein injuries or (2) in cases in which there has been a delay greater than 6–8 hours between injury and repair. If fasciotomies are not performed at the initial operation, careful observation must be maintained for development of tightness in the fascial compartments or loss of sensation in the extremity.

XIII. Extremity **perfusion** must be assessed objectively in the operating room and during the early postoperative period. Return of a distal pulse is the most obvious sign of success. An intraoperative arteriogram with 20–30 ml of contrast material is the standard means of imaging the site of reconstruction and distal run off. A sterile continuous-wave Doppler is also helpful in auscultating distal arterial signals. A sterile blood pressure cuff may also be used to monitor distal pulse volume recordings. If the arteriogram demonstrates obvious distal arterial spasm, a direct intraarterial dose of papaverine (1 ml of papaverine mixed in 9 ml of normal saline) into the affected extremity will often alleviate the vasoconstriction.

XIV. **Anticoagulation** is avoided in patients with multiple systemic injuries. Small doses of regional heparinized saline can be instilled down the distal arterial tree during operation.

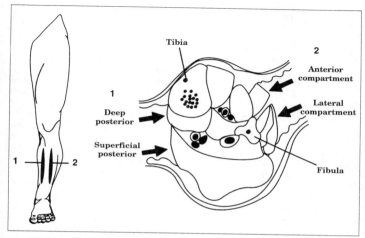

Fig. 24-2. Fasciotomy for compartment syndrome of the leg. All four muscle compartments of the leg can be decompressed through leg incisions. A longitudinal lateral leg incision (2) is made approximately halfway through the tibia and fibula. This incision allows decompression of the anterior and lateral fascial compartments. Care must be taken to avoid injury to the superficial peroneal nerve in the distal portion of the longitudinal leg incision. The superficial and deep posterior fascial compartments are decompressed by a medial leg incision (1) made approximately one fingerbreadth medial to the tibia.

However, doses in excess of 2,000–3,000 units of heparin may result in serious systemic anticoagulation and bleeding in other body sites (i.e., head or intraabdominal injuries).

Postoperative Care

Since patients with arterial trauma often have other major systemic injuries, they are generally observed in an intensive care unit. The following specific guidelines should ensure continued success of the vascular repair.

I. **Peripheral pulses** should be monitored frequently for any sign of thrombosis. If one has difficulty ascertaining the presence of a peripheral pulse, a continuous-wave Doppler unit should be used to ausculate peripheral arterial signals.

II. Continued surveillance for signs of **compartment syndrome** is critical, especially in the first 6–12 hours after operation. Muscles that were initially soft and not tense in the operating room may subsequently swell following reperfusion. The most common symptoms and signs of serious compartment syndrome are leg or forearm pain associated with tense, tender muscle groups. The patient may also complain of numbness in the extremity. Pulses may actually be present when significant compartment pressure has occurred. As pressure rises within a muscle compartment, tissue perfusion declines progressively and at a level of above 20–30 mm Hg becomes impaired. If clinical symptoms and signs cannot be assessed adequately, compartment pressure should be measured.

The preferred technique for lower-extremity compartment syndrome is a **four-compartment fasciotomy**. The anterior and lateral compartments can be decompressed through a lateral incision placed along the fibula. Care must be taken during anterior compartment fasciotomy to avoid injury to the superficial peroneal nerve. The superficial and deep posterior compartments can be decompressed by a single medial leg incision (see Fig. 24-2).

III. If extensive muscle injury has occurred, the patient may develop **acute renal failure** from myoglobinuria. Myoglobin will generally cause a dark discoloration (cola appearance) of the urine. When myoglobinuria is anticipated or diagnosed, intravenous hydration is critical. It is also helpful to add mannitol (e.g., 25 g to 1 liter of intravenous fluid) and to alkalinize the urine with 50 mEq of sodium bicarbonate in each liter of fluid. Persistent myoglobinuria usually indicates that further debridement of necrotic muscle will be necessary.

Results

Rapid transport of trauma patients by helicopter or ambulance to major surgical centers has decreased the average time from injury to treatment for most vascular injuries. The majority of patients currently arrive at trauma centers within 4–6 hours of initial injury. Most delays occur at the scene of the accident where the patient may not be discovered for a period of time, especially at night. Blunt trauma causes the most severe vascular injuries and accounts for most amputations (80–90%) and deaths (70–80%). Nearly all blunt trauma patients have serious associated injuries of other organs. Although blunt trauma counts for approximately 40% of vascular injuries, the remaining 60% are due to penetrating wounds. Penetrating vascular injuries account for approximately 10% of all amputations due to vascular trauma and result in 20% of the deaths related to arterial or venous injury.

The overall mortality rate for vascular trauma is currently in the 5% range. Blunt vascular trauma, however, carries a mortality risk of approximately 9–10%, while penetrating injuries are associated with a mortality rate of 1.5–3%. Overall amputation rate for all vascular injuries is about 7–10% currently. Ligation of a major-extremity artery will result in a 50% amputation rate, which has been lowered significantly in the past 40 years with arterial repair. Injuries of the popliteal artery continue to reflect the highest amputation rate following arterial repair (20–30%). Although arterial and venous injuries can frequently be successfully repaired in an extremity, the limiting factor for many severely traumatized patients is associated major nerve disruption. Such patients often develop causalgia or reflex sympathetic dystrophy of the injured extremity.

Selected Reading

Flanigan DP, Schuler JJ, Meyer JP (eds). *Civilian Vascular Trauma*. Philadelphia: Lea & Febiger, 1992.

Humphrey RW, Nichols WK, Silver D. Rural vascular trauma: A twenty-year review. *Ann Vasc* 8:179, 1994.

Perry MO. Vascular Trauma. In WS Moore (ed), *Vascular Surgery: A Comprehensive Review* (4th ed). Philadelphia: Saunders, 1993. Pp. 630–647.

Rich NW, Spencer FC. *Vascular Trauma*. Philadelphia: Saunders, 1978.

Wind GG, Valentine RJ. *Anatomic Exposures in Vascular Surgery*. Baltimore: Williams & Williams, 1991.

Appendix

Drugs Commonly Used in Adults

Drug	Oral	Intramuscular	Intravenous
Adenosine (Adenocard)			6-mg rapid bolus; may repeat with 12 mg 9½ min × 2
Aminophylline			Loading dose: 6 mg/kg over 30 min; maintenance: 0.5–0.9 mg/kg/hr
Amrinone (Inocor)			0.75 mg/kg bolus; then 5–10 μg/kg 1 min
Aspirin (enteric-coated)	80–325 mg bid (antiplatelet effect)		
Atenolol (Tenormin)	50–100 mg qd		
Atropine		0.4 mg	0.4–2.0 mg push
Bretylium			Loading dose: 5 mg/kg IV plus 10 mg/kg to maximum 30 mg/kg; maintenance: 5–10 mg/kg q6h IV
Calcium chloride			200 mg–1 g slowly
Calcium gluconate			10-ml slow push
Captopril (Capoten)	Initial dose: 25–50 mg bid or tid; maintenance: 25–150 mg tid		
Cefadroxil (Duricef)	500 mg bid		

Drug	Oral	Intramuscular	Intravenous
Cefazolin sodium (Ancef)		500 mg–1 g q6–8h	500 mg–1 g q6–8h
Cefoxitin sodium (Mefoxin)			1–2 g q6–8h
Chlordiazepoxide hydrochloride (Librium)	10–25 mg tid–qid		Initial dose: 25–50 mg; maintenance: 25–50 mg q2–6h prn
Cimetidine (Tagamet)	300 mg qid pc and hs		300 mg q6h
Clindamycin (Cleocin)	150–300 mg q6h		300–600 mg q6h
Clofibrate (Atromid-S)	500 mg qid		
Clonidine hydrochloride (Catapres)	0.1–0.4 mg bid		
Dexamethasone (Decadron) (1 mg = 30 mg cortisone)	0.75–9 mg qd (in 2 divided doses)	Initial dose: 10–20 mg; maintenance: 2–4 mg q6h	Initial dose: 10–20 mg; maintenance: 2–4 mg q6h
Diazepam (Valium)	2–5 mg bid–qid	2–5 mg q4h	For sedation: 2–5 mg q4h prn; for seizures: 5 mg push prn
Digoxin (Lanoxin)	Digitalization: 1.5–2.0 mg (in divided doses); maintenance: 0.125–0.250 mg qd		Digitalization: 1.0–1.5 mg (in 4–6 divided doses); maintenance: 0.125 mg bid
Diltiazem (Cardizem)	30–90 mg tid–qid		
Dipyridamole (Persantine)	As antiplatelet drug, 50–75 mg bid–tid		

Dobutamine hydrochloride (Dobutrex)		1 ampule = 250 mg in 500 ml D5W (500 µg/ml) at 2.5–15.0 µg/kg/min
Dopamine HCl (Intropin)		1 ampule = 200 mg in 500 ml D5W (400 µg/ml) at 2–3 µg/kg/min up to 20–50 µg/kg/min
Enalapril (Vasotec)	Initial dose: 5 mg in 1 dose; maintenance: 5–40 mg qd or bid	
Epinephrine		0.5–5.0 µg/min; 1 ampule = 1 mg in 250 ml D5W at 7–70 microdrops/min
Esmolol (Brevibloc)		Load with 0.5 mg/kg 1 min; then 5–10 mg/hr
Furosemide (Lasix)	20–80 mg bid	10–40 mg push
Gentamicin sulfate (Garamycin)	3–5 mg/kg qd (in 3 divided doses)	3–5 mg/kg qd (in 3 divided doses)
Haloperidol (Haldol)	2–5 mg q4–8h	2–5 mg q4–8h
Heparin	Not recommended	Loading dose: 1–2 mg/kg or 5,000–10,000 units; maintenance: 750–1,250 units/hr
Hydralazine (Apresoline)	100–200 mg qd (2–4 divided doses)	10–20 mg q4–6h

Drug	Oral	Intramuscular	Intravenous
Hydrochlorothiazide	50 mg qd–bid		250–500 mg q6h
Ibuprofen (Advil/Motrin)	200–400 mg q4–6h		250–500 mg q6h
Imipenem-cilastatin sodium (Primaxin)			
Isoproterenol (Isuprel)	50 mg qd–bid		1 ampule = 1 mg in 500 ml D5W (2 μg/ml) at 0.5–5.0 μg/min; titrate to effect
Labetalol (Normodyne, Trandate)	200–1,200 mg in 2 doses		20 mg over 2 min (40–80 mg q15min to 320 mg)
Levarterenol (Levophed)			1 ampule = 4 mg in 500 ml D5W (8 μg/ml) at 2–10 μg/min; titrate to effect
Lidocane HCl (Xylocaine)		100 mg (2% solution)	Initial dose: 50–200 mg push; maintenance: 1–4 mg/min continuous infusion
Lisinopril (Prinivil, Zestril)	5–40 mg qd		
Lorazepam (Ativan)	1–2 mg bid or tid	0.05 mg/kg (maximum: 4 mg)	0.044 mg/kg (total 2 mg)
Mannitol			12.5–25 g push
Methyldopa (Aldomet)	500 mg qd–qid		
Metoprolol (Lopressor)	50–100 mg bid		250–500 mg q6h

Drug			
Minoxidil (Loniten)	10–40 mg qd (in divided doses; plus a diuretic)		
Nadolol (Corgard)	Initial dose: 20 mg; maintenance: 80–160 mg in 1 dose		
Naloxone hydrochloride (Narcan)		1 ampule = 0.4 mg; push 1 ampule	1 ampule = 0.4 mg; push 1 ampule
Nifedipine (Procardia)	10–30 mg tid		
Nitroglycerin*	0.3–0.6 mg prn sublingually		60 mg in 500 ml D5W at 10–40 µg/min; titrate to effect
Nitroprusside sodium (Nipride)			1 ampule = 50 mg in 500 ml D5W (100 µg/ml) at 0.5–10.0 µg/kg/min
Phenoxybenzamine hydrochloride (Dibenzyline)	10–30 mg bid		
Phenylephrine hydrochloride (Neo-Synephrine)			1 ampule = 10 mg in 500 ml D5W (20 µg/ml); titrate to effect
Phenytoin sodium (Dilantin)	100 mg tid		Initial dose: 100–300 mg push; maintenance: 100 mg q4h
Prazosin hydrochloride (Minipress)	Initial dose: 1 mg bid; maintenance: 2–20 mg qd (in divided doses)		

Drug	Oral	Intramuscular	Intravenous
Procainamide hydrochloride (Pronestyl)	250 mg q3h	100–200 mg q3h	20–50 mg/min up to 1 g
Propranolol hydrochloride (Inderal)	40–480 mg qd (in 2–4 divided doses)		1–3 mg in incremental doses of 0.1–0.2 mg (continuous ECG monitoring)
Quinidine gluconate (Quinaglute)	330 mg q8h		
Ranitidine (Zantac)	150 mg bid		50 mg q8h
Streptokinase			Initial dose: 250,000 IU over 30 min; maintenance: 100,000 IU/hr up to 72 hr
Sucralfate (Carafate)	1 g qid		
Terbutaline sulfate (Brethine)	2.5–5.0 mg tid	0.25 mg SQ	
Triazolam (Halcion)	0.25–0.5 mg hs		
Trimethaphan camsylate (Arfonad)			500 mg/500 ml D5W via infusion pump at 3–4 mg/min
d-tubocurarine (Curare)			0.6 mg/kg push
Urokinase			Initial dose: 2,000 units/lb body wt over 30 min; maintenance: 2,000 units/lb/hr

Vancomycin (Vancocin HCl)

500–1000 mg q12h

Verapamil (Isoptin, Calan)

40–120 mg tid or qid slow
release (SR) 240 mg qd

Initial dose: 5–10 mg over 2–3
min; repeat in 30 min.
IV infusion: 0.375 mg/min
for 30 min; maintenance:
0.125 mg/min

Warfarin sodium (Coumadin)

Initial dose: 10–15 mg qd;
maintenance: 2–15 mg qd
(Check prothrombin time-INR)

INR = international normalized ratio.
*Nitroglycerin ointment should be applied to the skin in a 1- to 2-inch dose q3–4h.

Index